PROCESS VALIDATION IN MANUFACTURING OF BIOPHARMACEUTICALS

Guidelines, Current Practices, and Industrial Case Studies

PROCESS VALIDATION IN MANUFACTURING OF BIOPHARMACEUTICALS

Guidelines, Current Practices, and Industrial Case Studies

edited by
Anurag Singh Rathore
Gail Sofer

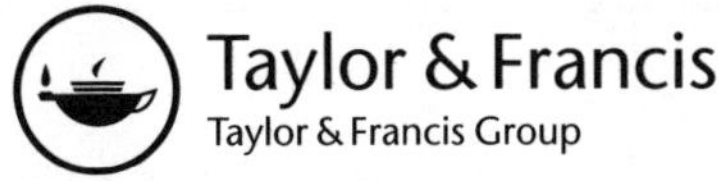

Taylor & Francis
Taylor & Francis Group

Boca Raton   London   New York   Singapore

A CRC title, part of the Taylor & Francis imprint, a member of the
Taylor & Francis Group, the academic division of T&F Informa plc.

Published in 2005 by
CRC Press
Taylor & Francis Group
6000 Broken Sound Parkway NW, Suite 300
Boca Raton, FL 33487-2742

International Standard Book Number-10: 1-57444-516-2 (Hardcover)
International Standard Book Number-13: 978-1-57444-516-9 (Hardcover)
Library of Congress Card Number 2004065748

Library of Congress Cataloging-in-Publication Data

Process validation in manufacturing of biopharmaceuticals : guidelines, current practices, and industrial case studies / edited by Anurag Singh Rathore, Gail Sofer.
p. cm. -- (Biotechnology and bioprocessing series ; 29)
Includes bibliographical references and index.
ISBN 1-57444-516-2 (alk. paper)
1. Pharmaceutical biotechnology--Quality control. 2. Biotechnological process monitoring. I. Rathore, Anurag S. (Anurag Singh), 1973- II. Sofer, G. K. III. Series.

RS380.P76 2005
615'.19--dc22   2004065748

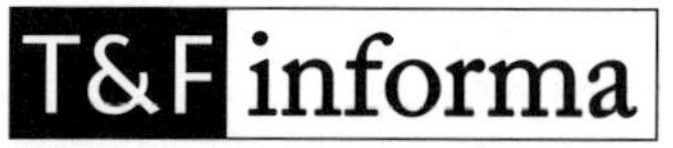
Taylor & Francis Group
is the Academic Division of T&F Informa plc.

**Visit the Taylor & Francis Web site at
http://www.taylorandfrancis.com**

**and the CRC Press Web site at
http://www.crcpress.com**

Dedication

To our family:
Bhawana, Payal, Bill, Gregg, and Douglas,
who contributed to this as much as we did.

Preface

Process validation continues to be a topic of much debate and confusion for biopharmaceutical manufacturers. It is usually perceived as a regulatory requirement and good business practice, since it can prevent failed batches when based on science and risk assessments. This book provides insights into the key aspects and current practices of process validation.

Chapter 1 addresses some of the current process validation concerns. In Chapter 2, the use of a risk assessment method (failure modes and effect analysis [FMEA]) is presented as a means to prioritize process parameters for further process characterization prior to validation. FMEA provides a logical approach that can aid in establishing critical parameters and ensure process robustness. Specific examples on the use of FMEA will aid readers to establish this method in their own organizations.

Process characterization is a prerequisite for process validation. In Chapter 3, a description of how to carry out thorough and consistent process characterization is presented. "Precharacterization" studies, which are used to help define the scope of the actual experimental characterization work, are also discussed. The discussions on timing of process characterization, needed resources, and a stepwise approach provide valuable insights. The importance of scale-down in process characterization is also addressed.

Accurately scaling down to mimic manufacturing processes is essential in several aspects of process validation. Chapter 4 provides further guidance and strategies for scaling down unit operations, including chromatography, chemical modification reactions, ultrafiltration, and microfiltration. In addition to general scale-down principles and parameters, the authors address specific problems and present some examples.

Prior to establishing a process that can be validated, it is essential to consider potential risks from adventitious agents, which include viruses, bacteria, fungi, mycoplasma, and transmissible spongiform encephalopathies. The potential sources of these agents and testing programs for them are described in Chapter 5. Examples of contamination events in biopharmaceutical manufacturing are presented. Bioburden assessment and sterility issues are also addressed, and a summary table describes adventitious agents, recommended tests, and stages at which to perform testing.

In Chapter 6, the life span of both chromatography and filtration media is addressed. There are discussions on the various factors that influence life span, along with experimental approaches for validation. The use of small-scale models for validation is discussed. The application of concurrent validation to provide life span data, an approach gaining more acceptance lately, is also discussed in this chapter.

Chapter 7 begins with an overview of filtration validation and a discussion of validation that can be performed in scaled-down studies as well as those aspects that require manufacturing scale. Next is a section on the validation of sterilizing-grade filters. Subsequent sections address validation of filters used for clarification and virus removal filters. Details of tangential-flow filter validation are presented. Also included are descriptions of specific validation issues in clarification of bacterial cell harvest and lysate clarification, mammalian cell clarification, and protein concentration and diafiltration. Cleaning validation for reusable membranes is also discussed.

It has been said that without assays, you have nothing. In Chapter 8, analytical test methods are discussed with a special focus on well-characterized biological and biotechnological products. Appropriate methods for testing raw materials and in-process samples during the various manufacturing steps are addressed. The authors also discuss Process Analytical Technology (PAT), which is being driven by the FDA as a means to better control processes. Another section of this chapter presents methods used for product characterization, release, and stability testing. Also included are the ever-problematic potency assay and strategies for choosing a quality-control testing scheme. Other topics discussed are the use of assays for demonstrating comparability, assay validation, dealing with out-of-specification (OOS) results, and assay revalidation.

In Chapter 9, the reader is provided with a regulatory perspective on facility design and validation issues. Written by two ex-FDAers, this chapter provides details on the regulatory requirements and the information that should be provided in a license application. Also presented are the requirements for cell inoculum suites and areas intended for fermentation/harvest, purification, and bulk filtration. In addition, support areas, such as those used for preparation of media and buffers, and the use of closed systems to reduce environmental classifications are discussed. There are extensive sections on utilities, cleaning, and environmental monitoring. Multiproduct facility issues are addressed. In the section on facility inspections, the authors provide insight into the current focus of inspections.

Chapter 10 discusses the importance of taking a risk-based approach toward computerized system compliance and how it adds value to the product and process that is commensurate with cost. It is concluded that a sound computer system validation (CSV) program encourages the introduction of new and exciting technologies with the ultimate promise of safer, more effective, and more affordable medicines.

In Chapters 11, 12, 13, and 14, many of the concepts described in the previous chapters are illustrated with case studies. First, we learn in Chapter 11 about process optimization and characterization studies for the purification of an *E. coli*-expressed protein product. Chapter 12 also addresses purification validation — in this case, for a therapeutic monoclonal antibody that is expressed and secreted by Chinese hamster ovary (CHO) cells. In Chapter 13, a matrix approach for process validation of a multivalent bacterial vaccine is described. Chapter 14 describes viral clearance validation studies for a product produced in a human cell line.

We hope this book will provide the reader with valuable insights into the current trends in process validation. Over the years, the biotechnology industry has advanced and we are now addressing concepts such as comparability and matrix approaches to validation. By sharing their knowledge, the authors have contributed to the biopharmaceutical industry's enhanced application of science- and risk-based approaches to process validation.

Anurag S. Rathore

Gail Sofer

Editors

Anurag S. Rathore is a scientist in Process Development at Amgen Inc., Thousand Oaks, CA. His group is responsible for support of process development, process characterization, scale-up, and production and process validation of late-stage products. Before Amgen, he had a similar position at Pharmacia Corp. He has authored more than 50 publications and presentations in these research areas. He also acts as the series editor of the "Biotechnology and Bioprocessing Series" and has recently edited *Scale-Up and Optimization in Preparative Chromatography* and *Electrokinetic Phenomena: Principles and Applications in Analytical Chemistry and Microchip Technology*. He also edits the "Elements of Biopharmaceutical Production Series" for Biopharm on issues that are routinely faced in process development and manufacturing of biopharmaceuticals. He has a Ph.D. in chemical engineering from Yale University.

Gail Sofer, after serving as the director of Regulatory Services at BioReliance for 6 years, has recently joined GE Healthcare (formerly Amersham Biosciences) as the director of Regulatory Compliance in a new consulting team. Her publications include numerous articles and book chapters on downstream processing, virus inactivation, and validation. She has also coedited and authored several books. She serves on the Science Advisory Board of PDA, the Editorial Advisory Boards of BioPharm, BioQuality, and BioProcess International, and the Scale-Up Advisory Board of Genetic Engineering News. She chairs a PDA task force on virus filters and is cochair of the ASTM subcommittee on Adventitious Agents for Tissue Engineered Medical Products. She holds an M.S. degree in biochemistry from the University of Miami.

Contributors

Chitrananda Abeygunawardana
Merck & Company
West Point, PA

Mark Bailey
Eli Lilly & Company
Indianapolis, IN

Jeffrey C. Baker
Eli Lilly & Company
Indianapolis, IN

Jeri Ann Boose
Bioreliance Corporation
Rockville, MD

Monica J. Cahilly
Green Mountain Quality
  Associates
Warren, VT

Jennifer Campbell
Millipore Corporation
Bedford, MA

Audrey Chang
Bioreliance Corporation
Rockville, MD

Lynn Conley
Process Sciences
IDEC Pharma Corporation
San Diego, CA

Michael L. Dekleva
Merck & Company
West Point, PA

Marshall G. Gayton
Merck & Company
West Point, PA

Ranga Godavarti
Drug Substance Development
Wyeth BioPharma
Andover, MA

John Haury
Amgen Inc.
Thousand Oaks, CA

Wayne K. Herber
Merck & Company
West Point, PA

Brian D. Kelley
Drug Substance Development
Wyeth BioPharma
Andover, MA

Ann L. Lee
Merck & Company
West Point, PA

John McEntire
Pharmaceutical Development
  Consultant
Bumpass, VA

John McPherson
Process Sciences
IDEC Pharma Corporation
San Diego, CA

Lorraine Metzka
Eli Lilly & Company
Indianapolis, IN

Valerie Moore
Bioreliance Corporation
Rockville, MD

Ray Nims
Bioreliance Corporation
Rockville, MD

Jon Petrone
Drug Substance Development
Wyeth BioPharma
Andover, MA

Carolyn Phillips
Bioreliance Corporation
Rockville, MD

Esther Presente
Bioreliance Corporation
Rockville, MD

Narahari S. Pujar
Merck & Company
West Point, PA

Michelle Quertinmont
Eli Lilly & Company
Indianapolis, IN

Anurag S. Rathore
Amgen Inc.
Thousand Oaks, CA

Nadine Ritter
Biologics Consulting Group, LLC
Alexandria, VA

Jeff Robinson
Drug Substance Development
Wyeth BioPharma
Andover, MA

Nancy Roscioli
Don Hill & Associates, Inc.
Silver Spring, MD

Michael Rubino
Eli Lilly & Company
Indianapolis, IN

James E. Seely
Process Development
Amgen Inc.
Longmont, CO

Robert J. Seely
Corporate Quality
Amgen Inc.
Boulder, CO

Gail Sofer
GE Healthcare
Piscataway, NJ

Jörg Thömmes
Process Sciences
IDEC Pharma Corporation
San Diego, CA

Susan Vargo
Don Hill & Associates, Inc.
Silver Spring, MD

William Wiler
Eli Lilly & Company
Indianapolis, IN

Richard Wright
Drug Substance Development
Wyeth BioPharma
Andover, MA

P.K. Yegneswaran
Merck & Company
West Point, PA

Contents

Chapter 13

Narahari S. Pujar, Marshall G. Gayton, Wayne K. Herber,
Chitrananda Abeygunawardana, Michael L. Dekleva,
P. K. Yegneswaran, and Ann L. Lee

Chapter 14

Michael Rubino, Mark Bailey, Jeffrey C. Baker,
Jeri Ann Boose, Lorraine Metzka, Valerie Moore,
Michelle Quertinmont, and William Wiler

1

Guidelines to Process Validation

GAIL SOFER

CONTENTS

1.1 INTRODUCTION

Much has already been written about process validation for biopharmaceuticals, and there are worldwide guidelines already established. Why, then, did we decide to produce yet another book on this topic? For starters, the guidelines addressing validation are usually purposefully broad to allow for the variability in products, manufacturing methods, analysis, clinical indications, patient populations, and doses for biopharmaceuticals. As a result, there is still much discussion related to validation approaches and specific issues that must be addressed to satisfy regulatory authorities and reproducibly produce safe and efficacious biopharmaceuticals. Furthermore, developing technologies, both analytical and manufacturing, can impact validation, and it is expected that sponsors of biopharmaceuticals will remain current with new developments.

Although validation is a regulatory requirement for licensed biopharmaceuticals, it also provides an economic value. By understanding a process and controlling it within realistic ranges, batch failures are minimized. A uniform approach to validation and avoidance of the pitfalls can provide further economic advantage. However, biopharmaceuticals encompass some vastly different products — not only therapeutic monoclonal antibodies and proteins produced by recombinant DNA technology but also gene and cell therapies. Is it possible to apply a consistent validation approach that is applicable to, for example, monoclonal antibody products produced in sources as diverse as cows' milk and *E. coli*? The answer in some respects is yes. Certain practical steps can be applied for all therapeutic products. A risk assessment is the starting point for determining how the manufacturing process should be designed so that it can, in fact, be validated. There must also be sufficient resources, both human and financial, applied to validation. Good science and common sense are essential, and basic regulatory requirements should be reviewed and followed.

1.2 CURRENT VALIDATION CITATIONS/PROBLEMS

The U.S. Freedom of Information Act (FOI) benefits the biotechnology industry as it tries to anticipate validation issues that are of concern, at least to the U.S. FDA. FDA approval letters, Form 483s, and warning letters can be useful in trying to make sense of the latest validation issues. This is not, however, the ideal way for industry to determine what is appropriate. Each product and its production method are unique in at least some aspects, and the risk assessment and good science should be the driving force in understanding validation requirements. However, reviewing recent regulatory citations can be an interesting beginning if we keep in mind that we do not have the full picture and that even reviewers writing 483s make mistakes. A review of 483 observations for 2003 accumulated as of June by BioQuality showed that validation comes in second when compared to investigations.[1] That is the good news, because validation used to be first. In a review of GMP warning letters from October 2001 to October 2002, it was observed that the most-cited GMP violation was validation.[2] Validation failures seem to fall into groups. Some are due to lack of resources and upper management buy-in. Those sponsors with multiple problems, many of which are related to a lack of thorough process validation, often appear to have an upper management that focuses on short-term profits and forgets that they or someone in their family might have to actually use the product. Employees with experience and good intent often have to do a really good internal selling job to ensure validation is performed properly.

Although the full story behind the regulatory comments is unknown, it appears that at least some of the observations are simply due to oversights. How could this occur? Take, for example, the observation that "validation studies are not given independent, final approval by QA." And "the same individuals plan, write, approve, and implement validation protocols, and they also write the final report and approve the validation. Validation studies are executed prior to approval of the protocol." This sounds like it is coming from organizations that did not have the structure to ensure that validation was performed according to regulatory requirements. For small, start-up biopharmaceutical companies and academic institutions, lack of understanding of the regulations and, often more importantly, lack of resources lead to such citations.

A process cannot be validated without validated analytical methods. So how did one sponsor think it could proceed with "no acceptance criteria for validating analytical methods, deleted data, and missing sections that made it impossible to assess the results"?

The rush to be first to market is always a challenge. And the shortage of experienced personnel also causes oversights that lead to process validation mistakes. Validation should be designed into the production process, but this requires time to understand risks associated with each unit operation, cell substrates, and raw materials, as well as the expected results from the fermentation/cell culture and purification processes that will minimize those risks.

Citations related to fermentation processes that were not properly validated include the comment that "production time limits had not been established for inoculum fermentation." Another comment in the fermentation area relates to hold times. In this case, there were "no microbiological data supporting specified hold time for autoclaved fermentation vessels." In another, it was observed that "the fermentation process was validated to last for a certain amount of time, but batches were terminated before the specified time due to contamination."

Bioburden control and related regulatory expectations in the manufacture of biopharmaceuticals have certainly raised concerns over the last few years. Some firms have claimed that a high limit, e.g., 100 CFU/ml, is acceptable when they have consistently found only 10 CFU/ml. If, in fact, one lot had 100 CFU/ml, it could overload process capabilities. Even if the bacteria are inactivated, residual unanticipated or unknown toxins might be copurified with the product. One has to wonder how a process could be validated for 100 CFU/ml if this had never been seen. Are spiking studies a realistic approach to solving this dilemma? Probably not, since it is likely not feasible to measure all potential contaminants and their by-products. Furthermore, the microorganisms introduced in manufacturing might be different from those used in the spiking study. However, a generic/family approach to validation of sanitization agent capability has proved to be valuable.[3] Such spiking studies, however, do not replace the need for validated in-process monitoring.

Comments on hold time studies, or the lack thereof, seem to indicate that this is an issue often cited. In addition to the previous comment for the autoclaved fermentation vessels, another reviewer noted that "there were no hold time studies for buffers and rinse solutions used in production." Hold times are clearly an essential element for ensuring consistent manufacturing, yet with no validation plan and minimal resources, they are sometimes overlooked.

Cleaning validation has been an issue cited during several inspections. Multiuse facilities and chromatography processes seem to draw the most concern. One sponsor had "no cleaning validation for cleaning critical manufacturing areas." Yet another was observed to have "no cleaning validation for laminar air flow hoods used for the preculture inoculation process." In another situation, it was observed that the manufacturer had "not conducted cleaning validation to demonstrate that a cleaning detergent/antifoam agent could effectively remove an unidentified substance that accumulated on a column resin and interfered with column packing."

The validation of chromatography remains a source of reviewer comments. Column lifetime, storage, and cleaning are all linked. An assessment of carryover and its risks are important elements that should be included in the validation plan. Validation of column storage times is a critical area, and it was observed at one manufacturer that there were "no column storage time studies including bioburden and LAL determination." In one postapproval inspection, the FDA reviewer commented that "the cleaning validation study was only conducted up to five uses of the column but the column could be used up to 46 lots based only on a laboratory study." In a review letter, a sponsor was asked to "please provide validation data to demonstrate there is no negative impact of extended use up to 150 production cycles on the efficacy of cleaning and regeneration of the column." Column packing has raised some comments such as "there were no studies on packing of purification columns." In another situation, it was observed that a column was "consistently out of specification for a test, and there was no evidence that validation was reviewed to verify performance within the specification."

Validation of filter reuse has also drawn some attention. In one case, SOPs were generated without validation data for the specification the operator was expected to meet. It was observed that "the SOP required filters to be replaced after a specified time or after a defined number of production runs. No data were generated to support the requirement for 200 runs." It is not uncommon to find that filtration needs to be repeated during manufacturing. Reprocessing of filtration requires validation, but one citation read "reprocessing (e.g., re-filtration) was performed without validated reprocessing procedures."

Small-scale studies can be invaluable for predicting resin lifetime. FDA spokespersons have noted that small-scale studies are useful for determining resin lifetime, but not monitoring during manufacturing is unacceptable. For other validation concerns, such as viral clearance, small-scale studies remain the only viable option at this time.

Viral clearance validation/evaluation studies have been problematic since the first biotherapeutics were produced. The reasons are manyfold. Among those reasons are safety issues, sensitivity and inhibition of infectivity assays, scale-down accuracy, effect of spike on process, cost of studies, and data interpretation. In the past, most sponsors have waited until they were almost ready to begin clinical trials to perform viral clearance studies. PCR now provides the process development scientist a more rapid, more sensitive, and less costly alternative that allows for the assessment of viral clearance capabilities during development. Clearance studies should also address sanitization studies. One sponsor was asked to "provide data that show complete removal of viral contamination prior to reuse of the system."

In the FDA's "Points to Consider in the Manufacture and Testing of Monoclonal Antibody Products for Human Use," it is noted that an appropriately conducted clearance study may be an acceptable substitute for lot-to-lot testing for potential contaminants and additives.[4] Validated clearance studies combined with final product testing on at least three production lots can significantly reduce quality control costs and expedite product release. However, it is essential that these studies be repeated when process changes with potential for changing clearance are made, since these clearance studies are often a critical element in ensuring patient safety. The capability to perform the validated assays used for the clearance studies must be maintained. This can be problematic during clinical studies, in the event that the one analyst who can perform the method leaves the company.

For clearance studies, scaled-down models must be validated to ensure that they reflect manufacturing results. For example, purity and impurity profiles should be the same at both scales. Viral clearance and microorganism sanitization studies must be done outside of the actual facility, often resulting in differences in operators, buffer preparation, and unit operations. All too often there is a disconnect between those who perform validation and clearance studies and personnel in manufacturing, leading to inconsistencies cited during regulatory review.

1.3 VALIDATION: TODAY AND TOMORROW

1.3.1 Today

Validation begins with good process development. It requires that process developers understand the necessity to design a process that will be capable of ultimately meeting predetermined specifications without being subject to deviations within a defined range of preset operating parameters. Development reports are invaluable when process changes are to be implemented and validated, but it has also been observed that companies usually put constraints on the time allotted for development, and the development reports are often not very effective. This is in spite of the fact that other companies find the development reports a means to expedite reviewer understanding of critical process parameters, which can lead to a reduced regulatory burden. In fact, the Common Technical Document requires a development summary.[5]

Technology transfer from process development to pilot or manufacturing is a challenge. The frustration level is high when a manufacturing process change is made that invalidates previously validated studies. It is a two-way process, however. The process developers must understand manufacturing capabilities. One frustrated manufacturing head noted that every process developer should spend a year in manufacturing.

Validation documentation is extensive and includes master validation plans, validation protocols, and validation reports. A master validation plan is a useful essential and is now specified in EU Annex 15 as a requirement.[6] This annex to the "EU Guide to Good Manufacturing Practice" provides an overview of several validation-related documents. You are less likely to overlook validation items that are specified in a plan. As noted by one CDER compliance officer, validation master plans and documentation will still be critical components of GMP compliance in the FDA's new GMP initiative. He went on to state that firms ought to start viewing process validation not just as a step in the manufacturing process, but as an ongoing activity from design to testing and continuous improvements.[7]

Validation protocols are also an essential basic. The protocol must state what will be done, how it will be done, and what the outcome must be for the validation to be a success. Validation cannot be just going back to a process step repeated three times and stating it is validated.

As noted previously, validation is an ongoing process. It is not a one-time effort that can then be ignored. For biotherapeutics, most validation is performed prospectively, i.e., prior to market approval. However, today there is more acceptance of also using concurrent validation for some aspects. For example, in the FDA's "Therapeutic Compliance Guide Program Guide 7341.001," it states, "There are situations where concurrent validation at the manufacturing scale may be more appropriate. Continued use may be based upon routine monitoring against predetermined criteria."[8] Certainly, data collected at the manufacturing scale can be more relevant provided that in-process analysis is sufficiently sensitive.

1.3.2 Tomorrow

New technologies and a risk-based approach applied to biopharmaceutical manufacturing are enabling more in-process monitoring. Process Analytical Technology (PAT) is being driven by the FDA, and although more commonly used for synthetic drugs, it is already being used by some firms producing biopharmaceuticals. Newer, highly sensitive, at-line, on-line, and in-line measurements allow more control of processes. Although unlikely to replace the need for prospective validation, it has the potential to reduce that effort. PAT has been used in fermentation control. Cell viability has been measured by NAD/NADH fluorescence; total cell counts by turbidity- and optical density-based sensors; product and nutrient concentration by HPLC, IC, NIR, and IR; and respiratory quotient by off-gas analysis with mass spectrometry, pH, DO_2, and DCO_2. In purification columns, PAT has been used to provide feedback of gradient control by NIR, UV, and conductivity. HPLC and a UV sensor have also been used to determine when to collect product.[9] As noted by Dr. Kathyrn Zoon, elements of PAT could be applicable even to traditional biologics, such as plasma derivatives. Dr. Zoon also commented that PAT could be used for online monitoring of adventitious agents found in biotech therapeutics.[10]

Another interesting validation approach is the use of generic or modular clearance studies. Several fairly recent publications have provided significant data that may lead to regulatory acceptance of these studies for viral clearance. A generic retrovirus low-pH inactivation study was performed, and it was shown that bracketed generic conditions were sufficient to inactivate X-MLV in cell-free intermediates produced in either NSO or CHO cell substrates. Both monoclonal antibody and recombinant protein processes were evaluated. In all cases, when the bracketed conditions were adhered to, a log reduction value of ≥ 4.6 $\log_{10}$ was obtained.[11] In another study with monoclonals, a generic/matrix chromatography virus-removal step was evaluated on Q-Sepharose Fast Flow. The column was operated in a flow-through mode so that the virus, not the product, would bind. The clearance of SV-40 was shown to be ≥ 4.7 $\log_{10}$ in three model antibodies with pIs ≥ 8.8.[12] Furthermore, the data were consistent in resins reused more than 50 times. These publications suggest that with data such as these, process development can begin with conditions that provide the likelihood of adequate viral clearance.

Caution should be taken, however, since this approach is not universally applicable. With other, more complex separation modes, the generic/matrix approach may not work, and at this time, the approach is not accepted by regulatory agencies.

The use of PATs and generic/matrix approaches can expedite validation strategies and ensure consistency in the production of biotherapeutics. These technologies, however, are also likely to enable approval of so-called follow-on biologics, also known as biogenerics.

REFERENCES

1. *BioQuality*, 8, 4–11, 2003 (biotech@pe.net).

2. Zaret, E.H., GMP notebook: A GMP report card from FDA, *Pharmaceut. Form. Qual.*, June/July, 54, 2003.

3. Hiraoka, M. and Broughton, C., Validating the sanitization of chromatographic resins: a sample case study, *BioPharm*, 14, 26–30, 52.

4. U.S. FDA, Points to Consider in the Manufacture and Testing of Monoclonal Antibody Products for Human Use, 1997.

5. *The Gold Sheet*, 37, 3–4, 2003.

6. Final Version of Annex 15 to the EU Guide to Good Manufacturing Practices, Qualification and Validation (http://pharmacos.eudra.org/F2/eudralex/index.htm).

7. *Validation Times*, 6, 2, 2003.

8. FDA's Therapeutic Compliance Guide Program Guide 7341.001 (http://www.fda.gov/ora/compliance_ref/).

9. *Validation Times*, 1, 6–7, 2003.

10. *Validation Times*, 6, 4, 2003.

11. Brorson, K., Krejci, S., Lee, K., Hamilton, E., Stein, K., and Xu, Y., Bracketed generic inactivation of rodent retroviruses by low pH treatment for monoclonal antibodies and recombinant proteins, *Biotechnol. Bioeng.*, 82, 321–329, 2003.

12. Curtis, S., Lee, K., Blank, G.S., Brorson, K., and Xu, Y., Generic/matrix evaluation of SV40 clearance by anion exchange chromatography in flow-through mode, *Biotechnol. Bioeng.*, 84, 179–186, 2003.

2

Applications of Failure Modes and Effects Analysis to Biotechnology Manufacturing Processes

ROBERT J. SEELY AND JOHN HAURY

CONTENTS

2.1 INTRODUCTION

Failure modes and effects analysis (FMEA) is a very powerful risk assessment tool widely used in a variety of manufacturing industries and business practices. Like many risk analysis procedures, FMEA provides a rigorous methodology for identifying, evaluating, and documenting potential modes of product or process failure [1,2,3]. In contrast to the other methods, an FMEA results in a numerical ranking of each potential failure, aiding the prioritization of follow-up investigations and implementation of corrections or controls to mitigate the failure [4]. FMEA is a useful tool in guiding and documenting the thinking process when operating parameters are evaluated for criticality or when a process is transferred to a different manufacturing site. It is a systematic, rigorous method for ranking parameters into (potentially) high-risk categories and for defining which variables need further process characterization [3].

The risk assessment is based on assigning a ranking of 1 to 10 (low to high), to three critical criteria: (1) the severity of a failure, (2) the expected frequency of occurrence, and (3) the likelihood of detecting the failure. The product of the three scores results in a risk priority number (RPN), which can vary between 1 and 1000. It is important to evaluate the potential failure with all three criteria because the effects may either multiply or offset one another. That is, a failure may be very severe, but if the occurrence is low and the detectability is high, the resulting RPN is low. The primary benefits of this tool are that it provides a rational approach to evaluating a process, and it generates a ranked order of parameters requiring characterization, hence a shortening of the total list of operating variables to be studied. In addition, it provides a sound documenting mechanism to record the group decision-making process.

2.2 RISK ANALYSIS METHODS

The concept of risk implies a degree of uncertainty regarding the outcome of an event, process, project, behavior, or decision.

To evaluate and measure this uncertainty requires a systematic framework involving the elements of probability, consequences, detectability, and recoverability or correctability. There are a wide variety of assessment methodologies available, ranging from risk avoidance to risk acceptance [5]. While they all share the common elements given previously, they have distinguishing characteristics that accommodate specific applications. For example, FMEA and Preliminary Hazard Analysis are inductive (or inferential). Inductive logic starts with particular instances and infers that the general cause exists (with a given probability). This logic is based on the question "Given a particular situation, what is the likely general system causing it?" FMEA, for example, allows the prioritization of those causes for preventive action. Other methods such as Fault Tree Analysis and Success Tree Analysis are deductive. They proceed from a general premise to derive or predict consequential results. Deductive logic asks the question "What general system components or scenarios must go right or wrong in order to cause a particular consequence?" Within these categories, some methods are qualitative, some are quantitative, and some rely heavily on probabilistic theory [4,5].

2.3 TWO APPLICATIONS OF FMEA

This chapter will describe a streamlined application of FMEA to two main aspects of bioprocessing: process characterization and process transfer. Process characterization is the portion of process development that examines the ranges to be specified in the manufacturing procedures, robustness of the process, and for a limited number of critical parameters, the edge of failure. In a recombinant protein process, there may be several hundred operational parameters and it is not practical, or necessary, to test the high and low value of every range. The FMEA method can be an effective tool to evaluate every variable, first as a paper exercise, then by follow-up study of the variables ranked as high risk if failure were to occur.

The transfer of a process from one site to another has been found to be another area where FMEA can provide a structured thinking process to help ensure success. Process transfers invariably involve some changes — in equipment, processing, raw material sources, water quality, personnel, and environmental conditions. Here the FMEA target is to identify any changes in the two processes, however slight. Many of the operational parameters will remain exactly the same as in the established process, and there may be a good deal of historical data to support their associated ranges. The variables that are identified by the group as being different or potentially different are the ones that should be subjected to the FMEA analysis, and the resulting high RPN parameters should be further evaluated. Additional lab studies performed by process development are often suitable for the evaluation.

These two applications of FMEA demonstrate a useable, value-added method to identify potential problems before they occur. The method is readily adaptable to a variety of other applications in the biotechnology industry and is simplified such that the readers can readily apply the techniques to their particular processes. In addition, FMEA is an effective mechanism for promoting teamwork and facilitating discussions throughout the development cycle and between departments. The benefits of such applications very much offset the man-hours required to execute the analysis [4,5].

2.4 FMEA WORKSHEET

The most efficient way to capture an FMEA exercise is the use of a simple spreadsheet, as shown in Table 2.1. The first column is to prospectively identify and list each and every parameter that is to be evaluated. For a recombinant protein production process, this list might be all the input variables for performing a manufacturing process. Here we list every control parameter specified in a Manufacturing Procedure (batch record), one spreadsheet for each unit operation, such as the setting of flow rate, temperature, mixing speed and time, pH, etc. These are the operating set points that are staged by an operator or by a computer controller to perform a specific unit operation, such as fermentation, centrifugation, and chromatography.

TABLE 2.1 Example FMEA Worksheet

Failure Modes and Effects Analysis				Page _____ of ____					
Process:									
Unit Op:									
Leader:									
Date:									
Operational Parameter	Failure Mode(s)	Cause(s)	Effect(s)	Follow-Up By	S	O	D	RPN	Recommended Follow-Up

Once this list is completed, and there may be several dozen variables for a given operation, the evaluation team begins to discuss and identify potential modes of failure and their respective causes and effects. Based on the causes and effects, the team can then decide on a numerical scoring of the severity of the (potential) failure, the possible frequency of occurrence, and the current ability to detect the failure (S, O, and D, respectively). These numerical assignments are somewhat subjective but are also based on historical experience with the process or related processes, scientific judgment, and an understanding of equipment capability [6,7]. Working definitions of the SOD criteria and examples are presented in the next sections.

The values for S, O, and D are arrived at by interactive discussions of an interdisciplinary team. It is critical to have the system experts present, as well as plant manufacturing personnel, development scientists, and scale-up engineers [3,7]. In addition, representatives from Quality Control and Quality Assurance may be called in for portions of the assessment that pertain to their roles. From the scores assigned, the RPN is calculated and the results can be graphically displayed as a Pareto chart [8]. Typically, the RPN values fall into clusters of very high, moderate, and very low. The RPN scale is 1 to 1000. At what point the "high" risk variables require further examination and additional characterization data need to be generated is often difficult to predetermine. This is due to factors such as the subjectivity involved in assigning S, O, and D values and team-to-team differences in consistently utilizing the definitions for SOD. Thus, rather than setting a prospective cutoff between "high" and "low" RPN, we rely on clustering of the values. The clustering can be readily seen in a Pareto chart, where an obvious set of high-ranking numbers can be visually distinguished from the obviously low values. Alternatively, one can choose to further evaluate the top-ranking 30% or 50% initially and evaluate some or all of the remaining variables as time and resources permit.

The purpose of the FMEA is to collectively evaluate potential failures, prioritize them on a consensus basis, and document the evaluation process. From there, the Process

Team must decide which of the variables require dedication of future efforts. As the top-ranking risk variables are investigated and corrected or controlled to reduce their risk of failure, individual follow-up reports will be written to document the actions taken.

2.5 EVALUATION CRITERIA: SEVERITY, OCCURRENCE, AND DETECTION

Table 2.2 gives some example definition for the levels, 1 to 10, of the three criteria. The definitions usually need to be modified to fit a particular FMEA application. Those for a medical device, where design needs and tolerances are fairly well established, are different from a biological process, where the effects of excursion of a manufacturing operating range may not be known. The definitions should be discussed as a team before the FMEA is begun. Even when a rating system is clearly defined, there may be disagreements as to the numerical values for SOD of a particular parameter. Further discussions, moderated by a trained facilitator, can bring consensus to the group [2,3,7]. Some examples of SOD assignments to manufacturing processes are given after the general discussions presented next.

2.5.1 Severity

The severity rating is a measure of the seriousness of a particular failure. The severity may be clear from previous experiences. Often it must be estimated based on what the outcome might be; e.g., yield loss, total batch loss, validation failure, or the need to perform an extensive investigation before further process or product release can occur. Out-of-compliance issues and patient safety are also major concerns. The examples given in Table 2.2 are generic and careful thought should be given to individual FMEA targets, especially for severity scoring. During the assessment of the final RPN ranks, items with very high severity rating should be considered for further study regardless of their overall RPN [7].

TABLE 2.2 Example Ratings for Severity, Occurrence, and Detectability

Scale	Severity	Occurrence	Detectability
10	Hazardous, without warning; may endanger machine or assembly operator; noncompliance with government regulation; fails final product specs >90% of the time; product lost or completely unrecoverable	>25 lots/yr >50% CpK <0.33	Almost impossible to detect; no known controls available to detect failure mode
9	Hazardous, with warning; may endanger machine or assembly operator; fails in-process performance parameters 100% of the time and final product specs 50% of the time; over 50% impact on step and overall yield	10–20 lots/yr ~25–40% CpK 0.33	Very remote likelihood that current controls will detect failure mode; occasionally we check for defects
8	Very high; major disruption to product line; 100% of product may have to be scrapped; fails in-process performance parameters ~75% of the time and final product specs >25% of the time; approx. 50% impact on step yield and over 25% impact on overall yield	6–9 lots/yr ~15% CpK 0.51	Remote likelihood current controls will detect failure mode; systematic sampling and inspection
7	High; major disruption to production line; product may have to be sorted and a portion scrapped; fails in-process performance parameters ~50% of the time; final product purity specs fail 10% of the time; 30–40% step yield and >20% overall yield impact	5 lots/yr ~10% CpK 0.67	Very low likelihood current controls will detect failure mode; all units are manually inspected

(continued)

TABLE 2.2 Example Ratings for Severity, Occurrence, and Detectability (Continued)

Scale	Severity	Occurrence	Detectability
6	Moderate; minor disruption to production line; may fail in-process performance parameters in ~25% of instances; may fail product specs 5% of the time; approx. 25% step yield and >10% overall yield impact	2–3 lots/yr ~5% CpK 0.83	Low likelihood current controls will detect failure mode; manual inspection with mistake-proofing
5	Low; minor disruption to production line; 100% of product may have to be reworked; runs on edge of in-process performance parameters and may fail these in ~10% instances; ~10% impact on step yield and ~5% impact on overall yield	1 lot per year ~2% CpK 1.00	Moderate likelihood current controls will detect failure mode; SPC monitoring and manual inspection
4	Very low; minor disruption to production line; measurable effect on in-process performance parameters, but will not exceed in-process control; measurable effect on step yield (5%)	1 lot every other year ~1% CpK 1.17	Moderately high likelihood current controls will detect failure mode; SPC with immediate reaction to special causes
3	Minor disruption to production line; a portion of the product may have to be reworked online; slightly measurable impact on in-process performance parameters; slight but measurable impact on step yield (<3%)	One lot every 3–5 years ~0.5% CpK 1.33	High likelihood current controls will detect failure mode; SPC with 100% inspection for special causes

(continued)

TABLE 2.2 Example Ratings for Severity, Occurrence, and Detectability (Continued)

Scale	Severity	Occurrence	Detectability
2	Very minor disruption to production line; in-process impact may go unnoticed	One lot every >5 years ~0.2% CpK 1.50	Very high likelihood current controls will detect failure mode; all units are automatically inspected
1	No effect on performance; not noticed	Never or > every 10 years CpK 1.67	Almost certain current controls will detect failure mode; defect is obvious and cannot affect anyone

Note: Occurrence here is based on 50 runs per year. CpK is the process capability index.
Source: D.P. Stockdale Associates. D. Stockdale, President. 10 Reata, Rancho Santa Margarita, CA 92688.

The severity of a failure can be assessed in several ways. Patient safety should always be a primary concern, but the severity may be a major issue before the product is ever released for distribution. In some instances, plant personnel safety might be the driving concern. Business issues such as cost or productivity, regulatory compliance, and consistent process control are other effects of operation failure. The FMEA may be geared toward one specific concern or a mixture as long as the target is agreed on by the FMEA team.

2.5.2 Occurrence

This is a measure of how frequently the failure might occur. If the excursion of a variable (operating temperature, for example) has occurred often in the past or may occur often at a new facility, additional controls may be needed. The occurrence is also assessed with respect to severity and detectability. If the severity is rated low and there are detection measures in place, the overall RPN may be low and this particular variable might not be studied until a later time in the development cycle. The examples for occurrence in Table 2.2 demonstrate that for a biological process, occurrence is somewhat easier to define than severity. The table offers three occurrence measurements: the failure rate based on number of lots per year, the percentage of batches, and the capability of the process [9].

2.5.3 Detectability

Detection is a significant criterion to include in the evaluation of risk. Even if a given failure has serious consequences and might occur often, if there are adequate detection modes in place that provide time for corrective action, the overall RPN might be low. However, there are several classes of detectability. The degree of detection just described is ideal; however, the failure may be detected but not in time for immediate correction. Often the batch of material is being processed at a later operational step before the failure, or excursion, is noticed. Detection may be noted from continuously logged data but no alarms are in place, or the results from analytical data require an extended period of time. Detection in these cases is still considered "good" and an intermediate rating of 4 to 6 might be appropriate. If the failure cannot be detected before the product is shipped — or even worse, before it is used — the rating should be very high.

2.6 EXAMPLE OF FMEA APPLIED TO PROCESS TRANSFER

An example of application of FMEA to process characterization has been presented previously [10]. An example of application to a validated, commercial process being transferred to a new manufacturing site is given in Table 2.3. The entries are not self-explanatory and the example is shown to illustrate a few noteworthy features. First, the spreadsheet is a

TABLE 2.3 Unit Operation

Unit Operation: Seed Train   Page____of____   Responsibility   Failure/Problem
Date:

Parameter	Follow-Up		Potential Failure Mode	Severity	Potential Cause of Failure	Occurrence	Current Controls	Detection	RPN
Shake platform throw	If throws are the same in both machines, no issue	I. L.							0
Shake temp controls	Temperature mapping studies will be performed	I. L.	Difference in growth profile	5	Different heat distribution profile could modify growth curve; potential to fail PV criterion	2	Temperature mapping studies	2	20
Tubing materials	Same material required by MP	J. M.							
Pumps	Will be same as B-7	J. M.							
Glassware same	Same as B-7	J. M.							0

Innoc. vial handling	Handling of vials from freezer to plant will be equivalent to B-7	B. D.						0
Fermentor R-0180 seal/ pressure		B. W.	Leakage	4	Design	2	5	40
				4	Assembly and maintenance			
				4	Utility failure			
		B. W.	Contamination	10	Design	2	5	100
				10	Assembly and maintenance			
				10	Utility failure			
				10	Inadeq. ster. cycle			

streamlined version of those provided in the references for the more "classical" FMEA applications. For biotechnology processes, there are so very many modes of potential failure that are largely unknown that it is the best use of the team's time to strive to quickly identify and rank the ones that are known. For a process transfer, as mentioned previously, the focus is on what aspects (processing variables, equipment, materials) are different from the site of origin to the site of transfer.

In the spreadsheet, it can be seen that several variables were identified as being possibly different but not known for certain at the time of the FMEA. A simple follow-up was noted with an associated responsible person (see Shake platform throw). If it is found that the item is indeed going to be different, then that person is responsible for investigating the degree of difference and the SOD it might have (off-line) and for defining what investigations or corrective action is necessary. The time may not be available to reassemble the team and review such follow-up activities.

A second feature of the table is shown by the fermentor seal/pressure. Here it was noted that the shaft seal will be of a different material and it may fail by not holding pressure in either direction. If the seal fails to prevent incoming air, as compared to exhaust gas, the failure effect of contamination will be much more severe, leading to a Severity rating of 10. Further, the Detectability was given a 5 because, even though it would be detected very quickly during operation, it would necessitate an unacceptably long shutdown and replacement time. The corrective action to this item was to expedite delivery and field-testing to ensure the seal is adequate.

The example shown in Table 2.3 is a very small snapshot of the FMEA process for the particular transfer being made, but it does show that the FMEA concept is useful to quickly identify, catalog, and assign risk priorities to the variables that will be or are suspected of being different between two sites. It also affords a structured methodology for a cross-sectional team to (1) reevaluate the possible changes and help ensure nothing was overlooked in the transfer and (2) document that that was done.

2.7　NEXT STEPS

Once the initial FMEA exercise has been completed, there remains the critical part of follow-up. The FMEA has resulted in (1) documentation that every element of the process (for characterization or for transfer) has been evaluated by a team, and (2) a prioritization of parameters or issues that now need to be addressed. Based on the RPNs, as visualized in Pareto fashion, the team should agree on a cutoff value for studying the "high" RPNs first, and perhaps some or all of the others as time and resources permit. As previously mentioned, this cutoff can be made prospectively (although for a biological process, this may be difficult and is not necessary), or it can be made retrospectively based on the results. The cutoff can be based on criteria such as obvious clustering (the top 25%, 33%, 50%, etc.), or the follow-up studies can be performed one at a time, working from high to low, as time permits. Whatever the team decision is, it should be recorded in the FMEA report.

The report can now be written and the initial FMEA can be closed out. The follow-up items identified in the FMEA are to be addressed by the responsible person or team and should be documented in subsequent, separate technical reports. The closure of all these items may take several months and typically is done by individuals from different departments. Because of these factors, it is important to finalize the initial FMEA and get it into the hands of the team members who need to act on the identified issues and to the team leader who will be responsible for ensuring timely completion.

We find that the best person to write the report is the facilitator. Even though the facilitator may not be fully aware of the physical/chemical aspects of the operating parameters discussed, he or she will have been present during the entire meeting. Other team members may come and go as the topics of expertise change. Also, it is crucial to the success of an FMEA to make it as easy as possible on the team and team leader. By assisting in organizing and moderating the FMEA, including defining SOD and writing the initial report, the facilitator can assume many tasks from the team and leader.

The report is essentially the "minutes" of the FMEA meeting and should contain the following elements:

- FMEA scope and date
- List of team members, by name and organization
- Definitions of SOD determined by the team
- Cutoff RPN, if known
- Completed worksheets
- Pareto charts
- Future work — a reminder that the identified individuals are to further investigate the items assigned to them and write subsequent technical reports

It may be useful to write one final report, once all items are closed, to summarize all the follow-up reports, listing them by title, author, and report number and perhaps including a brief outline of the issue and corrective action taken. For a process characterization FMEA, the final report could list the final key parameters and a discussion of why some were determined to be nonkey and thus need not be validated. Such summaries will aid in retrieval for nonconformance investigations, proposed process changes, or questions that might arise during an inspection or other regulatory review. The resulting compilation of documents, and the resolution of potential problems before they occur, should represent a body of work that was value-added and can be utilized for the life of the product.

REFERENCES

1. DeSain, C. and Sutton, C.V., *Risk Management Basics*, Advanstar, Cleveland, 2000.

2. Kieffer, R., Bureau, S., and Borgmann, A., Applications of failure mode effect analysis in the pharmaceutical industry, *Pharm. Technol. Europe*, Sept., 36–49, 1997.

3. McDermott, R.E., Mikulak, R.J., and Beauregard, M.R., *The Basics of FMEA*, Productivity, Portland, OR, 1996.

4. Shani, A., Using failure mode and effect analysis to improve manufacturing processes, *Med. Device Diagn. Ind.*, July, 47–51, 1993.

5. Ayyub, B.M., *Risk Analysis in Engineering and Economics*, Chapman & Hall/CRC, Boca Raton, FL, 2003.

6. Clemen, R.T., *Making Hard Decisions*, 2nd ed., Duxbury Press, Pacific Grove, 1995, pp. 5–8.

7. Stamatis, D.H., *Failure Mode and Effect Analysis; FMEA from Theory to Execution*, 2nd ed., ASQ Quality Press, Milwaukee, 2003, p. 39.

8. Burr, J.T., *SPC Tools for Everyone*, ASQ Quality Press, Milwaukee, 1993, pp. 8–12.

9. Kieffer, R.G., Validation, risk-benefit analysis, *PDA J. Pharm. Sci. Technol.*, 49, 249–252, 1995.

10. Seely, J.E. and Seely, R.J., A rational, step-wise approach to process characterization, *BioPharm Int.*, 16, 24–34, 2003.

3

Process Characterization

JAMES E. SEELY

CONTENTS

3.1 INTRODUCTION

Although considered to be a significant time and resource commitment from Process Development, process characterization has been shown to be valuable in ensuring validation and manufacturing success. Given the expense of producing biopharmaceuticals at large scale, process characterization gives an excellent return on investment over the lifetime of a product or process. Inadequate process characterization can result in costly lot failures and incidents, failed validation runs, and difficult inspections [1].

The overall goal of adequate process characterization for commercial manufacturing processes is to ensure efficient and successful process validation and the assurance of consistent process performance [2]. More specifically, process characterization provides:

- An understanding of the role of each process step, such as an understanding of where impurities are cleared during a particular purification step
- An understanding of the impact of process inputs (operating parameters) on process outputs (performance parameters) and identification of key operating and performance parameters
- Assurance that process delivers consistent product yields and purity within all operating ranges
- Acceptance criteria for in-process performance parameters

In addition, although not a primary reason for doing process characterization, these studies will frequently uncover areas for subtle process improvements in terms of process consistency, product yields, or product purity.

In this chapter we present an outline and some examples for how to carry out thorough and consistent process characterization. The proposed methods could provide a framework for carrying out this work. A good portion of this chapter will describe "precharacterization" studies. These studies are used to help define the scope of the actual experimental characterization work. They also lay the foundation for the experimental studies by demonstrating the adequacy of scaled-down process models and analytical methods. A framework and examples for doing experimental process characterization work will also be presented.

Finally, we will discuss future directions and challenges as our approach to process characterization evolves.

3.2 RESOURCES AND TIMING FOR PROCESS CHARACTERIZATION STUDIES

The driver for the timing of process characterization is the start of conformance/validation lots. Process characterization should be completed in time such that the information gained from these studies can be used to support operating ranges and acceptance criteria for validation protocols. Thorough process characterization may add as much as a year to the overall process development time, so the completion of commercial process development work and initiation of process characterization studies should be timed with this factor in mind [2]. Thorough process characterization requires a fully integrated process characterization team (~8–12 people) including upstream and downstream processing, analytical departments, and representatives from pilot and full-scale manufacturing. Resource planning from the analytical departments is especially important, since a single characterization run may generate several samples for analysis.

3.3 PRECHARACTERIZATION WORK

There are three key aspects to precharacterization work: (1) historical data review and risk assessment, (2) scale-down model qualification, and (3) analytical method qualification.

3.3.1 Historical Data Review and Risk Assessment

Retrospective review of historical data and risk assessment analysis can be used to determine operating parameters that need to be examined experimentally as part of process characterization. Lab notebooks, technical reports, process histories, run summaries, manufacturing records, and a list of the operating parameters and the provisional operating ranges for each unit operation can be used by the process characterization team to determine knowledge gaps in the process. Information from the operating ranges tested during process development can help identify those parameters that are most likely to impact the process [2–4]. In particular, experimental design studies (DOE) from the commercial process development work can be useful for identifying key parameters or even in determining operating ranges in certain instances, since these experiments are carried out over a range of operating parameters and may yield information about operating parameter interactions.

Once data mining is completed, a risk assessment analysis can be carried out on each unit operation where the effect and likelihood of an excursion from each operating parameter range is addressed. Hazard Analysis and Critical Control Points (HACCP) [5], Failure Mode and Effects Analysis (FMEA) [6–9], cause-and-effect diagrams [10], and other risk assessment tools can be used for these purposes. The FMEA tool assigns a numerical rating to the *severity* of an excursion of an operating parameter, the *frequency* of an excursion, and the *ability to detect* the excursion before it has an impact on the product [6–9]. The combined risk factor (Risk Priority Number or RPN) is a multiple of these three variables, giving a rating scale from 1 to 1000 if a 1–10 numerical rating is used [6–9]. This data is usually presented in the form of a Pareto chart [6–10], and those operating parameters below a predetermined threshold are considered non-key and will not be examined in the characterization experiments. It is a good idea to involve not only scientists who developed the process in the FMEA exercise, but also quality and plant engineers since they can bring insight into the likelihood of certain process excursions and the ability to detect them. There may be significant differences between the commercial and first-in-human processes, and there may be relatively little historical data on the commercial process. Therefore, it may be important to draw on any development and historical data from both the first-in-human and commercial processes.

Probably the biggest challenge in doing FMEA is coming up with a consistent and not totally subjective risk category definition system that everyone can agree on. There are a number of generic risk category definitions available [6–9,11]. A custom-made risk category definition system that we have used is shown in Table 3.1. One way to better define the rating system for FMEA is to consider the preferred operating range for each operating parameter in manufacturing. For example, although it may be possible to run a process at ±0.1 pH units, operationally the process may be more robust if it can be run at ±0.2 units. Examples of some preferred operating ranges for different operating parameters are shown in Table 3.2. For the FMEA exercise, we can improve the signal-to-noise ratio of our analysis if we assume that we are considering the severity of running the process approximately 3 times outside the normal operating range for a given operating parameter. For considering the operating parameter excursion frequency and the ability to detect them, we can increase our sensitivity by considering excursions that are just outside the tightest controllable operating range (Table 3.2).

Case Study 3.1

FMEA analysis for removal of a detergent from a protein preparation using an ion-exchange chromatography method is shown in Table 3.3. Scientists who developed the process determined the severity of an excursion approximately 2–3 times outside the preferred operating range. Manufacturing and plant engineers determined the frequency of excursions outside of the tightest operating range. Quality control and manufacturing provided information about the ability to detect these excursions

TABLE 3.1 Custom-Made Risk Category Rating Definitions for FMEA

1–10 Scale	Severity	Occurrence	Detection
10 "Bad"	Fails final product specs >90% of the time or product lost or completely unrecoverable	>50% >25 times per year	No way to detect defect
9	Fails in-process performance parameters 100% of the time and final product specs >50% of the time, or over 50% impact on step and overall yield	~30–40% 15–20 times per year	Unit sampling and inspection; defect not detected until after impact on process
8	Fails in-process performance parameters ~75% of the time and final product specs >25% of the time, or approx. 50% impact on step yield and over 25% impact on overall yield	~20% 10 times per year	Unit sampling and inspection; defect can be detected prior to impacting process
7	Fails in-process performance parameters ~50% of the time; final product purity specs failed 10% of the time, or 30–40% step yield and >20% overall yield impact	~10% 5 times per year	All units are manually inspected; defect not detected until after impact on process
6	May fail in-process performance parameters in ~25% of instances; may fail final product specs 5% of the time, or approx. 25% step yield and >10% overall yield impact	~5% 2–3 times per year	All units automatically controlled; defect not detected until after impact on process

(continued)

TABLE 3.1 Custom-Made Risk Category Rating Definitions for FMEA (Continued)

1–10 Scale	Severity	Occurrence	Detection
5	Runs on edge of in-process performance parameters and may fail these in ~10% instances, or ~10% impact on step yield and measurable impact on overall yield (~5%)	~2% Once a year	All units automatically controlled with secondary manual inspection; defect not detected until after impact on process
4	Measurable effect on in-process performance parameters but will not exceed in-process control limits, or more measurable effect on step yield (~5%)	~1% Once every 2–3 years	All units manually inspected; defect detected prior to impact on process
3	Slightly measurable impact on in-process quality attribute parameters or slight but measurable impact on step yield (<3%)	~0.5% Once every 5 years	All units automatically inspected; defect detected prior to impact on the process
2	Measurable effect on non-key, nonquality attribute in-process performance parameter (i.e., pool volume, peak position)	~0.2% Once every 10 years	All units automatically controlled with secondary manual control; defect detected prior to impact on the process
1 "Good"	Not noticed; no effect on performance	Never	Defect is obvious and would always be detected prior to starting process

TABLE **3.2** Examples of Tightest and Preferred
Operating Ranges (±) for Operating Parameters

Parameter	Tightest Operating Range	Preferred Operating Range	Range for FMEA Severity and Screening
pH	0.1	0.2	0.3 or 0.4
Time	5%	10%	15–20%
Temperature	1°C	2°C	3 or 4°C
Flow rate	5%	10%	15%
Volume	2%	5%	10%
OD	5%	10%	15%

Note: FMEA considers the severity of an excursion that is 2–3
times outside the preferred operating range. The test range for
initial screening experiments is ~1.5–2 times outside the preferred
operating range.

as well as, perhaps more importantly, the ability to react
to this excursion before it has product impact. For column
loading, the frequency and detection scores were quite
low and were the same whether loading was too high or
too low. However, with regard to severity, too high of a
loading was deemed to have a much greater severity since
it had the possibility of resulting in inadequate detergent
removal. This resulted in a much lower RPN score for
underloading than overloading. Likewise, high and low
flow rates have the same frequency and detection level,
but high flow rates can lead to inadequate removal of
detergent resulting in protein aggregation, giving it a
higher overall RPN score. For those parameters that do
not have a specified range (such as stop collect in this
instance), some judgment has to be made as to how much
of an excursion would have a serious impact. In the case
of this chromatography step, missing the stop collect by
a significant amount could result in detergent breakthrough, again resulting in potential product aggregation
and loss of activity.

A Pareto plot of the different operating parameters versus
their respective RPN scores is shown in Figure 3.1. In
most cases with this chromatography step, those with the
highest severity impact had the highest RPN scores and

are the parameters that warrant further study. However, another outcome of this exercise may be the identification of more redundant controls in manufacturing that can serve to either increase the ability to detect an excursion or decrease its frequency. For example, adding a pH check of the column eluate post-equilibration can give us extra assurance that the column is adequately equilibrated and decrease the frequency of equilibration errors by increasing our ability to detect them. In this case, it might bring the frequency and detection scores both down to "2" and perhaps make it unnecessary to examine equilibration pH in our process characterization studies. Likewise, having an additional way of checking the elution flow rate could increase our ability to detect an excursion here and, hence, decrease its frequency. However, the potential severity of running at too high of a flow rate makes this excursion something we would want to investigate as part of our characterization studies, in any case.

3.3.2 Scale-Down Model Qualification

The development of a representative scale-down model of each unit operation is the Achilles' heel of good process characterization work. If we cannot mimic, to a reasonable degree, the large-scale manufacturing process with our small-scale studies, any bench-scale process characterization work becomes meaningless [2]. Some unit operations, such as homogenization and centrifugation steps, are much more difficult to scale down and typically have to be run in a pilot plant setting. Other operations, such as chromatography, ultrafiltration, and microbial fermentation operations, can usually be run at a bench scale or smaller scales.

In general, the approach to scale-down model qualification is to run all operating parameters at the center of the operating range used for clinical/large-scale manufacturing. If the process has yet to be run in clinical manufacturing, the operating parameters should mirror those of the largest pilot scale runs. If no appropriate large-scale data is available, data from an earlier manufacturing process may be used; however, the scale-down model has to give data consistent with the large-scale runs. It is a good idea to write a protocol that

TABLE 3.3 FMEA Analysis for Removal of Detergent from a Protein Using Ion-Exchange Chromatography (Case Study 3.1)

Operational Parameter	Function or Requirement	Potential Failure Mode	Potential Effect of Failure	Severity Score (1–10)	Potential Causes of Failure	Frequency Score (1–10)	Current Controls	Detection Score (1–10)	RPN
Ion exchange lot	Detergent retention	Bad resin	Insufficient removal of detergent	7	Poor supplier; QC failure	2	Monitored in QC; defect detected prior to use	2	28
Load volume	Remove detergent	<20 CVs	Loss of protein on resin	3	Miscalculation; operator error	3	MPs	3	27
Load volume	Remove detergent	>60 CVs	Detergent in product	7	Miscalculation; operator error	3	MPs	3	63
Start collect A280	Capture product	Too early start collect	Dilute pool	2	Poor PM; incorrect standardization	3	Calibration; SOP	5	30
Start collect A280	Capture product	Too late start collect	Lower yield	5	Poor PM; incorrect standardization	3	Calibration; SOP	5	75

Stop collect A280	Capture product w/o detergent	Too early stop collect	Lower yield	5	Poor PM; incorrect standardization	3	Calibration; SOP	5	75
Stop collect A280	Capture product w/o detergent	Too late stop collect	Detergent in product	7	Poor PM; incorrect standardization	3	Calibration; SOP	5	105
Flow rate	Remove detergent	Low flow rate	Longer process time, possible loss of product on resin	3	Pump failure; power outage; operator error; incorrect calibration	4	SOP; MP; calibration	3	36
Flow rate	Remove detergent	High flow rate	Inadequate detergent removal	6	Pump failure; power outage; operator error; incorrect calibration	4	SOP; MP; calibration	3	72

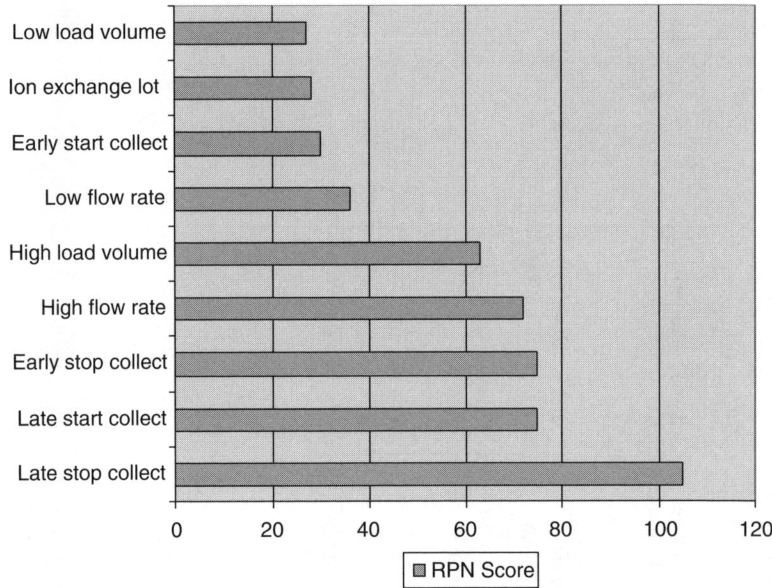

Figure 3.1 Pareto chart of RPN scores from detergent removal step (Case Study 3.1).

describes the scale-down model, how it is controlled, and acceptance criteria for each unit operation in terms of performance parameters. Generally, a numerical indication that the small-scale process is acceptable, such as a t-test tolerance interval or some other statistical means, should be used, or there may be a simple requirement that the mean of the data from the scale-down run be within the historical range of the large-scale data. Doing replicate runs can improve the level of statistical rigor for the scale-down model, since it is good to know something about the variability that occurs with the unit operation at small scale [3]. This can help in determining the number of replicates that are needed for the actual characterization studies.

The following chapter in this book provides points to consider and strategies for scaling down a number of different process steps, including chromatography, chemical modification reactions, ultrafiltration, microfiltration, and several other unit operations. Some points to consider for scaling down microbial fermentation and cell culture processes are described in the following section.

3.3.2.1 Scaling Down Fermentation and Cell Culture

Comprehensive characterization of microbial fermentation work requires many experiments and is usually carried out at the 10-liter scale with some supporting experiments run at larger scales. In our experience, outputs from 10-liter microbial fermentation experiments have been fairly representative of what we have seen at manufacturing scale. However, scaling down mammalian cell culture has proven to be more difficult. Although we have been able to determine the impact that a change in operating parameters might have on a cell culture process, we frequently have no good way of predicting the magnitude of that response from bench-scale data. Even so, process characterization experiments can still give insights into which operating parameters are the most important to control for cell culture processes.

Some of the points to consider when scaling down fermentation and cell culture processes include the following:

- Use the most current manufacturing procedures for scaled-down process.
- Use released GMP materials whenever possible. This includes master or working cell bank vials.
- Sterilization times of media and feed should match manufacturing scale. In some instances, it may be important to extend the heating time to make sure there is no effect of the sterilization on the media. Make sure media mass change from pre- to poststerilization is the same at both scales.
- Use same size and shape of shaker flask (baffled or unbaffled), as well as incubator conditions (shaker speed, throw, etc.).
- Maintain constant inoculum ratios for seed and production fermentation between scales.

- Operational parameters (pH, temperature, back pressure, dissolved oxygen [DO] set point, etc.) should be identical to those specified in the manufacturing process. Ensure that the DO calibrations are compatible.
- Total airflow should be scaled down on the scale factor to ensure similar sweeping of CO_2 from the fermentation. The overall oxygen control strategy should be equivalent to that used at scale (i.e., order of cascade, back pressures employed, etc.). A maximum agitation for the small scale should be selected that mimics as closely as possible power input limitations at scale. This might be accomplished with theoretical calculation or through equipment design.
- Addition order for all the ingredients should be the same at both scales. Also, make sure the hold times for all ingredients are within the same historical ranges.
- Antifoam strategy or total amounts of antifoam should match manufacturing scale. Antifoam usage typically increases with scale due to higher superficial gas velocities.
- Both scales should have the same feed rates and step times.
- Make sure you have good calibration of all DO probes, pH meters, spectrophotometers, etc., and that they match between scales.

Some of the key performance parameters to monitor include the following:

- Growth curves and final OD
- Growth rates
- Titer
- % solids
- Feed/acid-base usage
- Nutrient profiles
- Times (total seed fermentation time, main fermentation time, etc.)
- Genetic stability

- Cell viability
- Product quality

All of these are good to monitor as a part of the scale-down work, but the ones that are deemed critical may be on a case-by-case basis. Certainly, titer and product quality are two important performance parameters that should be considered. In addition, cell viability and percent solids could impact subsequent cell processing and purification steps. Therefore, it may be necessary to process one or two more steps downstream to determine the impact of these parameters on subsequent processing steps or product quality.

3.3.2.2 Analytical Methods Qualification

The analytical methods for process characterization studies should be robust and representative of what will be used for the commercial process. Ideally, the methods would be validated; however, for a product in early phase III clinical stage this may not always be possible. In these instances, the method should be qualified and developed to the point where there is a high degree of confidence that it can be validated at some point in the future. It is important, therefore, to allow enough time for method qualification prior to process characterization work. This can require anywhere from 3–12 months depending on the assay, the complexity of the protein and protein matrices, etc.

Points to consider for method qualification depend on what the assay is used for. For all assays, critical variables and nominal target values should be defined. For product quantification assays, the sample handling and preparation, particularly for in-process samples, should be established. There should be minimum interference from matrix components and adequate resolution. The linearity and range of the analysis should be determined, as well as the limit of quantification, if applicable. Reproducibility should be established based on a statistical equivalence between labs, and the relative standard deviation should be less than or equal to 5% for chromatographic methods, if possible. Any critical assay variables should be identified and the nominal target value defined. For product immunoassays, there should be minimal matrix interference and the antibody specificity should be confirmed. Linearity, precision, and ranges should be established on quantitative immunoassays for both product and process-related impurities (i.e., host cell proteins). For identification immunoassays, linearity and precision are not required, but the limit of detection and limit of quantitation should be confirmed.

As mentioned earlier, the analytical group supporting process characterization, whether in a process development department or in quality control, will be one of the hardest hit from a resource standpoint for characterization studies. A single purification run may produce as many as four or five samples for analysis. The analytical group supporting the characterization effort must be staffed appropriately so the sample turnaround does not become too much of a rate-limiting step for the completion of process characterization.

3.4 PROCESS CHARACTERIZATION STUDIES

3.4.1 Impurity Clearance

Much of this data may be available prior to the process characterization studies. An understanding of what each process step delivers in terms of yield, impurity clearance, or in-process pool quality should be an outcome of this work. In the case of cell culture, this may be a titer or some qualitative assessment of the product (such as the degree of glycosylation or sialylation). For a chromatography step, it would be not only what impurities are cleared during the step, but at what point are they cleared, i.e., in the wash step, before the product elution, after the product elution, during the regeneration step, etc. For a diafiltration step, one might examine conductivity or pH after different turnover volumes. The outcome of this work would be the identification of key performance parameters for each process step, which can help in the design of further characterization experiments. How these performance parameters are affected by excursions from the operating ranges will be the objective of the next set of characterization studies.

Case Study 3.2

This study was designed to track impurity clearance across a cation exchange capture/purification step for a recombinant protein made in *E. coli*. The impurities tracked included DNA, endotoxin, *E. coli* proteins (ECPs), product charge variants (measured by cation-exchange HPLC), and oxidized methionine (as measured by reversed-phase HPLC). The clearance of these impurities was tracked by collecting fractions starting with the load and going through the stop collect. (In some instances, we would also collect eluate from the regeneration step; however, all impurities had cleared prior to this step in this case.) Clearance of these impurities relative to the product peak is shown in Figure 3.2A–D. Endotoxin clearance was virtually identical to the DNA clearance and is not shown. From this data, we can provide a rationale for pool criteria. In addition, these studies can be used for addressing certain nonconformances, such as inadequate wash volumes, early pool collections, etc. This information is also used to identify the quality indicating performance parameters that should be monitored for this process step, which would include all of the impurities tested in this example.

3.4.2 Screening Experiments

Screening experiments are designed to eliminate the less critical parameters from further, more rigorous process characterization work. Experimental design (DOE) approaches can be used for these studies to easily screen a number of operating parameters [12,13], and there are a number of DOE software packages that can aid in the design and interpretation of these experiments [14,15]. Fractional factorial, Plackett-Burman, and D-Optimal DOE designs can be used for screening [2,12,13]. An example of a simple Resolution III fractional-factorial design for a fermentation process is shown in Table 3.4. In this design, only nine experiments are

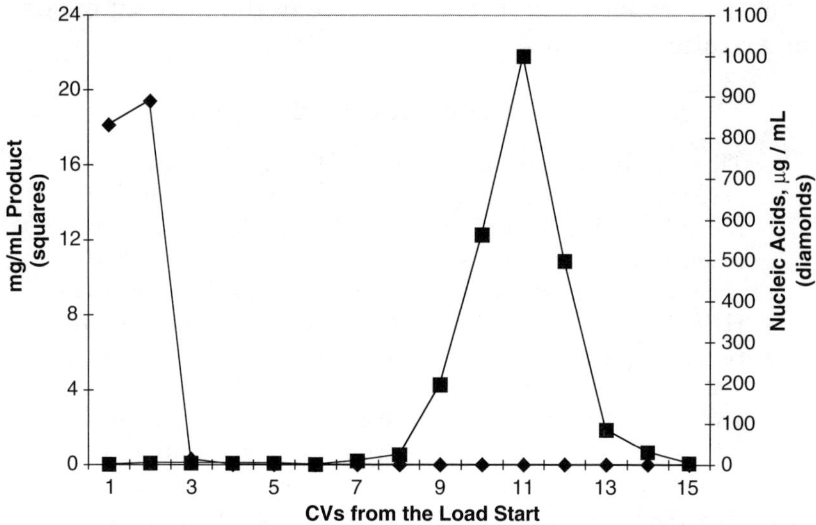

Figure 3.2 (A) Impurity clearance study (Case Study 3.2) examining the removal of DNA (A), *E. coli* proteins (B), reversed-phase impurities (C), and cation-exchange impurities (D).

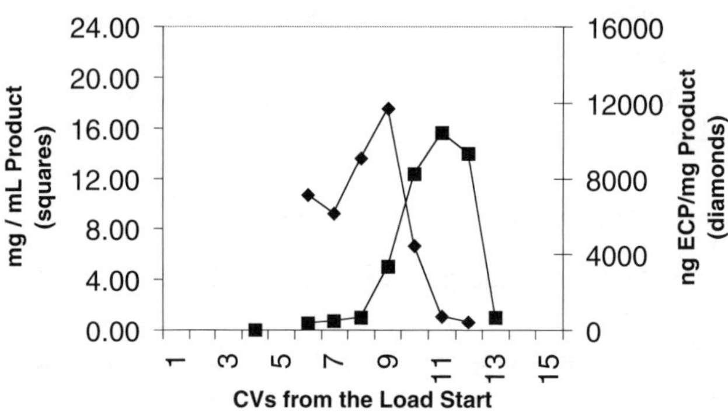

Figure 3.2 (B)

required to screen six operating parameters. Results can be analyzed using Pareto charts or regression analysis [12,13]. While these studies do not allow us to see interactions between parameters, they enable us to determine the main

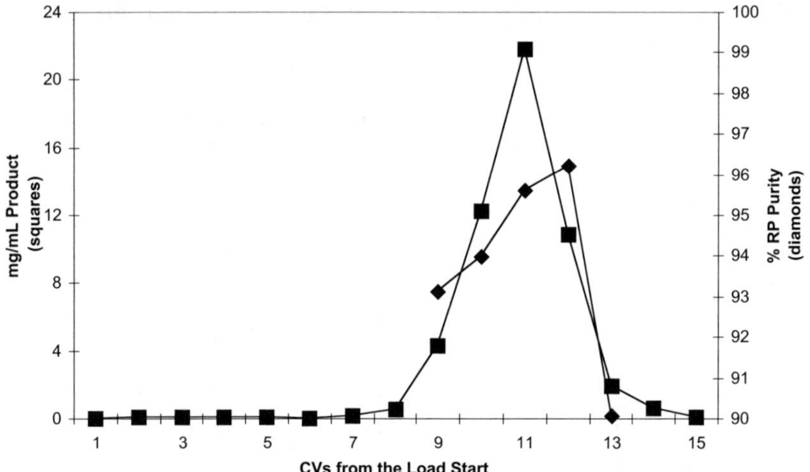

Figure 3.2 (C)

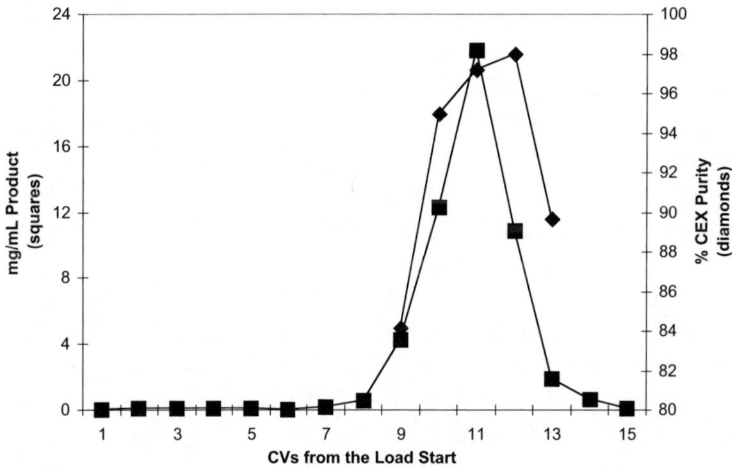

Figure 3.2 (D)

effects and identify what parameters have the greatest effect on key performance parameters. In some cases, it may be simpler to do "one-off" studies where only a single operating parameter is tested and all other parameters are held at their

TABLE 3.4 Resolution III Fractional-Factorial Design for a
Fermentation Process

Run	pH	Temp	Start Feed OD	Inducer Volume	Feed Rate (kg/h)	Induction Time (h)
1	6.7	27	17	9.6	97	17
2	6.7	27	23	10.4	72	13
3	6.7	33	17	10.4	72	17
4	6.7	33	23	9.6	97	13
5	7.3	27	17	10.4	97	13
6	7.3	27	23	9.6	72	17
7	7.3	33	17	9.6	72	13
8	7.3	33	23	10.4	97	17
9	7	30	20	10	84	15

center point. While this approach can require more experiments, it can give results that are more easily interpreted.

Typically, we assume that the performance response over
the operating parameter range tested will be linear; therefore,
only two-level (a high and a low value) studies are used for
these experiments. In addition, the two levels we prefer to test
are at approximately 1.5–2 times the *preferred* operating range
in manufacturing [2]. Of course, the "preferred" operating
range may be different for different unit operations and with
different processes. (Examples of these ranges for several commonly used operating parameters are shown in Table 3.2.) This
approach can enable us to get a clear indication of the effect
of an operating parameter on unit operation performance. The
range is wide enough to see an effect should one exist, yet not
so wide as to make a performance failure inevitable. Because
of this, it can give information on process robustness, i.e., the
ability of the process to run outside the prescribed operating
range. This can be useful for closing out manufacturing incidents and excursions from set operating ranges. In addition,
information from these studies can be used to tell manufacturing which parameters need tighter control or narrower
ranges and which require less attention. In some instances
they may be able to run at a more preferred operating range,
and in others they may have to tighten the range (Table 3.3).

Finally, these studies will clearly separate key from non-key parameters. If an operating parameter tested over this range has no significant effect on process performance, we may designate it a non-key parameter. However, even if excursions from these operating parameters have no product impact, we still may monitor them to ensure consistent process control. Those parameters that have a significant, measurable effect are identified as key parameters that should be tested in the next set of characterization experiments.

For some operations, particularly purification steps where several contaminants are removed, there will be more than one performance parameter, and some will be more important than others. For example, an operating parameter that has a large effect on pool volume and a minimal effect on product purity would be considered to be of less importance than a parameter where the reverse was true. In these cases, the impact of the operating parameters will have to be weighed relative to their effect on the different performance parameters.

Case Study 3.3

This study involves a reversed-phase column that is used to remove several product-related variants as well as host cell proteins from a recombinant glycoprotein. Risk assessment analysis determined that there were six potential key parameters that could affect the performance of the chromatography step: pH, bed height, column load factor, temperature, resin type (elutriated versus nonelutriated), and flow rate. A near-resolution IV fractional factorial design was set up to screen these operating parameters with regard to eight different process performance parameters, which included % yield, product variants 1, 2, and 3, host cell proteins, pool volume, retention time, and peak asymmetry (Table 3.5). (This experiment was a bit unusual in that the ranges tested were somewhat wider than what we usually test.) The relative impact of each operating parameter on each performance parameter was determined using Pareto plots, and the data is summarized in Table 3.6. The importance of the performance parameter was multiplied by the impact of the operating parameter (size of the effect) to give the rating for a given operating parameter/performance parameter pair (e.g., temperature/yield had a relative effect of $6 \times 2 = 12$). The total score for each operating parameter is the sum of the effect on all of the performance parameters (e.g., total score for pH was 21.0, temperature was 28.5, etc.). Another factor was added to account for the "ease of control" for each operating parameter to give the final adjusted score ("ADJUSTED SCORE"). From this analysis, it is evident that load factor has the largest overall impact on the process; pH, temperature, and bed height have some effect; and flow rate and resin type have a minimal role. Therefore, for our next set of experiments, we would only want to focus on load rate, pH, temperature, and bed height.

TABLE 3.5 Fractional-Factorial Screening Study to Examine Operating Parameters from a Reversed-Phase Column (Case Study 3.3)

Run No.	pH	Temperature	Protein Load	Resin Type*	Bed Height	Flow Rate
1	6	4	4	NE	3	50
2	6	4	4	E	15	100
3	6	4	20	NE	15	100
4	6	4	20	E	3	50
5	7.5	4	4	NE	3	100
6	6.4	7	8	E	8.5	75.5
7	7.5	4	4	E	15	50
8	7.5	4	20	NE	15	50
9	7.5	4	20	E	3	100
10	6	22	4	NE	15	50
11	6	22	4	E	3	100
12	6.4	7	8	E	8.5	75.5
13	6	22	20	NE	3	100
14	6	22	20	E	15	50
15	7.5	22	4	NE	15	100
16	7.5	22	4	E	3	50
17	7.5	22	20	NE	3	50
18	7.5	22	20	E	15	100
19	6.4	7	8	E	8.5	75.5

*E = elutriated, NE = non-elutriated.

TABLE 3.6 Impact of Operating Parameters on Different Performance Parameters from a Reversed-Phase Column (Case Study 3.3)*

Output	Relative Size of Effect (Pareto Plot)						Total Effect (Size of Effect X Importance)					
	pH	Temperature	Load	Bed Height	Flow Rate	Resin Type	pH	Temperature	Load	Bed Height	Flow Rate	Resin Type
Product purity (column pool)	1	1		1.5			6.0	6.0		9.0		
Yield		2			1			12.0			6.0	
Product variant 2	1	0.5	2	1.2			5.0	2.5	10.0	6.0	0.0	0.0
Product variant 1	1	1	2	1			3.0	3.0	6.0	3.0	0.0	0.0
Pool volume	1		2	1		1	3.0			6.0	3.0		3.0
Host cell protein	1		2.4				2.0	0.0	4.8	0.0	0.0	0.0
Peak position	1	2		1			2.0	4.0		2.0		
Peak asymmetry		1	1	1.5				1.0	1.0	1.5		

	pH	Temperature	Load	Bed Height	Flow Rate	Resin Type
TOTAL SCORE	21.0	28.5	27.8	24.5	6.0	3.0
Ease of control (1 = easiest)	1.5	1.5	3.0	2.0	1.0	1.0
ADJUSTED SCORE (score × control factor)	32	43	83	49	6	3
RANK	4	3	1	2	5	6
Include in next DOE?	Yes	Yes	Yes	Yes	No	No

* Relative importance of output parameters: product purity = 6, yield = 6, product variant 2 = 5, product variant 1 = 3, pool volume = 3, host cell protein = 2, peak position = 2, peak asymmetry = 1.

3.4.3   Interactions between Key Parameters (The Next Round of Process Characterization Experiments)

From the screening experiments, we know that the operating parameters being tested at this juncture have some effect on process performance. Therefore, we typically test these parameters only to the edge of their normal or preferred operating ranges. As in the screening experiments, a DOE approach may be used. Depending on the number of variables to be tested, a full-factorial, fractional-factorial, or other design could be used [12–15]. In general, however, we will want to use a design where the effect of any suspected interactions can be determined, which will necessarily mean a higher-resolution (IV or V) experimental design [12–15]. Although we typically assume the performance response to be linear over the operating ranges tested, some judgment has to be made as to whether or not this is a valid assumption. In those cases where nonlinearity is suspected, multilevel experimental designs should be used. In addition, we generally look for no more than two-factor interactions, since interactions with more than two variables are quite rare and would require extensive studies to detect. One of the outcomes of these experiments may be the identification of other process weak spots, due to interactions or additive effects between parameters that were not observed in the initial screening experiments. In some cases, certain operating ranges may have to be readjusted. The ultimate deliverable from this set of experiments is to provide assurance that the process provides consistent yields and product quality attributes within the confines of all combinations of the operating limits.

Case Study 3.4

In order to more accurately characterize the behavior of the chromatography experiment from Case Study 3.3 and to determine if there were interactions between key parameters that could result in process failure, we undertook a second, more rigorous DOE with the four key inputs identified from the DOE screening studies. An

TABLE 3.7 A 20-Run, Three-Level D-Optimal Design Study (Case Study 3.4)

Run No.	pH	Temperature	Protein Load Rate	Bed Height
1	5.8	3	5	4.5
2	7.0	3	5	10
3	5.8	3	5	15
4	6.4	3	10	15
5	7.0	3	15	4.5
6	6.4	3	15	4.5
7	5.8	3	15	10
8	7.0	3	15	15
9	7.0	7	5	4.5
10	5.8	7	5	15
11	5.8	7	10	4.5
12	6.4	7	15	10
13	6.4	11	5	4.5
14	5.8	11	5	10
15	7.0	11	5	15
16	7.0	11	10	10
17	5.8	11	15	4.5
18	7.0	11	15	4.5
19	7.0	11	15	15
20	5.8	11	15	15

experimental design with the fewest number of experiments that would provide a model capable of discerning nonlinear behavior and two-factor interactions was a 20-run D-optimal design with each of the four inputs set at three levels: low, intermediate, and high (Table 3.7). The input settings (high and low) were narrowed compared to those in the first study since we only wanted to test to the edge of the proposed operating ranges in this set of experiments. Column performance was monitored by seven output parameters: step yield, product purity, product variants 1 and 2, an additional assay for product variant 3, host cell proteins, and pool volume.

The results for the study are show in Table 3.8. Even though effects, some of them significant, were observed on most performance parameters, all (with the exception of host cell proteins) fell within the acceptable range. There were several instances where host cell proteins

TABLE 3.8 Results from D-Optimal Experimental Design Study for Reversed-Phase Column (Case Study 3.4)

Run No.	Yield	Pool Volume CVs	Product Purity	Product Variant 1	Product Variant 2	Product Variant 3	Host Cell Protein
1	38.6	2.2	90.5	0.57	0.81	0.5	2077
2	38.7	1.8	93.2	0.67	0.68	0.7	817
3	39.5	1.6	91.1	0.34	N/D*	0.3	1524
4	39.8	2.1	91.1	0.57	0.66	0.5	2596
5	43.2	5.3	90.1	1.29	0.93	1.3	10835
6	36.7	3.9	90.5	1.03	0.85	1.1	4599
7	39.0	2.7	90.1	0.72	0.80	0.8	3658
8	41.3	3.1	91.1	1.04	0.82	1.0	3357
9	41.9	2.4	91.3	0.86	0.78	0.9	265
10	37.0	1.5	91.8	0.27	0.57	0.3	938
11	38.2	2.6	91.0	0.72	0.78	0.8	256
12	36.2	2.7	91.8	0.92	0.80	0.9	5163
13	38.6	2.0	91.7	0.31	0.80	0.5	39
14	33.4	1.5	92.9	0.35	0.67	0.3	137
15	39.4	1.7	92.9	0.42	0.81	0.4	68
16	39.4	2.4	91.7	0.73	0.75	0.9	443
17	35.3	3.0	91.0	0.80	0.77	0.9	4138
18	38.9	4.5	91.8	1.14	0.80	1.4	4861
19	40.4	3.0	91.0	0.83	0.93	1.0	2506
20	33.1	2.2	91.6	0.31	0.86	0.4	4662
ctrl 1^	39.1	2.0	91.8	0.36	0.84	0.5	2653
ctrl 2^	37.4	2.2	91.7	0.53	0.80	0.5	3659
ctrl 3^	36.8	2.2	92.9	0.49	0.85	0.6	N/D*

exceeded the upper acceptance limit (~4000 ppm). Based on the Pareto plot for host cell protein (Figure 3.3), it is apparent that the main factor affecting host cell protein content in the product pool is the column load factor. In order to ensure that we are consistently below the historical upper limit for host cell proteins, we set the load factor at no greater than 10. With this new limit on load factor, we now have a process that will deliver acceptable yields and quality attributes within the confines of all operating ranges. The Pareto plots also gave some hints as to how we might improve step yields (increasing pH and decreasing temperature) or increase product purity (also by decreasing load).

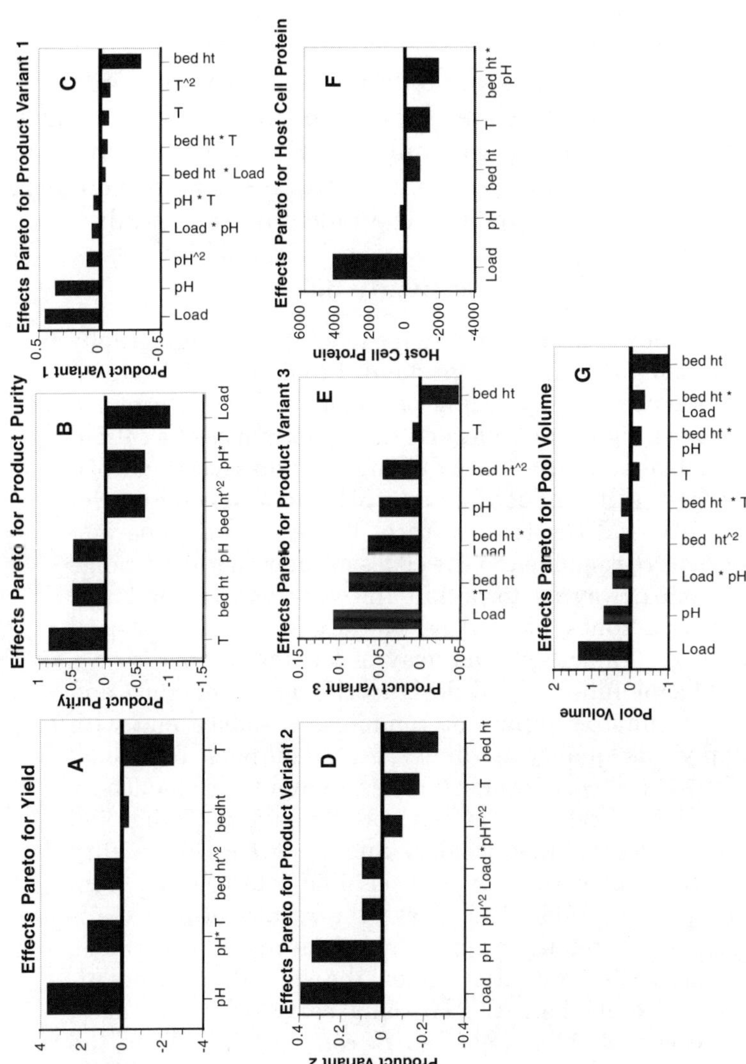

Figure 3.3 Pareto plots from D-optimal study of reversed-phase column (Case Study 3.4).

3.4.3.1 Combining Variables

In some instances, it may be possible to combine variables in such a way as to more quickly explore the "operating space" of a given unit operation [2,12]. This will greatly cut down on the amount of experimentation required. Sometimes, however, it may give you results that are difficult to interpret if there is a process failure and it only assumes that there are additive effects between operating parameters. We typically use this approach when we have some degree of confidence in our operating ranges and only need confirmatory information that the process will perform properly over these ranges. One example would be to combine pH and conductivity as inputs to an ion-exchange chromatography step. An even more extreme example is shown in the following case study.

Case Study 3.5

> This study was from a cation-exchange chromatography step using a linear salt gradient. From an initial screening study, seven operating parameters were determined to have a significant effect on the performance of a cation-exchange step: the low salt buffer conductivity and pH, the high salt conductivity and pH, the feed conductivity and pH, and the temperature. These operating parameters were combined to the edges of their operating range in such a way as to obtain the very earliest or latest retention times, as well as the largest or smallest pool volumes (Table 3.9). One way of looking at this is as a two-factor full-factorial design, with retention time and pool volume as inputs or combined variables and with step yields, quality attributes, etc. as outputs. Table 3.10 shows the effect of pool volume as an input variable. There is a slight effect on yield (but nothing outside of what had been observed historically) and no effect on quality attributes over the range of possible pool volumes from this process. Table 3.11 shows the results of an experiment where retention time is set up as an input variable. At the earliest retention times, the yield drops dramatically. Also, for both the late and early retention times, there is a slight increase in *E. coli* proteins. When the column feed pH and conductivity are kept at their center

TABLE 3.9 Combination of Operating Parameters for a Cation-Exchange Step to Obtain Earliest and Latest Retention Times and Minimum and Maximum Pool Volumes (Case Study 3.5)

Operating Parameter	Earliest Retention Time	Latest Retention Time	Minimum Pool Volume	Maximum Pool Volume	Control
Equil pH	Low	High	High	Low	Center
Equil conductivity	High	Low	Low	High	Center
Elution pH	Low	High	Low	High	Center
Elution conductivity	High	Low	High	Low	Center
Small ion capacity	Low	High	Center	Center	Center
Temperature	High	Low	Center	Center	Center
Feed pH	Low	High	Center	Center	Center
Feed Conductivity	High	Low	Center	Center	Center

TABLE 3.10 Effect of Cation-Exchange Pool Volume on Product Purity and Yields (Case Study 3.5)

Pool Volumes	Runs	Product Concentration	Pool Volume (ml)	% Yield	% RP Purity	% CEX Purity	*E. Coli* Proteins
Low	1	20.8	195.6 (1.47 CV)	102.2	95.3	95.1	3776
	2	20.8	194.6 (1.47 CV)	105.7	95.2	95.0	3878
Center	1	14.8	257.3 (1.94 CV)	95.7	94.4	95.9	3526
	2	14.6	259.3 (1.95 CV)	97.0	94.4	95.2	3833
High	1	11.2	313.1 (2.36 CV)	90.4	96.2	95.2	3144
	2	11.7	300.1 (2.26 CV)	89.8	94.7	96.3	3037

points, the yield effect is greatly reduced and there is a slight reduction in the amount of *E. coli* proteins (Table 3.12). We concluded from these experiments that to improve the robustness of this step we needed to lower the center point of the column feed pH by 0.1 units (maintaining the operating range at ±0.1 unit).

TABLE 3.11 Effect of Cation-Exchange Retention Time on Product Purity and Yield (Case Study 3.5)

Retention Times	Runs	Product Concentration (mg/ml)	% Yield	% RP Purity	% CEX Purity	*E. Coli* Proteins
Early	1	7.7	37.9	92.9	94.8	4682
	2	7.0	36.2	94.5	95.2	5195
Center	1	12.7	87.0	94.8	95.7	4068
	2	12.7	88.2	95.5	95.6	3387
Late	1	14.1	102.7	93.6	94.4	4289
	2	13.5	102.0	93.6	94.1	5085

TABLE 3.12 Effect of Cation-Exchange Retention Time on Product Yields and Purity when Column Feed pH and Conductivity Are Run at Their Center Points

Retention Times	Runs	% Yield	% RP Purity	% CEX Purity	*E. Coli* Proteins
Early	1	84.1	95.1	95.8	4590
	2	83.5	94.8	96.5	3788
Center	1	94.2	94.2	96.3	3229
	2	91.0	94.2	95.8	3520
Late	1	98.6	95.0	95.6	4050
	2	98.4	95.5	95.4	4519

The advantage of this study design is that with no more than six experiments we are able to explore the edges of the operating space for this unit operation. The disadvantage is that any nonlinear responses or significant interactions between variables could be lost. As with any design, one has to determine the risk-benefit of combining variables or using a lower-powered study.

3.4.4 Key and Critical Parameters

Operating parameters that have a significant effect on the performance of a unit operation are considered key parameters. More specifically, this would include those parameters from the initial screening experiments that have a significant, measurable effect on process performance parameters (particularly product quality attributes, impurities, or step yields). These parameters should be included as the key operating parameters for full-scale validation runs, although, in some instances, there may be additional parameters included in the full-scale validation runs as key parameters as well.

In addition to key parameters, there may be a subset of "critical" operating parameters that have an even greater effect on product quality. The FDA definition clarifies the definition of critical parameters as "process parameters that must be controlled within established operating ranges to ensure that the API or intermediate will meet specifications for quality and purity" [16]. Most parameters, even most key parameters, can be run slightly outside their prescribed operating range without resulting in a failed product or product intermediate specification. However, there may be a handful of operating parameters for a given process for which an excursion outside the prescribed range would result in such a failure. Generally, for a robust process there should be very few of these. Those that are identified as critical should be highly characterized in terms of defining their edge of failure and identification of any interactions with other operating parameters that could result in process or product failures.

3.4.5 Setting Acceptance Criteria for In-Process Performance Parameters: Using Feed Quality as a Process Input

A number of factors need to be considered for setting acceptance criteria for in-process performance parameters. Setting the criteria too stringently can lead to unnecessary validation failures. Setting the criteria too loosely may result in product that may ultimately fail the final product release specifications.

Statistical analysis of pilot, clinical, and commercial-scale manufacturing data is one of the most common ways of setting acceptance criteria on key performance parameters. Frequently, however, the data sets may not be representative (due to process differences between pilot and large scale) or there may be a limited number of manufacturing runs. In these cases, basing acceptance criteria on a historical range or a statistical evaluation of the data, such as three standard deviations or tolerance intervals [16], may not give the appropriate acceptable ranges for process performance parameters. Therefore, it is important to use process characterization data to determine the process capability and redundancy so that acceptance criteria are based on what the process can actually deliver.

In most process characterization studies, representative feed material should be used, whether this is material from a seed fermentor feeding a production fermentor, a column feed, or a feed material going into an ultrafiltration step. However, to really test the "top-to-bottom" robustness of the process, the effect of feed quality on each unit operation should be tested. This will give us an understanding of the downstream sensitivity to upstream process excursions. For fermentation, this might include different seed fermentor cell densities. For cell harvesting, it might include different fermentation media OD or viscosity. In the case of chromatography steps, the purity of product from the previous step or load factor should be considered (although we usually run all process characterization experiments at the upper end of the loading range). All other operating parameters (pH, temperature, etc.) are run at the center of their respective ranges, because the likelihood of having both an operating parameter excursion and a feed quality excursion is remote.

These experiments can be used to set performance parameter acceptance criteria for each unit operation. One way to address this is to run a unit operation under conditions where it fails to perform adequately. The pool from the failed unit operation is processed further downstream to see if subsequent process steps can make up for the poor performance from the failed unit operation and allow for the product to stay within specifications. These experiments give information on process redundancy with regard to different key performance parameters [2].

An example of this is shown in Figure 3.4. In this instance, column 1 is run in such a way that a product-related

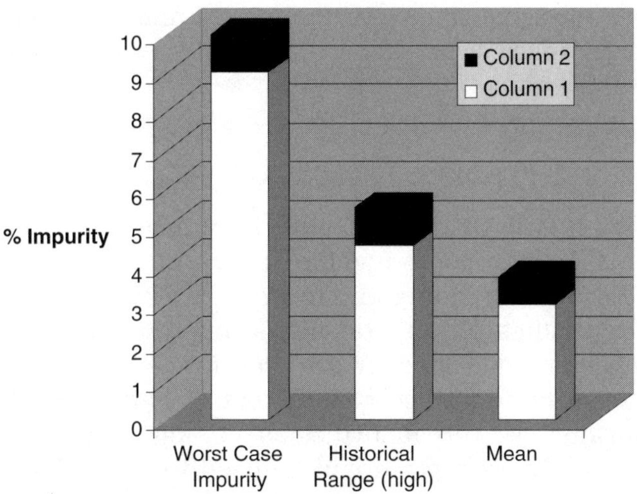

Figure 3.4 Impurity clearance showing process redundancy between columns 1 and 2.

variant was present at values higher than the historical range. When this column 1 pool is processed through column 2, however, the amount of this variant falls within the historical range for the column 2 pool. Therefore, rather than setting the acceptance criteria for the column 1 pool based on historical ranges for the product-related variant, a wider acceptance criteria can be set due to the process redundancy between columns 1 and 2. There may be other instances where a pool has to be processed through more than one additional step downstream to determine the process redundancy, but the principle is the same. This method of setting acceptance criteria is scientifically based and can give a more realistic indication of what the process can actually deliver than statistical analysis of historical data (standard deviation, tolerance intervals, etc. [17]), particularly since at the time the process characterization is carried out there may be very little if any historical data to set a statistically valid acceptance criteria. Setting the acceptance criteria for process validation studies based on what the process can actually deliver will result in fewer validation failures due to acceptance criteria being set incorrectly. Of course, as the process matures and more lots are run, the acceptance criteria can more easily be set based on statistical analysis.

3.5 FINISHING UP: REPORTS, FOLLOW-UP, ETC.

Process characterization reports should be written for each unit operation. These reports include the results from the clearance studies, the screening and interactions studies, and the feed quality studies. Key operating parameters and their respective ranges are identified, as are acceptance criteria for all key in-process performance parameters. A rationale for why certain parameters were identified as non-key is included as well. Data from these reports will be used to support the validation studies, and the reports should be completed prior to writing the validation protocols.

After the characterization work is completed, it may be valuable to go back and repeat the FMEA exercise. The severity factor for each operating parameter will be known at this point and this could, in some instances, dramatically change the outcome of the risk priority number. In this way, plant engineers can best devote their time to those unit operations and operating parameters that require the greatest control and detection.

3.6 FUTURE CHALLENGES

Process characterization requires a significant commitment of time and resources, but the payoff in terms of better process understanding, improved success rate in manufacturing, and avoidance of costly regulatory delays makes it a very worthwhile investment. The approaches described in this chapter can provide information used for setting operating ranges and performance parameter acceptance criteria and can give an indication of overall process robustness.

There are a number of challenges that we continue to face in process development and in other departments involved in carrying out process characterization studies. Some of these include the following:

- Developing appropriate scale-down models for cell culture, centrifugation, and other difficult-to-scale upstream steps. Finding a representative scale that will still be amenable to the high run number generally required for thorough process characterization work can be a real challenge. For cell culture, one approach may be to use small-scale bioreactors to identify key operating parameters and then to use larger, more representative bioreactors for confirming ranges or studying interactions between key parameters. Even so, this entails a great deal of work and may still give information that is of marginal value.

- Use of appropriate analytical methods and analytical method turnaround time. Having "mature" analytical methods available in time for starting process characterization studies can be a real problem. The availability of more generic analytical method platforms so that methods can be more easily qualified would help ensure that process characterization studies are started at the appropriate time. In the absence of this, analytical resources will have to be spent "at risk" earlier in the product development cycle in order to ensure timely qualification of analytical methods. Also, since sample analysis can be a major bottleneck for completing process characterization work, development of more rapid and automated methods can help in sample turnaround time and in planning of subsequent process characterization experiments.

- Appropriate resources for process characterization. Many companies are still dialing in the appropriate resource requirements for process characterization. It is important to tailor the process characterization requirements for each product to key business drivers in order to have the most efficient use of resources. All products will have certain requirements with regard to regulatory commitments, such as providing data that the process will provide consistent yields and product quality attributes within the normal operating ranges. For products with less intensive run rates or fewer cost-of-goods issues, broader yield ranges or higher process excursion rates may be acceptable. In these instances, it may be possible to reduce the scope of some of the characterization work by reducing the number of variables to examine or by testing only to the edge of the normal operating range for certain parameters. Another problem encountered is how to deal with products that have accelerated development timelines that may not allow time for thorough characterization studies. In these cases, a more "bare-bones" approach to characterization might be used prior to conformance runs, with more thorough studies being carried out later (but still in time for the BLA filing).

It is hoped that we will be able to better address these and other challenges as the strategies for doing process characterization continue to evolve in the biopharmaceutical industry.

ACKNOWLEDGMENTS

The author wishes to acknowledge Steve Rausch, David Dripps, Carl Richey, and David Smiley for input and discussion on this manuscript.

REFERENCES

1. Bobrowicz, G., The compliance costs of hasty process development, *BioPharm*, 12, 35–38, 1999.

2. Seely, J. and Seely, R., A rational, step-wise approach to process characterization, *BioPharm Int.*, 16, 24–34, 2003.

3. Gardner, A. and Smith, T., Identification and establishment of operating ranges of critical process variables, in *Pharmaceutical Process Validation*, Sofer, G. and Zabriskie, D., Eds., Marcel Dekker, New York, 1999, pp. 61–76.

4. Rathore, A.S., Johnson, G.V., Buckley, J.J., Boyle, D.M., and Gustafson, M.E., Process characterization of the chromatography steps in the purification process of a recombinant *Escherichia coli*–expressed protein, *Biotechnol. Appl. Biochem.*, 37, 51–61, 2003.

5. Armbruster, A. and Feldsien, T., Applying HACCP to pharmaceutical process validation, *BioPharm*, 13, 170–178, 2000.

6. Kieffer, R. et al., Applications of failure mode and effects analysis in the pharmaceutical industry, *Pharm. Tech. Europe*, Sept., 36–49, 1997.

7. Nobel, P., Reduction of risk and the evaluation of quality assurance, *PDA J. Pharm. Sci. Technol.*, 55, 235–239, 2001.

8. Sahni, A., Using failure mode and effects analysis to improve manufacturing processes, *Med. Device Diagn. Ind.*, July, 47–51, 1993.

9. McDermott, R. et al., *The Basics of FMEA*, Productivity, Inc., Portland, OR, 1996.

10. Burr, J.T., *SPC Tools for Everyone*, ASQC Quality Press, Milwaukee, 1993.

11. Rath and Strong Consultants, *Six Sigma Pocket Guide*, Division of Aon Worldwide, Lexington, MA, 2001, pp. 26–31.

12. Kelley, B., Establishing process robustness using designed experiments, in *Pharmaceutical Process Validation*, Sofer, G. and Zabriskie, D., Eds., Marcel Dekker, New York, 1999, pp. 29–60.

13. Haaland, P., *Experimental Design in Biotechnology*, Marcel Dekker, New York, 1989.

14. Juran, J.M. and Godfry, A.B., *Juran's Quality Handbook*, 5th ed., McGraw-Hill, New York, 1999, pp. 47.1–47.77.

15. Montgomery, D.C., *Design and Analysis of Experiments*, 5th ed., John Wiley & Sons, New York, 2001.

16. FDA Guidance for Industry: Manufacturing, Processing or Holding of Active Pharmaceutical Ingredients, August 1996.

17. Seely, R., Munyakazi, L., and Haury, J., Statistical tools for setting in process acceptance criteria, *BioPharm*, 14, 28–34, 2001.

4

Scale-Down Models for Purification Processes: Approaches and Applications

RANGA GODAVARTI, JON PETRONE,
JEFF ROBINSON, RICHARD WRIGHT,
AND BRIAN D. KELLEY

CONTENTS

4.1 INTRODUCTION

The U.S. Food and Drug Administration (FDA) defines *process validation* as "establishing documented evidence that provides a high degree of assurance that a specific process will consistently produce a product meeting its predetermined quality attributes" [1]. Regulatory agencies have published general guidelines to aid in developing validation strategies [2,3]. A complete process validation package is a major component of any regulatory filing. The process validation package consists of systematic documentation of protocols, reports, and results from well-planned studies. A key to successful process validation studies is ensuring strong scientific rationale in their design and interpretation while maintaining cGMP (current Good Manufacturing Practice) compliance.

Process validation studies are typically performed at full scale. However, oftentimes scale-down models are used for validating processes. Scale-down systems are laboratory scale models used for developing a purification process, which are subsequently scaled up to pilot, and eventually production scale. Alternatively, they are used prospectively as useful tools designed to mimic a large-scale process. In the case of validation of virus inactivation/removal by a purification process, use of appropriate scale-down models prevents the introduction of virus in manufacturing facilities. In addition to being used in viral clearance studies, scale-down models have been used to evaluate removal of host cell-derived impurities such as nucleic acids and host cell proteins, evaluate removal of media additives, determine useful life of chromatographic resins, etc. For licensed processes, scale-down models could play an important role in supporting process changes, establishing process comparability, and supporting manufacturing investigations. A more detailed discussion of the various applications of scale-down models is provided later in this chapter.

Figure 4.1 shows a flow diagram for a typical manufacturing process. The fermentation or bioreactor process involves the addition of multiple media additives, which will need to be removed by the purification process. The cells are separated from the harvested conditioned medium through centrifugation, microfiltration, or other cell removal techniques. For a process where the protein of interest is expressed intracellularly, one would have to incorporate a cell disruption step followed by a refolding step, if the expressed protein is insoluble. For a process where the expressed protein is secreted, the cell-free fluid may be concentrated and diafiltered prior to loading the capture purification step. The purification process typically consists of a capture chromatographic column followed by multiple purification/polishing steps. The process could also include viral inactivation steps such as low-pH incubation, solvent-detergent addition, etc. A nanofiltration step may be included to provide additional viral clearance if warranted. The product is finally concentrated and diafiltered into the formulation buffer followed by final filtration to generate bulk drug substance. Each of the unit operations described has unique principles involved in designing scale-down models. The International Conference on Harmonization (ICH) viral safety document [4] states: "The level of purification of the scale-down model should represent the production scale as closely as possible." This chapter is intended to provide a perspective on the general scale-down principles, critical parameters, and primary end points used in the design of scale-down models for a variety of unit operations used in downstream processing.

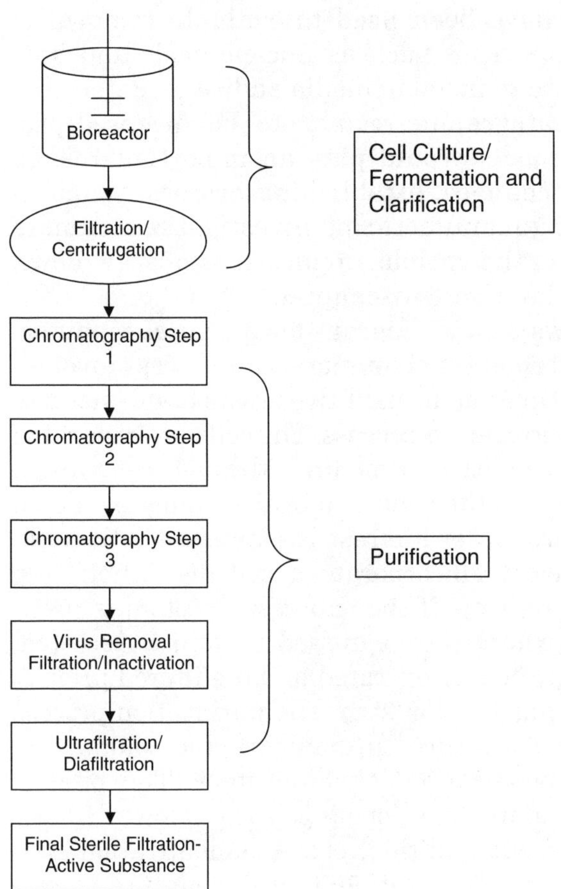

Figure 4.1 Typical biopharmaceutical manufacturing process flow diagram illustrating cell culture, cell separation, and purification steps. Multiple bioreactors can be processed per batch. The actual number or sequence of steps depends on the individual processes. Some processes may or may not include additional ultrafiltration/diafiltration steps. Viral inactivation steps may be incorporated where appropriate or necessary.

4.2 DESIGN OF SCALE-DOWN SYSTEMS

4.2.1 Principles

Prior to conducting any process validation studies, it is very important to ensure that the scale-down model system appropriately reflects the performance of the unit operation at full scale. Several parameters may need to be considered in designing a scale-down model. As an example, for chromatographic-based separations these parameters would include column dimensions and bed height, linear flow rates, buffer conditions, etc. For membrane-based separations, these parameters would include flux, transmembrane pressure, and loading per membrane area. It is important to identify the key parameters, scaling principles, and appropriate end points for each unit operation prior to designing the scale-down model that is intended to model the production scale unit operation.

4.2.2 Evaluation of Scale-Up before Scale-Down

Data from laboratory-scale development studies are used to scale-up the process to pilot or full-scale production, and data from these scale-up runs are in turn used to demonstrate the equivalence of scale-down models. Therefore, the first indications of the appropriateness of scaling principles are available upon scale-up. If differences in performance are observed between the scales, the scale-down models should then be refined. One could encounter numerous problems upon scale-up, some of which could be related to equipment differences. Also, the impact of hold times on product should be evaluated, as there could be longer hold times upon scale-up when large volumes are processed. Longer hold times could lead to differences in product quality such as deamidation, aggregation, etc., which could consequently lead to changes in product quality such as lower activity. A spectrum of analytical tools may be needed to establish the equivalence of the two scales.

4.2.3 Scale-Down Model Limitations: Equipment

A scale-down model not only represents the unit operation itself but also includes the ancillary equipment, such as pumps, temperature controllers, agitators, etc. Any equipment limitations that could potentially lead to differences in performance between small scale and large scale should be noted. As an example, for a chromatography unit operation, differences in UV monitors between small scale and large scale could lead to slightly different chromatograms or peak volumes if the peak volume is based on a percent of UV absorbance at peak apex. Another potential difference between the two scales could be the length and volume of tubing and other fittings, which could lead to a shift in elution times or altered resolution. Column frits or precolumn filters could absorb product or impurities and should therefore be of comparable materials of construction at both scales to avoid differences in performance [5]. Different design of pumps at large scale could introduce shear effects and potentially lead to product denaturation or aggregation. Equipment for temperature control and mixing may also be different between scales and could lead to differences in performance.

4.2.4 Scale-Down Model of an Entire Process Train

Scale-down models are typically designed for a single unit operation. However, it is often necessary to have a scale-down model for an entire process train. These models are especially useful while evaluating cell culture or fermentation process changes or troubleshooting deviations in commercial manufacturing processes. Another application could be in designing process characterization and robustness studies where the robustness of a step is evaluated for its impact on the performance of downstream steps. Most often, a scale-down model for an entire process train is not necessarily identically scaled-down models operated sequentially. This is due to possible difference in scales such that the amount of product eluting from the first scale-down model may not provide a sufficient amount of load following sampling to the subsequent step's scale-down model. In such instances, a scale-down model for the subsequent step with a greater scale-down factor may need to be qualified. Establishing a scale-down model for an entire process train could prove to be a valuable tool in mimicking large-scale manufacturing processes or in supporting laboratory-scale bioreactor experiments used in evaluating process options or robustness studies.

4.3 EXAMPLES OF SCALE-DOWN MODELS

The guidelines and principles governing scale-down of various unit operations have both unique and common features. The following sections describe examples of various unit operations currently used in industry, focusing on general guidelines and critical parameters affecting scale-down and primary end points used to assess the performance of the scale-down model. A critical parameter is defined as any parameter that would have an impact on process performance and product quality, if allowed to vary outside its control range.

4.3.1 Chromatography

4.3.1.1 Description of Chromatographic Techniques

Chromatography is one of the most widely used unit operations in downstream purification processes. The principle of chromatographic separation is based on the differential interactions between the product and impurities for a chromatographic medium. Chromatographic columns are typically operated such that the product binds the column while impurities are recovered in the unbound fraction (for weaker binding impurities) and in the column regeneration (for stronger binding impurities). Alternatively, the column could be operated in a flow-through mode whereby the impurities bind to the column while the product flows through. In size exclusion chromatography (SEC), there are no binding interactions involved, as products are separated from impurities on the basis of their size.

A variety of chromatographic techniques are employed in purification processes to achieve the purity required for biopharmaceuticals, enzymes, diagnostics, and plasma products. These techniques exploit differences in properties of proteins such as size, surface charge, surface hydrophobicity, and binding specificity. Examples include affinity chromatography, ion-exchange chromatography, hydrophobic interaction chromatography, metal affinity chromatography, and size exclusion chromatography. A typical purification process would comprise a combination of the aforementioned chromatographic steps with complementary separation mechanisms. Chromatographic steps can be optimized to yield a high-resolution purification method.

The separation of proteins by chromatography involves multiple interactions between the solute, solvent, and solid chromatographic support matrix. Separation can be influenced by factors such as nature of ligand and matrix, solvent pH, temperature, size of the beads and pores, etc.

4.3.1.2 General Scale-Down Principles and Parameters

Chromatographic steps are typically operated as a batch operation using clarified cell culture fluid. In such operations, entire product pools from the previous process step are applied to the chromatographic column steps either directly or after some sample manipulation such as concentration, diafiltration, pH/salt adjustments, or dilution, and a single product pool is generated. In some instances, product pools from multiple cycles on a single chromatographic step may be loaded onto the next step. An emerging technology that has been applied recently for protein separation is expanded bed technology, which is operated in batch mode but does not require a clarified feed stream [6,7]. Some continuous chromatographic methods, such as simulated moving bed, are also used for protein purification [8].

4.3.1.2.1 Scale-Down Validation of Column Chromatography Systems

The fluid distribution system of a column such as tubing, frits, monitors, column hardware, etc., plays a crucial role in separation. These elements, though difficult to maintain with identical geometry and materials of construction between large scale and small scale, should be kept as similar as possible. One example of common equipment differences would be the use of stainless steel pipes and columns in large-scale manufacturing compared to plastic tubing and columns at small scale [5].

Table 4.1 summarizes the scale-down parameters for chromatography systems. Typical scale-down column diameters range from 0.5 cm to 1.6 cm while the maximum diameter for manufacturing scale columns may be as large as 2.0 m or higher. Therefore, the scale-down factors for chromatography steps may range from 1:100 to over 1:100,000. Residence time of the product is a critical parameter and must be maintained while scaling down the process step. This is achieved by maintaining the bed height and linear velocity and decreasing the column diameter [9]. All process solution volumes are normalized to column volumes and must be the same between the two scales. In some cases, residence time has been maintained by changing both the bed height and linear velocity [10]. However, the European Union's Committee for Proprietary Medicinal Products (CPMP) has listed column bed heights as one of the parameters to be compared to show validity of a scale-down model [11]. One consideration to keep in mind when scaling down column diameter is wall effects, which could impact chromatographic performance, potentially for column diameters less than 1.0 cm. Yields and product purity between the two scales must be compared [5].

Procedures for preparation of buffers and solutions for scale-down studies should be according to established protocols used in large-scale manufacturing, since subtle changes in ionic strength or pH could lead to altered elution and purity profiles. Further, the quality of buffers and salts used for

TABLE 4.1 Scale-Down Parameters and Assessment Methods for Chromatographic Steps

Scale-Down Parameters[a]

Bed height
Buffer volumes (bed volumes)
Linear flow rate
Column loading (g product/l of resin)
Elution pool collection criteria
Solution pH, conductivity, protein concentration, composition
Temperature

Assessment Methods and Techniques

HETP and asymmetry factor	Solution spike (UV, conductivity)
Product yield	Product concentration (UV, HPLC, activity)
Total protein yield	Total protein concentration (Bradford, UV, HPLC)
Chromatographic profile	Chromatographic profiles for UV, conductivity/pH should be within manufacturing experience.
Product purity	SDS-PAGE, HPLC, specific activity
Impurity levels	SDS-PAGE, ELISA, SEC-HPLC, DNA
Product isoform distribution	specific tests
	HPLC, iso-electric focusing (IEF)

[a] Within manufacturing range unless otherwise specified.

preparing solutions for scale-down studies should also be consistent with those used in manufacturing. For chromatographic resins, the base matrix, functional groups, and ligand densities should be similar to large-scale manufacturing since these parameters could have an impact on impurity removal. Resins with the same functional group but differences in base matrices or porosities have yielded different levels of virus and DNA removal, respectively [5].

Temperature is another variable that could affect the retention time of proteins on chromatographic resins. Scale-down models should be run at the same temperatures as large-scale manufacturing. Fluctuations in temperature could lead to changes in pH and conductivity of certain buffers, which could affect retention of proteins. Among the various chromatographic techniques, hydrophobic interaction chromatography has been reported to be especially prone to changes in performance due to temperature variations, which could give rise to large changes in product retention or selectivity [12].

4.3.1.3 Primary End Points

Several important control variables such as solution pH, conductivity, temperature, and protein concentrations of the load should be measured prior to initiating scale-down runs to verify that they are comparable to large scale. Very often, column packing can play an important role in the chromatographic separation. Differences in column packing at the two scales may have an impact on the separation and be visualized as differences in the chromatograms. It is therefore important to evaluate the quality of column packing as a tool for comparison at different scales. Height-equivalent-to-a-theoretical-plate (HETP) and asymmetry factor (A_s) are typically used to evaluate quality of column packing [13]. A small volume of a concentrated salt solution such as sodium chloride or a UV-absorbing molecule such as benzyl alcohol is injected into a column. The resulting conductivity or UV peak typically is used to calculate the HETP and A_s values [14]. A range of acceptable values is determined during development and can be compared to values from large-scale columns. When comparing packing quality at the different scales, it is important to pay careful attention to factors such as test sample volume, linear flow rate, chart recorder speeds, and equipment differences (tubing length and diameter, monitors, pumps), among others.

Several outputs are used as end points to assess the performance of the scale-down model relative to large-scale manufacturing (Table 4.1). One of the primary end points used in assessing the performance of a scale-down qualification model is an evaluation of chromatograms to include a qualitative comparison of UV, pH, or conductivity profiles. Other outputs include product yields (often a quantitative comparison to large-scale runs using appropriate statistical methods such as a t-test), product purity (measured by specific activity or other methods), and impurity levels (SDS-PAGE, RPHPLC, or other methods).

Elution pool volumes are determined by the pooling criteria for elution pools. The method of pooling will have an impact on pool volumes and possibly on product purity. Collection of the product pool is typically initiated and controlled by use of a UV absorbance detector. The pool collection is usually initiated when the UV absorbance increases above baseline or attains a set absolute absorbance as the product starts to come off. The end of pool collection could be defined in different ways: (1) fixed number of column volumes, (2) when the UV absorbance returns to a certain predetermined level, or (3) when the UV absorbance has returned to a certain proportion of the UV peak maximum. Each of these methods has particular advantages and disadvantages. The use of a set number of column volumes makes the peak collection independent of the UV signal. This method of collection would be desirable if the UV signal of the product pool goes beyond the linear range of the UV detector during elution or if it is important to limit the volume of the elution pool. The disadvantage of this method is the potential for varying yields or product quality with varying loads to the column. Higher loads with larger elution pools might result in a lower yield. Low loads with narrower elution profiles might include more undesired, late-eluting impurities in the product pool. The second method also controls the end of pool collection when the absorbance maximum goes beyond the linear scale but can allow variation of the product pool volume depending on load. In addition, the purity of the product pool can vary if significant levels of impurities are present in the tailing portion of the peak. The third method of pool collection has a greater likelihood of maintaining consistent composition of the elution pool through varying load levels but will allow relatively greater variation in elution pool volume. However, it requires that absorbance be in the linear range of detection throughout the elution.

An example of a successful qualification of a scale-down chromatographic step is provided in the following section.

4.3.1.3.1 Example of a Scale-Down Validation of a Chromatographic System in Batch Mode

In this study, a cation exchange process step used in the purification of a therapeutic protein with a basic pI was scaled down. This protein is produced by expression as a neutral fusion protein in *E. coli*. The fusion protein is selectively released from the cells and is partially purified. The purified fusion protein is then chemically cleaved and the product stream is exchanged into a low ionic strength buffer. This load contains the therapeutic protein, an acidic fusion protein partner, uncleaved fusion protein species (which are neutral), and miscellaneous *E. coli* proteins. Purification of the target protein from these impurities is achieved by the use of a cation exchange step in product-binding mode. This column step was scaled down so it could be used to validate the removal of trace DNA and host cell proteins using radiolabeled tracers and to validate hold times for process intermediates by processing upstream pools.

For the scale-down system, the column diameter was reduced from 63 cm to 1 cm and the bed height was maintained, resulting in a scale-down factor of 1:4000. HETP and asymmetry measurements were made of the scaled-down columns to ensure that they were adequately packed and representative of the full-scale process (Table 4.2). The scaled-down system was run in triplicate, keeping the linear flow rate and column volumes of buffers and process load stream the same as the full-scale process. The load feed stream for the scale-down qualification was from a single representative process batch. An in-line filter upstream of the scaled-down column was employed using membranes with the same materials of construction as the process scale.

Evaluation of the scale-down model included qualitative and quantitative comparisons with the goal of determining whether there were any meaningful differences in column performance between the two scales. The UV and conductivity profiles from the scale-down model are comparable to the profiles from manufacturing scale (Figure 4.2). SDS-PAGE

TABLE 4.2 Comparison of Scale-Down and Manufacturing Scale Yields and Purities

Manufacturing and Prospective Scale Comparison Parameters		Scale		Means Test p-Value
		Manufacturing	Prospective	
% yield	Mean	76	76	0.92
	Standard deviation	4.8	3.6	
Mean purity	Mean	97	96	0.48
	Standard deviation	1.2	0.4	
Reduced HETP	Mean	2.7	7.7	0.07
	Standard deviation	1.5	1.7	
Asymmetry factor	Mean	1.2	1.3	0.26
	Standard deviation	0.3	0.1	

purity analysis on product pools from the scale-down model and manufacturing scale show similar banding patterns and removal of *E. coli* proteins (Figure 4.3). Comparison of quantitative outputs between scales employed a Student's *t*-test to compare the product yields, purity by reversed-phase high-performance liquid chromatography (RPHPLC), and column HETP and asymmetry (Table 4.2).

One should be careful in applying the t-test in scale-down processes when a single lot of load material is applied to the column. Replicates at the small scale give a good estimate of the variability of the small-scale system, but manufacturing processes may vary more due to changing feed streams. A more detailed discussion on evaluation of the suitability of scale-down models is provided in Section 4.4.

4.3.1.4 Scale-Down Validation of Expanded Bed Chromatography

Typical purification processes consist of an initial cell-separation step such as centrifugation or microfiltration to remove whole cells or cell debris. The purpose of this step is primarily solid–liquid separation, and it is usually followed by a capture

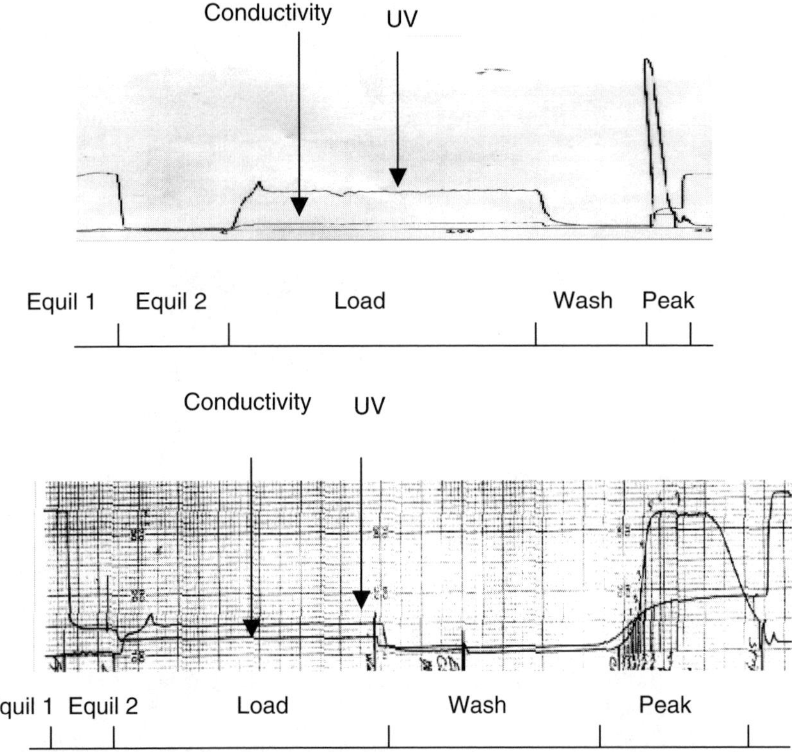

Figure 4.2 Comparison of UV and conductivity traces of scale-down and manufacturing scale runs. (top) UV and conductivity traces for the scale-down system. The line below the chromatogram indicates the points of application of the buffers. (bottom) During the manufacturing run, the chart speed in the horizontal direction was 0.33 mm/min for all segments up to elution. From elution onward, the chart speed was 10 mm/min. The vertical axis units are 0 to 50 mS/cm for conductivity and 0 to 5.0 absorbance units at 280 nm. During product elution, the product pool concentration goes beyond the linear range of the absorbance detector, which would explain the differences in the shape of the elution peaks. The line below the chromatogram indicates the points of application of the various buffers to the column.

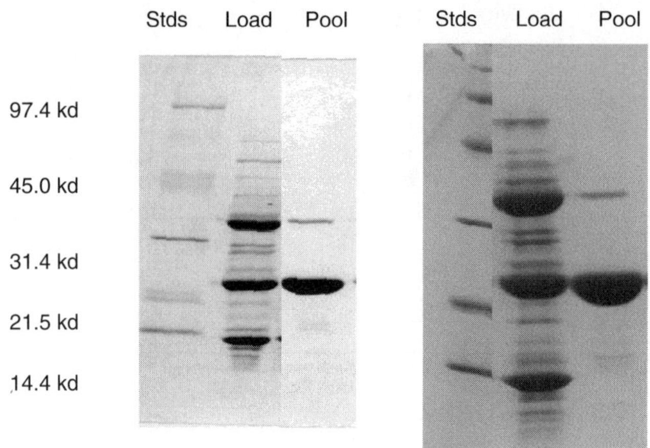

Figure 4.3 SDS-PAGE purity analysis on product pools from the scale-down model (left) and manufacturing scale (right). Nonreducing, 10–20% SDS-PAGE gel of the step loads and pools using a modified Laemli method followed by staining with Coomassie Blue.

Lane	Sample
1	BioRad low-range-molecular-weight standards
2	Load
3	Product pool

chromatographic step for purification. Expanded bed chromatography or adsorption (EBC or EBA) is an attractive cost-effective alternative since it combines clarification and purification operations into one operation [6]. The primary difference in the setup of EBC compared with traditional chromatographic columns is that the top flow adaptor is appropriately positioned such that the bed is allowed to expand upward in the direction of the liquid flow. Process streams containing solids can be applied directly, and the product is typically eluted in the packed bed mode, similar to traditional chromatography.

With a goal of employing EBC technology at industrial scale, columns with diameters from 20 cm to 1.2 m have been used [15]. At smaller scale, operations have been performed using 2.5- and 5-cm-diameter columns [16,17]. More recently,

EBC columns have been scaled down successfully 25- and 100-fold from the 5-cm-diameter scale to 1.0- and 0.5-cm-diameter columns [6] and similarly from 2.6- and 1.6-cm-diameter columns to 0.8-cm-diameter columns [7]. The settled bed height was maintained for all the runs.

For EBC, bed expansion is a critical parameter to control, and it is important to ensure that the mixing and expansion behaviors of scale-down systems are representative of large-scale systems. Several factors can affect bed expansion, such as liquid velocity, liquid viscosity, and particle diameter, among others. It has been reported that degree of expansion does not depend on the sedimented bed height or column diameter but is strongly affected by density and diameter of particles [7]. To obtain high column efficiency, liquid–liquid mixing and excessive movement of the solid absorbent should be minimized, and therefore the factors affecting bed stability and flow distribution should be controlled [6].

HETP measurements should be used to ensure that the column has been scaled down appropriately for EBC systems, similar to batch mode chromatography systems. Parameters such as flow rate, settled bed height, column diameter, and temperature do not significantly impact HETP measurements in EBC systems, suggesting similar mixing profiles [7]. Output variables used as end points for batch chromatography systems should be applicable for EBC systems. It is also important to monitor the extent of cell removal and cell lysis.

4.3.2 Protein Modification Reactions

Some unit operations involve the chemical or enzymatic modification of proteins to generate the final form of the product. The example in the previous section described the scale-down of a chromatographic step for purification of a fusion protein. In the case of expression of fusion proteins, the gene coding the protein of interest may be fused to a suitable partner for a variety of reasons including increased expression, improved product stability, and efficient purification by affinity chromatography [18]. However, the fusion protein could pose a challenge in downstream purification since the fusion partner has to be cleaved off and removed. Several chemical and enzymatic methods for cleavage of proteins have been studied [18]. Other examples of protein modification reactions include remodeling of glycoproteins [19], enzymatic modifications, and addition of poly(ethylene glycol) PEG or PEGylation for increased pharmacological properties. Design of scale-down models for such postbiosynthesis modification reactions of proteins presents unique challenges. Some examples of scale-down of protein modification reactions are discussed subsequently.

4.3.2.1 Hydroxylamine Cleavage Reactions

In cases where the recombinant protein of interest is to be cleaved from its fusion partner, linker regions can be engineered with specific cleavage sites. These sites can be designed for proteolytic or chemical cleavages. This discussion will focus on chemical cleavage with hydroxylamine, but many of the principles for both cleavage methods are similar.

Cleavage with hydroxylamine requires the linker region between the fusion pair to have an asparagine–glycine dipeptide site. When paired with glycine, and to a lesser extent leucine [20], cyclization of the asparaginyl side chains can occur forming cyclic amides, which are susceptible to nucleophilic attack from hydroxylamine. Reaction conditions such as pH, time, temperature, and concentration of reactants must be established and controlled in order to maximize cleavage efficiency and minimize unwanted side reactions. These side reactions can include aggregation, oxidation of methionines, hydroxylation of glutamine and asparagine, or deamidation of asparagine into an uncleavable iso-asp form [21].

4.3.2.1.1   General Scale-Down Principles and Critical Parameters

Table 4.3 summarizes the critical scale-down parameters for hydroxylamine cleavage reactions. Hydroxylamine cleavage steps are typically carried out at elevated pH and temperature [22]. The reaction is performed in stirred vessels to ensure thorough mixing of reactants and homogeneous control of pH

TABLE 4.3 Scale-Down Parameters and Assessment Methods for Hydroxylamine Cleavage Steps

---

Scale-Down Parameters[a]

Temperature profile (includes set points and ramp-up and cool-down rates)

pH (reactants, reaction hold point, neutralization buffer, neutralization hold, and end point)

Mixing[b]

Cleavage reactant concentration(s) (cleavage buffer, fusion protein solution, neutralization buffer)

Cleavage hold time

Cleavage buffer to fusion protein volume ratio

Cleavage buffer and neutralization buffer feed rate

Assessment Methods and Techniques

Cleavage efficiency	RPHPLC, SDS-PAGE
Cleavage rate	RPHPLC, SDS-PAGE
Product modifications	SDS-PAGE, hydroxymate assay, oxidized methionine (RPHPLC), deamidation (IEX)
Precipitation events	Turbidity (UV-VIS spectrometry), Bradford assay

[a] Within manufacturing range unless otherwise specified.

[b] Nonlinear scale-down; evaluate mixing time and compare to process; evaluate effects on yield and reaction rate.

and temperature. This is also important when the cleavage reaction is stopped at a predetermined time, which is typically done by lowering the temperature or pH. The ramp-up of the solution temperature at the start of the cleavage reaction and the cool-down at the end should be performed at a steady and controlled rate equivalent to the full-scale operation to ensure consistency. The scale-down reaction model could employ a simple system such as a jacketed beaker with a stir bar for mixing and attached to a temperature-controlled water bath. In such a system, heat-up and cool-down rates can be controlled manually so that they mimic the rates achieved at production scale. Monitoring temperature can be done with thermometers with data recorded at regular intervals or with thermocouples for continuous data recording.

The solution pH should also be monitored off-line in at least a semicontinuous fashion with a pH meter. This can be especially significant if the reaction is terminated with a combination of pH neutralization/titration and a cool-down phase. Buffering components in neutralization solutions may be temperature dependent. If a temperature-sensitive buffer is used, a bolus addition of a titrant at a high temperature may cause the pH to drop to levels well below the intended target until cool-down temperature set points are reached. In these types of systems, the neutralization buffer should be added in such a manner as to maintain the reaction pH until the low-temperature set point is reached. At that point, a bolus that has been predetermined to achieve target pH can be added. To achieve this type of pH control, continuous pH measurement is required during cool-down.

Scale-down factors in this type of system can be large but may be limited by the ability to control the system to mimic production scale characteristics. As mentioned previously, rates of temperature change could impact the final output of cleavage efficiency, and the level of pH control can influence undesirable side reactions. Practical considerations of sufficiently controlling these input parameters could limit the level of scale-down. Another factor in deciding the cleavage reaction scale-down factor is that in some instances it may be desirable to further process the neutralized cleavage product through other scale-down models of subsequent steps in the purification train. In these cases, the neutralized cleavage mixture must provide an appropriate volume to the subsequent step and the scale-down factor should be set accordingly.

Mixing of the reaction can be another complicating factor. Though the rates of mixing in impeller or stir bar systems can be quite rapid, shear forces can be quite different. Depending on the characteristics of the fusion protein and the cleavage products, the environment of the cleavage reaction could promote precipitation events. Shear forces could exacerbate this situation. Differences in shear due to mixing methods may need to be considered especially if precipitation occurs and the extent of precipation will be an output for assessing the scale-down system. Some assurance of the similarity in mixing times in the scale-down and production-scale systems should also be shown.

4.3.2.1.2   Primary End Points

The scale-down validation should demonstrate that the critical input parameters of pH, temperature, reaction time, reactant concentrations (both fusion protein and cleavage buffer), and rates of addition and mixing of various solutions to the reaction vessel are within the pre-established production-scale ranges. Output variables should include those typically determined for the production-scale step. Table 4.3 summarizes the primary end points to be measured and the assessment techniques. Total protein recovery by such methods as the Bradford assay can show that protein loss due to precipitation events is similar at both scales. The extent of precipitation should also be determined by turbidity or spectroscopic measurements. An assessment of cleavage efficiency should also be made. Minimally the final conversion efficiency at the end of the process step should be compared. Additionally, the rate of conversion through the reaction steps could also be compared by measuring the extent of cleavage in samples at various time points. SDS-PAGE analysis can be performed to qualitatively compare the relative distribution of the fusion protein and cleavage products (and other clipped species) in the neutralized cleavage mixture in both production and scale-down systems.

Other useful output parameters can be the extent of undesirable side reactions. Since many of these reactions can be pH, temperature, or reactant concentration dependent [21], the level to which side products accumulate can test the suitability of the scale-down system. The formation of hydroxymates and oxidized methionine as well as uncleavable species due to deamidation and additional cleavage at Asn-Leu sites can all be measured and compared between scales.

4.3.2.2 Enzymatic Cleavage Reactions

Insulin is a polypeptide hormone that consists of two separate peptide chains, A chain and B chain, that are linked together by disulfide bonds. It is typically expressed in its precursor form, proinsulin, where the two chains are connected by a third peptide C. Recombinant human insulin has been manufactured for over two decades; however, efforts to make efficient manufacturing processes are continuing. The various methods of insulin production in different expression systems have been reviewed elsewhere [23]. Current methods include manufacturing proinsulin as a single chain and subjecting it to modifications such as enzymatic cleavage of the C peptide or transpeptidation followed by hydrolysis, to yield human insulin [23]. Most of the scale-down parameters and assessment methods described in Table 4.3 for hydroxylamine cleavage are applicable for enzymatic cleavage reactions, too.

For the enzymatic cleavage reaction, careful attention must be given to maintaining control of the ratio of enzyme to substrate concentrations. Factors affecting kinetics of reaction such as pH, temperature, protein concentration, and time of cleavage reaction are also important to control. The cleavage efficiency or extent of conversion should be assessed. The levels of any undesirable side products should be monitored and compared between the scale-down and large-scale systems.

4.3.2.3 PEGylation

Covalent coupling of PEG to proteins (PEGylation) has been a very successful approach toward improving the pharmacological and biological properties of proteins [24]. PEG conjugation can shield antigenic epitopes of the polypeptide and thus reduce recognition by the immune system and reduce degradation by proteolytic enzymes. PEG conjugation also increases the apparent size of the polypeptide, thus reducing renal filtration and altering biodistribution [25].

Several factors related to the coupling reaction could affect the aforementioned properties. These include the number, molecular weight, and structure of PEG chains attached to the protein, the location of the PEG sites on the protein, and the chemistry used to attach the PEG to the protein [25]. These factors may also affect scale-down reactions and would need to be similar at the two scales. Most of the scale-down parameters and assessment methods described for hydroxylamine cleavage reactions are applicable here as well. Other parameters that may need to be controlled in scale-down reactions include pH, temperature, ratio of PEG to protein, addition rate of PEG, and extent of reaction, among others.

One of the methods widely used for PEG conjugation of proteins is to activate the PEG for reaction with lysine residues on proteins. Since multiple lysine residues are typically present on all proteins, a heterogeneous mixture is produced that is composed of a population of several PEG molecules attached per protein molecule. The extent of modification is important in determining the pharmacological properties of the conjugated protein. The heterogeneity in lysine substitution and in PEG molecular weights is of some concern for PEG–protein pharmaceuticals, and it is generally necessary to demonstrate that the conjugation for a particular pharmaceutical can be characterized and is reproducible [25].

4.3.3 Precipitation

4.3.3.1 Description of Precipitation Techniques

Fractional precipitation may be used to concentrate proteins, remove broad classes of impurities, or provide modest increases in product purity. Alternatively, precipitation steps may be designed to keep the product soluble, forgoing any product concentration but providing concomitant removal of impurities in the solid phase. A precipitation process step entails manipulation of the feed solution to favor protein or impurity precipitation, mixing of the vessel contents as the precipitation takes place, and subsequent solid–liquid separation to separate the two phases [26–28].

Typically, a precipitation step is performed on process streams at the beginning of a purification process. While not a high-resolution purification method, precipitation steps are commonly used in plasma protein fractionation, where variations on the Cohn-Oncley process are used to generate products including clotting factors (Factor VIII, Factor IX), albumin, immunoglobulins, and antithrombin III, among others. The classic Cohn-Oncley process employs manipulation of pH, temperature, ionic strength, and ethanol and protein concentrations [29]. Other methods for protein precipitation include addition of high concentrations of polymers such as polyethylene glycol, raising salt concentrations (salting-out), lowering salt concentrations (salting-in), addition of solvents, and exposure to extremes of pH.

The precipitation of proteins is a complex phenomenon involving protein–protein, protein–solvent, and protein–excipient interactions. While protein solubility is governed by thermodynamic principles, kinetic effects may prevent reaching an equilibrium state, and other nonidealities can arise from coprecipitation of multiple proteins or over precipitation due to mixing limitations [28].

4.3.3.2 General Scale-Down Principles and Critical Parameters

Table 4.4 summarizes the critical scale-down parameters for precipitation reactions. Precipitation steps are most often performed in batch operation, using simple tanks employing a single impeller for mixing, and jackets or heat exchangers for temperature control. Given the simplicity of the equipment used for this unit operation, it would seem to be quite easy to scale down. However, complexities arise from various phenomena described subsequently. Some processes employ continuous or semicontinuous operation, using static in-line mixers [30,31], which would require special care in design and qualification of scale-down systems. Translation from continuous to batch operation in concert with scale-down would appear possible, provided sufficiently quantitative performance end points can be defined to ensure that the same extent of precipitation has occurred for both soluble and insoluble species. In some cases, changes in the level of precipitant required were observed when moving from continuous to batch operation [28]. The subsequent solid–liquid separation of the precipitate from the supernatant may be performed by

TABLE 4.4   Scale-Down Parameters and Assessment Methods for Precipitation Steps

Scale-Down Parameters[a]

Mixing[b]
Final precipitant concentration
Precipitant stock concentration
Precipitant to feed volume ratio
Precipitant feed rate
Solution pH, conductivity, protein concentration, etc.
Solid/liquid separation[c]
Temperature

Assessment Methods and Techniques

Product yield	Product concentration (UV, HPLC, activity)
Total protein yield	Total protein concentration (Bradford, UV, HPLC)
Product purity	SDS-PAGE, HPLC, specific activity
Impurity levels	SDS-PAGE, ELISA, SEC-HPLC
Precipitate yield or phase ratio	Gravimetric, volumetric measurement
Supernatant turbidity	UV-VIS spectrometry, nephelometry

[a] Within manufacturing range for all parameters, unless otherwise specified.
[b] Nonlinear scale-down (evaluate mixing time and compare to process, and evaluate effects on yield and purity).
[c] Centrifugation may be used to model filtration; if filtration is used, match filtration area to volume ratio.

either depth filtration (often with Celite or other filter aids) using filter presses, ultrafiltration, or centrifugation using continuous-flow tubular bowl, disc stack, or other centrifuge designs.

The scale-down factors for precipitation steps may range from 1:100 to over 1:100,000 [32]. Because mixing is commonly employed during precipitation steps, and mixing parameters such as tip speed, power input, and average shear are scale dependent [33], a very large scale-down factor will necessitate significant changes in some of these parameters. Unlike the simpler mixing problem of achieving homogeneity in a homogeneous solution, the influence of mixing on the heterogeneous, dynamic system of a precipitation reaction requires more care in scaling. A measurement of the mixing time of the small-scale vessel should be evaluated to confirm that the vessel contents are well mixed over the timescale of precipitant addition. (Generally, small vessels with adequate mixing times are not difficult to design.) Equipment design features that will influence mixing include the ratio of the impeller to tank diameter, presence or absence of baffles, impeller speed, and impeller type. Given the fact that so many scale factors will inevitably change upon scale-down, the need to maintain exact geometric similarity with the process vessel may be relaxed. The Camp number, which is related to the power input per unit volume, has been used in scaling correlations for some precipitation steps as a means of ensuring adequate particle strength [34]. However, as scaling laws for mixing steps are not universally established for all precipitation methods [35], an empirical evaluation of stirrer speed and impeller diameters may be needed to closely match performance at full scale.

The operating temperature is an important variable for some precipitation steps and is often controlled to within a few degrees of set point. For solvent precipitation, the heat of solution released upon mixing the aqueous and organic solutions must be removed through the vessel walls in a batch operation. Fortuitously, temperature control of small-scale vessels is not difficult and can be achieved by heating blocks or water baths.

The precipitation conditions must remain constant between scales, with regards to the protein concentration and final precipitant concentration or solution conditions [36]; one should be cognizant of the tolerance or operating range allowed in manufacturing. The same stock solution concentration of precipitant should be used for both full-scale and small-scale processes to ensure the same overall dilution factor. Careful control of relevant solution variables of pH, ionic strength, protein concentration, and other parameters is important, as "small changes in the prerequisites or conditions of the manufacturing process can influence the efficacy of the process to inactivate or remove viruses" for precipitation steps [37]. Later, during virus removal validation studies, a worst-case condition may be tested (for instance, a lower limit of final precipitant concentration and contact time for cases where the product remains in the supernatant [38]).

The rate of precipitant addition should also be held constant, which in some cases will occur over many hours (the rate of addition can affect floc size and subsequent centrifugation [28]). The total contact time for precipitation is typically held constant, although it is possible that slight differences in kinetics between scales may be evident. Ideally, the same steady state (not necessarily equilibrium) will be reached in both systems. During the aging process, some overprecipitated proteins generated by contact with elevated levels of the precipitant stock solution prior to complete mixing may redissolve, thus potentially impacting the purity of the precipitate.

Following the precipitation step, a solid–liquid separation must be performed. Filtration steps are generally straightforward to scale down, provided filtration equipment of the appropriate area is available. The ratio of filter aid to solution should be held constant to maintain similar filter cake properties, although due to scaling limitations, the use of oversized filters is not uncommon. In some cases, filtration steps are modeled at small scale by centrifugation, and their equivalence was demonstrated in actual virus removal validation studies using both techniques [32,39]. Centrifugation steps may be difficult to scale down [40,41], and often changes in equipment design or even the mode of separation are adopted in the translation to small scale. Batch centrifugation is the method of choice for lab-scale operations, with g-force, sedimentation distance (solution volume), and time being the most important variables governing performance of the small-scale system. The practical impact of this change in centrifugation conditions may be hard to interpret. For instance, there is the potential for a slight solution carryover in a product in the solid phase to impact viral validation studies, if the virus were to strongly partition to the solution phase. Temperature control is important for the solid–liquid separation step as well to prevent any redissolution, which could occur upon heating. Jacketed filter funnels or refrigerated centrifuges allow temperature control during this final step. Washing steps, if used in the manufacturing process, should employ the same ratio of wash to precipitation solution.

4.3.3.3 Primary End Points

Table 4.4 summarizes the primary end points of a precipitation step and the techniques used for their measurement. The critical control variables of pH, conductivity, final precipitant concentration, and temperature should be verified by measurement in the small-scale system [42]. Output variables should include those measurable parameters, which could conceivably vary with improperly scaled processes. These would include product purity (measured by specific activity or chromatographic methods), product and total protein yield, and impurity levels (assessed by SDS-PAGE or the degree of product polymerization). Examples of scale-down system performance assessment using comparisons of some of these output variables to full-scale manufacturing can be found in the literature [32,43–45]. Additional measurements could include measurement of ion concentrations (sodium content), turbidity of the supernatant to gauge the extent of precipitate removal, and the phase ratio or fraction of solids in the precipitate. The kinetics of precipitation are generally not measured or followed, but in the case where a significant discrepancy exists between the operating scales, more subtle analyses such as precipitation kinetics, floc size distribution, etc., may be valuable in refining the design of the scale-down system to more accurately reflect full-scale performance.

Precipitation is recognized as a relatively difficult unit operation to scale down and qualify [46]. However, with the appropriate equipment design and attention to detail, control of critical parameters including temperature and mixing, and the assessment of appropriate performance parameters including product yield and purity, one can establish an adequate degree of assurance that the full-scale precipitation operation has been modeled by laboratory equipment.

4.3.4 Microfiltration

4.3.4.1 Description of Microfiltration Techniques

Microfiltration (MF) membranes can be used to harvest cells from mammalian and bacterial cell culture to provide cell-free conditioned medium (containing the product) to the downstream purification steps. The pore sizes of typical MF membranes range from 0.1 to 0.8 microns. MF membranes retain cells and cellular debris by a sieving mechanism at the membrane surface. Pressure is applied to the feed stream to force permeate through the membrane. Proteins and small-molecular-weight species (media salts) pass through the membrane and are collected in the permeate stream. MF separations and system design considerations have been reviewed in several publications [47–50].

MF separations can be conducted with the feed flow directed in a normal or tangential direction to the membrane surface. An example of normal flow filtration (NFF) would be dead-end or cartridge filters where cells are retained at the membrane surface or within the membrane structure. As cells build up at the membrane surface, the filtration rate, or flux, decreases as the resistance to permeate flow through the membrane increases. In tangential flow filtration (TFF), the feed solution is passed tangentially over the membrane surface. Cells build up on the membrane surface as permeate flows through the membrane and are swept off the membrane and recirculated back to the feed tank [51]. The cells are concentrated to a target volume concentration factor (VCF = initial feed volume/final feed volume). The concentrated feed may then be diafiltered to recover additional product. The number of diafiltration wash volumes (DV) is calculated by dividing the permeate volume collected during the diafiltration by the feed volume at diafiltration.

The membrane pore size can affect the capacity and separation performance of the MF system. Larger pore size membranes allow higher capacity, and hence higher yields can be achieved. However, membranes with smaller pore sizes may provide a cleaner permeate that will require less polishing filtration area to protect the downstream unit operations. The increased capacity of the more open membranes must be balanced with the required clarity of the resulting permeate stream.

4.3.4.2 General Scale-Down Principles and Critical Parameters

Table 4.5 summarizes the critical scale-down parameters for MF systems. The efficiency of NFF cell separations can be influenced by operating parameters including nominal pore size distribution, filter structure (fibrous, graded pore density, or uniform pore), additives such as diatomaceous earth, operating pressure, flow rate, and temperature. The ratios of the load volume and chase volume to surface area are also important scale-down parameters. The efficiency of cell separation with MF systems operated in TFF mode can be influenced by several key operating parameters including feed channel height or lumen diameter, cross-flow velocity, transmembrane pressure, operating flux, and temperature. The feed side fluid path length, load volume to surface area, and the number of diafiltration wash volumes are also important scale parameters in TFF systems [52]. The MF feed material is often characterized by cell concentration, viability, susceptibility to shear (cell age), and permeate streams by spun-down supernatant turbidity.

The feed pumps used on TFF MF systems must provide sufficient cross-flow to sweep the membrane surface while not damaging the shear-sensitive mammalian cells. Flow restrictions such as valves and tortuous paths are minimized to prevent cell damage in the feed path. Low-shear pumps such as rotary lobe pumps are commonly used for feed recirculation. Typical operating pressure for mammalian cell harvest MF systems is 5–15 psig, with transmembrane pressure (TMP = [feed pressure + retentate pressure]/2 – permeate pressure) of 0.1–2 psig. Sensitive pressure monitors are used to measure these low pressure differentials. MF operations are often operated initially at a constant flux for mammalian cell harvests. Flux control is typically achieved by restricting the permeate flow. At low permeate flow rates, a peristaltic pump

TABLE 4.5 Scale-Down Parameters and Assessment Methods for Microfiltration Steps

Scale-Down Parameters[a]

All MF[b] steps
  Load volume to surface area ratio
  Solution pH, conductivity, protein concentration, etc.
  Temperature
NFF[b]-specific systems
  Feed flow rate
  Feed pressure
  Chase volume to surface area ratio
TFF[b]-specific systems
  Crossflow rate per feed channel (or lumen)
  Flux
  Channel height (or lumen diameter)
  Number of modules connected in series or feed side path length
  Transmembrane pressure
  Number of diafiltration wash volumes

Assessment Methods and Techniques

Product yield	Product concentration (UV, HPLC, activity)
VCF[c] target	Volumetric measurement
DV[c] target	Volumetric measurement
Permeate pool turbidity	UV-VIS spectrometry, nephelometry
MF[b]-generated cell lysis	Lysis measurement (lactate dehydrogenase, DNA, etc.)
Permeate pool filterability	Filter-specific capacity

[a] Within manufacturing range for all parameters, unless otherwise specified.
[b] Abbreviations: MF, microfiltration; NFF, normal flow filtration; TFF, tangential flow filtration.
[c] Abbreviations: VCF, volume concentration factor; DV, diafiltration volumes.

can be used to restrict and control the permeate flow. With MF systems that have large permeate flow rates, control valves or rotary lobe pumps are used. Temperature and the permeate turbidity are often monitored.

MF systems have been used to harvest mammalian cell cultures with volumes of 12,500 liters [53]. As mentioned previously, it is important to maintain the membrane path length, or number of modules connected in series, during scale-down. The small-scale system area is determined by the number of modules in series multiplied by the area of the smallest device available from the vendor at the same path length as the production-scale module. Scale-down factors of 1:10 to 1:200 are achievable for MF systems. This is a low range for the scale-down factor, which significantly limits MF scale-down flexibility. A typical lower limit for membrane area is about 1–2 m^2 to process 100–200 l of conditioned media, and a higher limit for membrane area could be in the range of 50–200 m^2.

The minimum recirculation volume required to operate the scale-down MF system to prevent air entrainment on the suction side of the pump may be an issue. This may limit the VCF that may be achieved and thus not provide information about operating at the highest cell concentration. Peristaltic or small rotary lobe pumps are used with small-scale MF systems. These pumps may not appropriately mimic the large-scale production pumps with regard to shear, slip, and cell damage.

4.3.4.3 Primary End Points

A successful scale-down of an MF system will provide cell-free conditioned medium with similar permeate quality (turbidity and filterability) and product yield as the large-scale system. The feed flow rate and permeate flux are generally controlled during the MF operation. The pressure of the feed, retentate, and permeate streams and the TMP are monitored throughout the process. Temperature control is important for these systems and temperature profiles should be monitored. The permeate flux and TMP profile should mimic the production system performance as the processing objectives of VCF target and DV targets are achieved.

Table 4.5 summarizes the primary end points to be measured and the techniques used for their measurement. TMP profiles and quality of permeate are monitored over the run. The permeate quality can increase the particulate burden on the downstream operations and can affect the downstream prefiltration performance. The final VCF and diafiltration performance will affect the overall recovery from the step. Following cell harvesting, the MF membrane and system are cleaned to remove residual cells, protein, and foulants from the membrane surface. The ability to restore the membrane permeability to its initial value using cleaning agents should be demonstrated, if a small-scale system is to be reused.

4.3.5 Ultrafiltration

4.3.5.1 Description of Ultrafiltration Techniques

Ultrafiltration (UF) is a membrane-based separation that is used to concentrate or diafilter (buffer exchange) protein solutions. UF is a pressure-driven process where permeate is forced through a semipermeable membrane. UF membranes can also be used to fractionate protein solutions using high-performance tangential flow filtration (HPTFF) [54]. UF operations are typically conducted in a tangential flow filtration (TFF) mode where the feed solution is recirculated over the membrane and then returned to the feed vessel. Macromolecules such as proteins are retained by the membrane and low-molecular-weight species such as buffer salts and water pass through the membrane into the permeate stream. UF membranes are available in nominal molecular weight limits of 1000 to 1,000,000 Daltons. UF separations and system design considerations have been reviewed in several publications and books [48,55–57].

UF systems consist of a feed pump, recirculation vessel, and connecting piping and valves. A separate pump is used to add diafiltration buffer to the recirculation vessel. The control parameters include feed and retentate pressure (the permeate pressure is usually atmospheric for UF applications), temperature, and the feed flow rate per feed channel. The permeate flow rate is monitored over the concentration and diafiltration operations. The time average flux is used to predict system performance and to determine the required membrane area of production systems.

4.3.5.2 General Scale-Down Principles and Critical Parameters

Table 4.6 summarizes the critical scale-down parameters for UF systems. These include membrane material and pore size, feed channel geometry (turbulence-promoting screen or open channel), device configuration, cross-flow rate per feed channel (or feed side pressure drop), transmembrane pressure (TMP), and the number of UF modules connected in series [58]. The feed protein concentration, ratio of volume processed to total surface area, temperature, and buffer composition also affect UF performance. Scale-down UF systems are used to predict or mimic the flux (permeate flow rate normalized to membrane area and often expressed in units of liters per

TABLE 4.6 Scale-Down Parameters and Assessment Methods for Ultrafiltration Steps

Scale-Down Parameters[a]	
Channel geometry	
Crossflow rate per feed channel or lumen (or feed side pressure drop)	
Number of modules connected in series or feed side path length	
Transmembrane pressure	
Solution pH, conductivity, protein concentration, etc.	
Temperature	
Load volume to surface area ratio	
Number of diafiltration wash volumes	

Assessment Methods and Techniques	
Product yield	Product concentration (UV, HPLC, activity)
VCF target	Volumetric measurement
Diafiltration wash volume target	Volumetric measurement
Extent of buffer exchange	Changes in pH, conductivity, excipient concentration
Contaminant removal	HPLC, impurity-specific measurement
Aggregate generation	SEC, light scattering, UV-VIS spectrometry

[a] Within manufacturing range for all parameters, unless otherwise specified.

square meter per hour [LMH]) performance and product rejection of full-scale operation.

Production-scale UF systems may operate with 5 to more than 100 square meters of membrane area. The smallest UF devices have areas of 10–50 cm^2. Scale-down ratios of 1:100–400 [58,59] have been reported and scale-down ratios of 1:20,000 may be achievable, depending on the process. The ability of UF scale-down systems to operate at low working volumes allows UF scale-down factors to be much greater than for MF scale-down systems.

The operation of scale-down UF systems can have limitations in the ability to achieve high volume concentration factors (VCF = initial feed volume/final feed volume) due to minimum working volumes required to eliminate air entrainment at the pump suction. Typical holdup volumes for 50-cm^2 devices are in the range of 10–50 ml. Shear and air–liquid interfaces can cause protein denaturation and aggregation [60–62]. Another complication is that production systems typically use rotary lobe pumps to provide the recirculation flow rate at feed pressures of 40–80 psi. Rotary lobe pumps that are capable of operating at the very low feed flows (<50 ml/min) of 50-cm^2 systems are not availabale. Typically peristaltic pumps are used at the small scale. These pumps can provide the low flow rates but arc subject to the pressure limitation of the tubing (25 psi typically). Therefore, scale-down systems are often operated at lower transmembrane pressures than the production system. In such cases, the flux can be normalized to the transmembrane pressure, and the resulting permeability (in units of LMH/psi) can be compared for the two operating conditions. Process time is longer as a result; if process time is critical, larger areas can be used. Another complication is that small-scale systems may not mimic the performance of large-scale membrane holders with respect to internal pressure drops and flow distribution uniformity, which could be significant [59].

Scale-down UF systems are required to process the same volume-to-surface-area ratio as the large-scale system and to achieve the volume concentration factor and diafiltration wash volume targets. The scale-down system should operate with the same feed channel geometry, path length, feed flow per channel (or feed side pressure drop), transmembrane pressure, and temperature as the large-scale system. At the scale-down conditions, the flux and product retention are measured over the concentration and diafiltration operations.

4.3.5.3 Primary End Points

Table 4.6 summarizes the primary end points to be measured for evaluating the scale-down performance of ultrafiltration steps and the techniques used for their measurement. The UF step recovery can be determined using HPLC or product-specific assays. When the UF step is operated with relatively pure proteins (>95%), UV absorbance at 280 nm (A_{280}) can be used for yield measurements. Temperature control is important and the process fluid temperature should be monitored. Calculating a mass balance is useful to determine if losses are into the permeate stream, left behind in the holdup volume, or irreversibly bound to the membrane. The membrane performance is also judged by comparing the process flux trend over the concentration and diafiltration operations. The average flux over the UF step is used to size production-scale equipment. The efficiency of the buffer exchange can be shown by pH and conductivity measurements. In the case where the objective of the diafiltration is contaminant removal, analytical techniques such as HPLC and ion chromatography can be used to monitor the washout of low-molecular-weight species. The generation of high-molecular-weight species or aggregates can be monitored using SEC or light-scattering techniques.

Following the protein processing steps, the UF membrane and system are cleaned to remove residual protein and foulants from the membrane surface. The ability to restore the membrane permeability using cleaning agents should be demonstrated, if the system and membranes are to be reused.

4.3.6 Centrifugation

4.3.6.1 Description of Centrifugation Techniques

Centrifuges are used for solid–liquid or immiscible liquid–liquid separations based on differences in phase densities. They are manufactured in basket, tubular, and stacked-disc configurations [63]. Solid–liquid separations include harvesting bacterial or mammalian cell cultures, particulate capture, or fractionation. For the harvesting of bacterial and mammalian cells, stacked-disc centrifuges have been used [64]. The cell culture solution is continuously fed to the outside of the centrifuge and flows through the spaces between the stacked discs toward the center of the centrifuge. Cells and particles are thrown radially outward by the centrifugal force toward the underside of the upper disc and slide down the disc surface to the sediment-holding space. The collected solids are either continuously or discontinuously discharged from the centrifuge. The liquid flows continuously to the top of the centrifuge and is discharged under pressure [65].

The principle of the centrifugal separation is that particles (or the denser liquid) migrate through the continuous lighter liquid phase under the acceleration of centrifugal force [66]. This migration must be in a direction other than parallel to the continuous phase to be useful. The centrifugal field varies in proportion to the distance from the center of rotation [66]. Particles settle faster as they move outward from the rotational center.

The sedimentation rate of a particle is proportional to the liquid flow rate through the centrifuge (Q) divided by the quantity sigma (Σ), which can be demonstrated to be the area of a simple gravity settling tank of equivalent sedimentation characteristics to that of the centrifuge. Theoretically, the performance of two centrifuges processing the same feed material will be equivalent if the Q/Σ value is kept constant [67].

4.3.6.2 General Scale-Down Principles and Critical Parameters

Table 4.7 summarizes the critical scale-down parameters for centrifugation steps. The centrifuge is operated by controlling the feed flow rate, centrifuge RPM (creating the centrifugal force), and system backpressure. The temperature and pressure of the feed and centrate are monitored over the run.

The scale-down of centrifugal separations can be achieved by reducing the number of active discs in the centrifuge or by using smaller equipment. The separation performance of a disc-stack centrifuge has been examined with

TABLE 4.7 Scale-Down Parameters and Assessment Methods for Centrifugation Steps

Scale-Down Parameters[a]

Feed flow rate[b]
RPM or centrifugal force[c]
System back-pressure
Solution pH, conductivity, protein concentration, etc.
Temperature

Assessment Methods and Techniques

Product yield	Volume and product concentration (UV, HPLC, activity)
Centrate turbidity	UV-VIS spectrometry, nephelometry, particle size distribution
Centrifuge generated cell lysis	Lysis measurement (lactate dehydrogenase, DNA, etc.)
Centrate filterability	Filter-specific capacity
Centrate and solids temperature rise	Thermocouple or thermometer

[a] Within manufacturing range for all parameters, unless otherwise specified.
[b] Scaled with the equivalent sedimentation area (sigma) to provide constant Q/Σ (where Q is flow rate).
[c] Scaled with the feed flow rate to provide constant Q/Σ.

respect to the number of active discs, active disc location, and the feed flow rate [65]. Blank aluminum inserts were placed into the centrifuge to reduce the available separation area to 10% of the centrifuge capacity. This still requires a significant amount of feed material. Lab-scale centrifuges have also been used to predict disc-stack centrifuge performance for polyvinyl acetate particles and yeast cell debris [68]. The smallest disc-stack centrifuges available for scale-down have Σ values of 1800 m² and can process feed volumes of 2–20 l at flow rates of 10–60 l/hr with a solids-holding volume of 0.5 l. Production-scale disc-stack centrifuges are made with sigma values as high as 130,000 m². Thus, scale-down factors of 70-fold are achievable.

However, in many commercial applications, centrifuge efficiency does not approach 100% [67]. Some of the reasons for this deviation arise from turbulent or transitional flow in regions of the disc stack that can cause re-entrainment of settled solids into the carrier fluid, uneven solids distribution at the entrance to the disc, and disproportionate fluid flow within the disc spacing [65,69]. Other factors that can complicate the centrifuge scale-down include differences in acceleration and deceleration times between scales [68] and the fact that following solids discharge it may take seven to eight bowl volume changes before steady state is achieved [70].

4.3.6.3 Primary End Points

The quality of the feed material can be measured in terms of cell concentration, cell viability, packed cell volume, and the spun-down supernatant turbidity of the feed (Table 4.7). The centrifuge control parameters include feed flow rate, RPM, and system pressure. The step performance can be measured by step yield, the clarity of the centrate, filterability of the centrate, particle size distribution, and amount of generated cell lysis [64]. The clarity of the centrate can be measured using particle counters, UV-VIS spectroscopy, or turbidity measurements.

4.3.7 Viral Inactivation

4.3.7.1 Description of Inactivation Techniques

Processes used for production of therapeutic proteins derived from human plasma or mammalian cell culture may incorporate steps designed for virus inactivation. These steps expose the process stream to conditions that kill or inactivate virus, by a variety of techniques, either by addition of chemicals, acid, or heating, followed by an incubation for a predetermined time period under controlled temperature. The solution may or may not be mixed during this incubation period, but it is assumed that the solution is homogeneous throughout the incubation period.

Examples of dedicated virus inactivation methods include addition of solvent and detergent to inactivate enveloped virus, addition of caprylate or B-propiolactone, low pH, and heat treatment or pasteurization [71–75]. Virus removal filtration, sometimes called nanofiltration, is a virus removal step and is treated in its own section in this chapter.

4.3.7.2 General Scale-Down Principles and Critical Parameters

Viral inactivation methods that add chemicals or acid to the product solution are carried out in stirred vessels to ensure that every fluid element is contacted with the inactivation chemicals. Once a homogeneous solution is generated, the solution is often transferred to a second vessel, which may or may not be agitated (the use of two vessels in this fashion introduces a viral inactivation barrier between two processing areas, clearly segregating the preinactivation from postinactivation equipment, thus preventing cross-contamination). Heat treatment may be carried out in the final product container or in bulk, as may be the case for albumin production. Temperature control would be maintained by a jacket or heat exchanger on the contacting vessel, or in a vat containing circulating, tempered water, which would bring product vials up to temperature. Table 4.8 summarizes the critical scale-down parameters for virus inactivation reactions.

TABLE 4.8 Scale-Down Parameters and Assessment Methods for Viral Inactivation Steps

Scale-Down Parameters[a]	
Temperature	
Mixing[b]	
Contact time	
Final inactivation chemical concentration(s)	
Inactivation chemical stock concentration	
Inactivation chemical to feed volume ratio	
Inactivation chemical feed rate	
Solution pH, conductivity, protein concentration, etc.	

Assessment Methods and Techniques	
Product modifications	SDS-PAGE, ELISA, SEC-HPLC
Supernatant turbidity	UV-VIS spectrometry, nephelometry
Solution composition	Various methods (GC, LC, pH, etc.)

[a] Within manufacturing range for all parameters, unless otherwise specified.

[b] Nonlinear scale-down (evaluate mixing time; compare to process and evaluate effects on yield and purity; measure final levels of inactivating chemicals).

The scale-down factors for these types of virus inactivation steps may be very large, as there is little limitation to designing a temperature-controlled contacting vessel, which simply needs to maintain a well-mixed solution. Test tubes or small vessels may be used if they are immersed in a temperature-controlled heating block and mixed either before or during contact. The level of the heating solution should be above the liquid level in the test vessel to ensure that all the test solution contents have reached the target temperature. Measurement of the heat-up and cool-down cycles may also be recorded, and while this information may not be critical to the virus inactivation validation studies performed later (the virus will be spiked in the solution when the incubation temperature is reached), differences in performance parameters could conceivably arise from the more rapid approach to the hold temperature typically seen for smaller vessels. A special case of heat treatment employs high-temperature short-time inactivation through the use of microwaves to rapidly heat a solution in a continuous-flow heat exchanger, followed by the rapid cooling of the product [76]. Such a system requires a very careful scale-down using a miniature model of the process equipment, which could limit the scale-down to more modest ratios. An alternative approach to minimizing the volume of product required for the scale-down process is to introduce a short pulse of the product into the feed stream to the full-scale process heat exchanger using a shunt [77].

The mixing of the vessel contents should be confirmed, especially for solvent–detergent inactivation, as dispersion of the colloidal suspension must be complete [78]. Standard mixing studies may be employed [79], although there could be complications at very small scale arising from sampling limitations. The measurement of the kinetics of virus inactivation is required by regulatory agencies [80]; the mixing time should be rapid enough to include time points that may be as early as 2 minutes [81] or even 30 seconds [82]. The same stock solution concentration should be used for both scales to ensure that the same dilution factor is achieved and to avoid complications of mixing more viscous, higher-concentration stock. The addition rate of the inactivation chemicals should match the manufacturing process, and the final target concentrations of solvent and detergent, acid, etc., should be the same as full scale.

As the virus inactivation may be a function of solution pH, solution composition, and protein concentration, these variables should be maintained within manufacturing ranges.

4.3.7.3 Primary End Points

The scale-down process should verify that the following controlled variables are maintained in range throughout the inactivation process: pH, temperature, contact time, and the final inactivation chemical concentrations [83]. Temperature control may be demonstrated by monitoring a mock solution, which is adjacent to the test solution heating block and handled in the same fashion as the test solution [84]. Agitation during contacting, if required, should be maintained at set point levels of impeller or stir bar speed.

There are not many process performance variables that may need to be measured and compared to full scale (Table 4.8). In some processes, a pH drift will occur, and this should be confirmed to be comparable at small scale. In other cases, the product may be modified during the process step, e.g., albumin polymerization and aggregation during heat treatment [85] or protein modification by propiolactone [44], and this should be measured for the small-scale system to show similar effects. Some inactivation chemicals are unstable and hydrolyze during processing (propiolactone, for instance), and it may be crucial to assessment of virus inactivation during validation studies to show that the inactivating chemical concentration profile is consistent between scales. If the solution becomes turbid during treatment, then the turbidity levels should be compared between scales.

4.3.8 Virus Removal Filtration

4.3.8.1 Description of Unit Operation

Virus removal filtration (VRF) is a unit operation widely used in plasma fractionation or mammalian cell culture processes. In plasma fractionation processes, use of VRF steps reduces the risk of potential for blood-borne viral contaminants and significantly improves the safety profile of plasma products. Mammalian cells such as Chinese hamster ovary (CHO) and hybridoma cell lines frequently release retrovirus-like particles [86,87]. Regulatory agencies require that steps be employed to reduce the levels of viruses in purification processes [1–4].

VRF is a pressure-driven process where permeate is forced through a semipermeable membrane with typical pore sizes in the range of 15–50 nm. The pore size distributions allow for passage of the product and buffer ingredients, while retaining viral particles. In most cases, VRF devices are used once and then discarded. VRF separations and design considerations have been reviewed in several publications [88–90].

4.3.8.2 General Scale-Down Principles and Critical Parameters

VRF separations can be affected by the membrane material and pore size, feed flow rate for TFF operation, flux, operating pressure, and the molecular weight of the protein product (Table 4.9). The feed protein concentration, ratio of volume processed to total surface area, buffer chase volume (or amount of diafiltration), the buffer pH and ionic strength, temperature, and the presence of high-molecular-weight species can also influence the VRF performance [91–93].

VRF membrane devices can be operated in TFF or NFF mode. For VRF applications using TFF devices, the equipment used is similar to that used for UF systems (see Section 4.3.5.2). A UV detector is often included in the permeate line to monitor the passage of protein during the process. For VRF applications using NFF devices, the system can be operated either at constant flux or at constant pressure. For constant-flux NFF applications, the control parameters include feed flow rate and temperature. The feed pressure and accumulated permeate volume are monitored over the load and chase operations. For constant-pressure NFF applications, the control parameters include feed pressure and temperature. The permeate flow rate and accumulated flow are monitored over the load and chase operations. A UV detector is often included in the permeate line to monitor the passage of protein during the process.

Production-scale VRF systems may operate with 0.1 to 4.0 m^2 of membrane area. The smallest VRF devices have areas of approximately 10 cm^2. Scale-down ratios of 1 to $\geq$ 2000 may be achievable, depending on the process. Small-scale VRF devices are used for process robustness (or limits) testing as well as validation studies to demonstrate the removal of actual viruses spiked into the load material. It is required that VRF devices have an integrity test that is correlated to virus removal performance. The manufacturer generally provides this correlation.

The operation of scale-down VRF systems can present complications. When using multilayer membrane discs for

TABLE 4.9 Scale-Down Parameters and Assessment Methods for Virus Removal Filtration (VRF) Steps

---

Scale-Down Parameters and Scaling Rules[a]

All VRF steps
  Load volume to surface area ratio
  Solution pH, conductivity, protein concentration, etc.
  Temperature
  Channel geometry[b]
NFF-specific systems
  Feed flow rate
  Feed pressure
  Chase volume to surface area ratio
TFF-specific systems
  Crossflow rate per feed channel (or lumen)[c]
  Flux
  Channel height (or lumen diameter)
  Number of modules connected in series or feed side path length[b]
  Transmembrane pressure
  Number of diafiltration wash volumes

Assessment Methods and Techniques

Product yield	Product concentration (UV, HPLC, activity)
VCF target	Volumetric measurement
Diafiltration wash volume (or chase volume) target	Volumetric measurement
Aggregate generation	SEC, light-scattering, UV-VIS spectrometry

[a] Within manufacturing range for all parameters, unless otherwise specified.

[b] Within manufacturing range, if possible. Small-scale devices may have different feed geometries than the production scale modules.

[c] Within manufacturing range, or using manufacturer's recommendation to provide equivalent shear rate when geometries differ with scale.

evaluation, specifically designed holders may have to be used to provide the required sealing between the membrane sheets to prevent feed material from bypassing layers. Scale-down VRF devices may have the same membrane in the production-scale devices, but the feed side flow geometries of the scale-down devices may not be consistent with the production modules. Feed side path lengths may not be consistent and feed flows may have to be adjusted to provide equivalent shear forces at the membrane surface. Similar to UF application, air–liquid interfaces should be minimized to prevent protein denaturation and aggregation.

Scale-down VRF systems are required to process the same volume-to-surface-area ratio as the large-scale system and to achieve the volume concentration factor (or load challenge) and diafiltration wash volume (or chase volume) targets. The scale-down system should operate with the same feed channel geometry, path length, feed flow per channel (or feed side pressure drop) for TFF applications, feed pressure for constant-pressure applications, flux for constant-flux applications, and temperature as the large-scale system. For constant-flux operations, the TMP (or feed pressure) profile, permeate UV trace, product passage, and accumulated permeate volume are monitored over the run. For constant-pressure operations, the flux profile, permeate UV trace, product passage, and accumulated permeate volume are monitored over the load and buffer chase operations.

4.3.8.3 Primary End Points

The VRF step recovery can be determined using HPLC or product-specific assays (Table 4.9). When the VRF step is operated with relatively pure proteins (>95%), UV absorbance at 280 nm (A_{280}) can be used for yield measurements. Creating a mass balance is useful to show if losses are left behind in the system volume or irreversibly bound to the membrane. The membrane performance is also judged by comparing the process flux trend (or pressure increase for constant-flux operations) over the concentration and diafiltration (or chase) operations. The average flux over the VRF step is used to size production-scale equipment. The purity of the product stream can be measured using SDS-PAGE or HPLC techniques. The potential generation of high-molecular-weight species or aggregates can be monitored using SEC or light-scattering techniques.

4.3.8.4 Example of a Scale-Down Validation of an NFF Virus Removal Filtration System

In this study, a virus removal filtration (VRF) process step was scaled down in the purification process for a therapeutic antibody for validating the removal of model viruses. The antibody is produced in a Chinese hamster ovary (CHO) cell culture. Following cell separation and three chromatographic steps, the antibody is processed through a VRF device. The VRF step is operated at a constant flux in a normal flow filtration (NFF) mode where the antibody product passes through the membrane and is collected in the permeate stream. Noninfectious retrovirus-like particles (RVLPs) and potential adventitious viruses are retained by the membrane. The VRF step consists of system and membrane equilibration with buffer, processing of the load through the membrane, a buffer chase of the system and membrane to recover additional product, membrane cleaning, and a post-use integrity test.

The VRF device was scaled down 2000-fold by reducing the membrane area. The scale-down process was run in triplicate keeping the flux, load volume (L/m^2), and buffer chase volume the same as the full-scale process. The process load material was taken from a single representative process batch. All devices were post-use integrity tested to confirm that the membrane devices were integral throughout the step.

The evaluation of the scale-down model included qualitative and quantitative comparisons to determine whether there were any meaningful differences in the membrane performance between the two scales of operation. The overlay of the UV profiles of the three scale-down runs is shown in Figure 4.4 (top). The overlap of the UV traces indicates consistent antibody passage during the load and chase operations. The scale-down UV traces are comparable to a representative manufacturing scale process run shown in Figure 4.4 (bottom). For a quantitative comparison, a student's t-test was performed to compare the product yields by absorbance at 280 nm (A$_{280}$) at the two scales (Table 4.10).

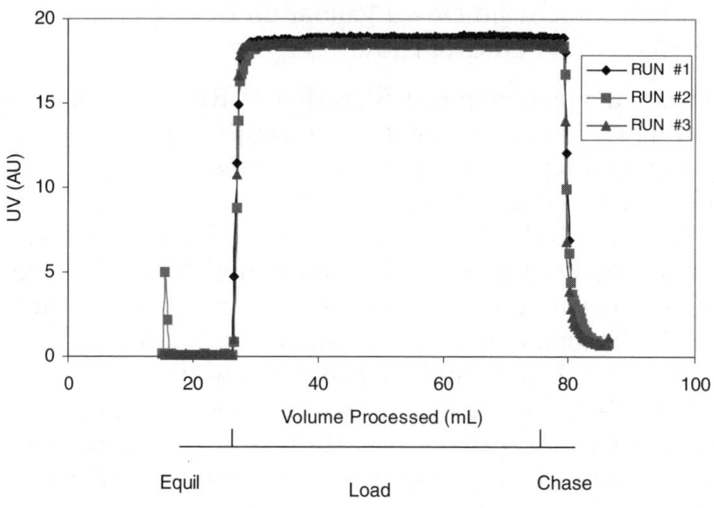

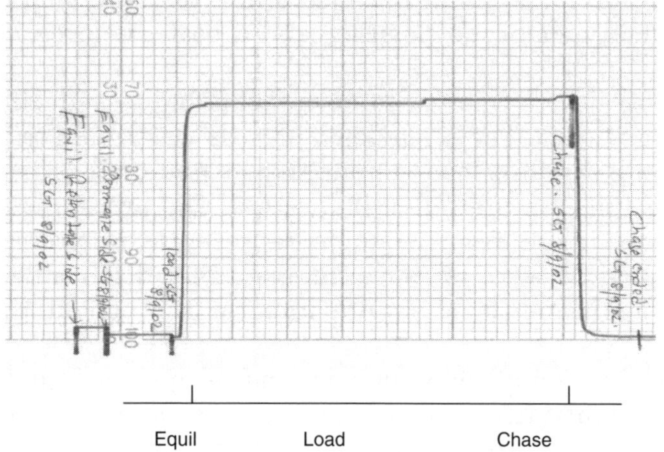

Figure 4.4 (top) Overlay of UV traces of VRF system permeate streams for scale-down model; (bottom) UV trace of VRF system permeate stream at manufacturing scale. The line below indicates the beginning of various steps in the run.

The difference in the yields was not significant at the 95% confidence level.

TABLE 4.10 Comparison of Scale-Down and Manufacturing Scale Yields

Virus Removal Filtration Run	A_{280} Yield (%)
Run 1	107.9
Run 2	99.7
Run 3	97.3
Scale-down mean (± 1 SD[a]; n = 3)	101.6 ($\pm$ 5.6)
Manufacturing scale mean (± 1 SD; n = 3)	98.9 ($\pm$ 2.8)

[a] SD = standard deviation.

4.4 EVALUATION OF SUITABILITY OF SCALE-DOWN SYSTEMS AS MODELS OF FULL-SCALE OPERATION

For process validations that are used to support product licensure applications for therapeutic proteins, the evaluation of the performance of the small-scale system (also called the qualification of the small-scale model) must be conducted according to cGMP validation guidelines. This requires that a qualification protocol be written that describes the qualification studies to be conducted and should include preapproved acceptance criteria for key performance parameters. The description of the scale-down system should include detailed information regarding potential scale-related variables so that the qualification of the scale-down system will still hold for studies conducted years later on equipment that may need to be reassembled or which will have changed slightly. Typically, three runs are performed during qualification scale-down studies, which will allow an assessment of the reproducibility of the scale-down process and provide a more meaningful comparison to full scale. The data from the key process parameters from the scale-down process should be compared to the full-scale process. Depending on the type of analysis, the comparison may be qualitative or quantitative.

Qualitative comparisons may be used for evaluation of data from complex analytical methods (product impurity or isoforms assessment by SDS-PAGE banding patterns or peptide maps). These evaluations should use direct, side-by-side comparisons of the two scales of operation to avoid introducing artifacts from the analysis (adjacent lanes on SDS-PAGE gels should be used to compare two samples, for instance). Other outputs are qualitative as well, such as chromatograms from a process chromatography step. While some portions of chromatograms may be evaluated using quantitative measures (elution peak asymmetry and HETP, for instance), it is more often the case that the chromatogram is used to confirm that the appropriate buffer transitions have taken place at the correct times, by recording column effluent conductivity, pH, and UV absorbance.

For quantitative variables, statistical analyses may be used to more rigorously compare performance at the two scales. A comparison of the means for the laboratory and process systems can be conducted using a t-test, although there may be limitations to this methodology. A confidence limit must be set, which is typically 95%. Complications arise when the process data set is very large; in this case, even a small difference in means may be judged to be statistically significant by a t-test. One approach is to review the moving average of the larger data set and confirm that the scaled-down data set falls within the range from the process data set [94].

Although a comparison of the variability of the two scales is possible using an F-ratio test, this is seldom of value unless there is a concern over the consistency of the small-scale data set. Often the scaled-down data set displays less variability than the process data set, as the runs are typically conducted with identical equipment over a short time span, using the same lots of raw materials, and the product peaks are typically analyzed together. The load material used to perform the qualification runs will influence the process outputs, and a direct comparison to the full-scale process run derived from the same lot starting material may be useful, although this weakens the statistical evaluation by artificially reducing the variability in the scale-down system outputs. Outlier analysis may be needed when one of the scaled-down qualification runs is markedly different from the other two, and several outlier tests can be performed and their outputs compared [95]. When an outlier is suspected, an investigation into the root cause should be conducted; if an explanation for the deviant result can be established, the questionable run should be eliminated from the data set and another completed. In some cases, a root cause for the inconsistency may not be identified, in which case one or more additional runs will be needed to confirm the stability of the scale-down system's performance.

When discrepancies between scales are detected, potential causes should be identified and corrected. This investigation is an important and necessary response to the detection of significant differences between scales, as it may highlight design flaws that could improve the small-scale model. The investigation should be documented, and the data from both the original and improved scale-down model should be included in the report to the qualification protocol. As an example, in our experience this type of investigation was triggered when a chromatographic step yield was significantly different between scales. It was discovered that the UV detector flow cell path length was incorrect; when the correct path length was used, the difference in step yields was greatly reduced and was no longer found to be statistically significant.

In some cases, there may be differences in performance observed between the scale-down and process systems (only in rare instances are the means of two data sets exactly identical). For quantitative variables, these would have to be statistically significant in order to warrant further investigation, and the appropriate statistical tests should be completed to make this assessment. With qualitative variables, a significant difference arises when the output is outside of the manufacturing experience derived from a representative sample of a sufficiently large data set to provide an accurate estimate of full-scale performance (leading to the acceptance criteria for qualitative or characterization data being within the standard range of manufacturing [96]). By using multiple lots of load material for the triplicate qualification runs, it is more likely that the mean process performance of the small-scale system will approximate that of the full-scale system, but at the expense of accurate information about the run-to-run variability of the lab-scale system.

If no correction for the discrepancy between scales can be found, then adjustments may be made to the small-scale system to more closely match the full-scale process, even if these violate one of the scaling laws adopted for the scale-down process step design. As an example, if a scale-down centrifugation step fails to adequately clarify the process stream based on a calculation of the *g*-force, residence time, and settling distance of a process-scale unit, a longer centrifuge residence time may be tested. In addition, load samples for the small-scale system that are frozen for ease of operation may develop low levels of precipitate that can be removed by filtration before use, even if the full-scale product stream is never frozen or normally filtered at that point.

Finally, if performance differences between scales cannot be corrected, a judgment may be made as to the process significance of this difference. In some cases, the differences are relatively small and may not be likely to have any influence on the more relevant process outputs. As an example, the HETP of a small-scale column chromatogram may not uncommonly have a modest increase in plate height compared with the full-scale column; while this is important for delicate separations and size-exclusion chromatography, for most bind and elute modes of chromatography, this difference may not matter. In these cases, the small-scale system can still be used for prospective validation studies. Should the difference be judged to have process significance (a major shift in the product isoforms of chromatographic separations, the presence of new impurities or product isoforms, or large yield discrepancies), however, the small-scale system should not be used for process validation studies unless absolutely no other alternative exists. This may require more validation work at full scale using concurrent studies as a result.

A preliminary evaluation of the potential for success of a scale-down qualification may come from careful analysis of the scale-up of the steps following their definition based on small-scale process development studies. This scale-up is simply the application of the same scaling laws used for the design scale-down, but in the opposite direction. Parallel runs conducted using samples from the full-scale process, which are processed and analyzed at the same time as the full-scale batch, should minimize the potential for any surprises when the qualification studies are conducted under protocol. Careful analysis of several of these parallel runs may also identify subtle yet reproducible scale-related effects, which often require a larger data set than the three qualification runs in order to become statistically significant.

Flexible operations using small-scale systems with various scaling factors may be supported by qualifying a range of small-scale system sizes. The smallest would be the most efficient to use for studies that involve many runs, such as multivariable robustness or process characterization studies or chromatographic column reuse. Larger systems may be needed if multiple steps are used to model a full purification train, for instance. Because losses are incurred when peak pools are sampled for analysis or portions held as retains, the scale-down factor will by necessity increase as the product progresses through the purification train. Another factor that can have the same effect is the fact that small-scale systems often come in quantum sizes (i.e., chromatographic column diameters or filter sizes), which will result in a maximum scale factor for the process train based on the maximum scale factor for the limiting unit operation. When considering the qualification of multiple scales of operation, a bracketing strategy should be applicable if similar equipment is used for both the largest and smallest scales. Intermediate scales of operation would therefore be covered by the successful qualification of the minimum and maximum scales.

4.5 APPLICATION OF SCALE-DOWN SYSTEMS

Scale-down models are valuable tools during process development and beyond. As mentioned earlier, one of the primary applications of scale-down models is during process development for evaluating impurity removal. However, these small-scale models can also be used for evaluation of process robustness, resin cleaning, and resin lifetime, among others. Furthermore, they can also be used to support licensed commercial processes to address manufacturing investigations, postapproval process change for comparability, and evaluation of raw material changes postlicensure.

4.5.1 Clinical Development Phase-Process Validation

4.5.1.1 Assessment and Validation of Impurity Removal

Production processes for biologics give rise to a range of impurities that must be removed by the purification process. These impurities could be either host cell-derived, such as nucleic acids, host cell proteins (HCPs), and potentially viruses, or process-derived, such as cell culture medium components, leachables arising from the purification process, etc. It is very important to validate the clearance of these impurities, which could potentially cause adverse reactions in patients and thus pose a safety concern.

Host cell protein impurities have the potential to cause severe immunological responses in people. Several analytical techniques such as SDS-PAGE, ELISA, and HPLC are used in validating the removal of HCPs. ELISA is currently the industry standard for release testing of active substances as well as for testing in-process intermediates to evaluate the capacity of any purification step to remove HCPs as part of a concurrent validation protocol. However, the sensitivity of the assay may limit the use of ELISA for process validation of all chromatographic steps. In such instances, radiolabeled studies using scale-down models are useful to determine the capacity of any step to remove HCPs. This involves preparing a representative radiolabeled HCP sample, which could be achieved by growing cells in the presence of a null vector (i.e., lacking the product gene) and labeling the host cell proteins with [125]I. Spiking studies can be conducted either on individual chromatographic steps by treating them as single unit operations or on sequential unit operations. Spiking studies using scale-down models are also employed to validate removal of host cell DNA when analytical methods are not sufficiently sensitive to be used for concurrent validation [97]. Typically [^{32}P]-labeled DNA is added to the feed stream and its removal through the process is evaluated. For both HCP and DNA, a clearance factor is calculated by dividing the total radioactivity in the load by the total radioactivity in the product pool.

For products derived from cell culture processes using cell lines of human or animal origin, it is a regulatory requirement to demonstrate that the purification process has the capacity to remove viruses. Virus validation studies are conducted using scale-down systems. A panel of model viruses is chosen for spiking studies. The model viruses in the panel are chosen to reflect a range of different sizes and shapes and include both DNA and RNA viruses or enveloped or nonenveloped virus families.

Cell culture processes have several components that are added to either enhance productivity or maintain stability of cell lines. Some of these components could be potentially toxic, bioactive, or immunogenic in humans, and it may be required to demonstrate clearance of these additives by the purification process. Examples of cell culture additives include methotrexate, antibiotics, and growth factors. If assays for these components do not exist or are not sensitive enough, radiolabeled spikes of some of these components can be used with scale-down models to determine the clearance factors for the various steps. Using the starting amounts added to the cell culture and the clearance factors, levels of these components in active substance can be estimated and an assessment of safety can be performed.

Purification process-derived impurities include leached ligands from chromatographic columns such as protein A. It is required to demonstrate the removal of protein A by the purification process to low and consistent levels. Other examples of the use of scale-down models for impurity removal studies include validation of removal of endotoxins [98]. Endotoxins are pyrogenic lipopolysaccharides derived from bacteria such as *E. coli*. They could also be introduced through contaminated raw materials. If concurrent testing for protein A or endotoxin is not possible, scale-down models can be used to establish the removal capacity of the process step. This is especially useful for situations where the protein A or endotoxin challenge to the columns in the process is low.

4.5.1.2 Process Robustness

Process variability is inherent to complex manufacturing processes such as the manufacture of biopharmaceuticals. Process robustness studies, sometimes referred to as process characterization studies, are designed to provide information on the extent of process variability. These studies are typically conducted using scale-down models to demonstrate that the process performance is acceptable at the limits of operation.

Several factors could affect the performance of a step, and in most instances, it is not possible to test the effect of every factor. The number of factors is often reduced based on development studies. Alternatively, some factors may be combined and treated as a single variable [99]. Robustness runs could include running the process at extremes of operating ranges of conditions such as pH, conductivity, flow rate, temperature, etc. Most often, these runs are designed using a statistical approach to the design of experiments, such as fractional factorial designs. These studies can evaluate several control parameters at once, at the two levels representing the upper and lower control limits. Robustness studies are also useful in identifying whether combinations of certain variables could be optimized to maximize a process performance parameter [100].

In some instances, resin reuse and robustness studies have been combined into a single protocol [101]. A fractional factorial study was designed to use a single cation exchange chromatography column and included control runs to verify that column performance was not affected by reuse or robustness conditions. Results from the study found no differences in yield, impurity clearance, or column regeneration ability with either continued use (42 cycles) or different combinations of test variables.

4.5.1.3 Resin Capacity

The dynamic capacity of chromatographic resins for the product of interest is an important parameter as it has a direct impact on productivity. The amount of product that can be loaded per unit volume of resin is an important control parameter, and hence an accurate estimate of a column's dynamic capacity is necessary. Resin capacity is a function of several factors such as linear flow rate, bed height, residence time, load composition, and in some instances physical characteristics of the resin such as ligand density.

The capacity obtained by batch experiments (static binding capacity) will be higher than that obtained through column experiments (dynamic binding capacity), and the difference will depend on the residence time and other factors influencing mass transfer and column efficiency. Scale-down models may be used to perform breakthrough analysis to determine the dynamic binding capacity of resins. Dynamic binding capacities are typically calculated by loading the appropriate load material on scale-down columns up to the point where 5–10% of the product appears in the unbound fraction. It becomes more complicated to define a resin capacity when a column is operated in a flow-through mode, i.e., when the product of interest is in the unbound fraction and the impurities bind the column. In such cases, it may become important to determine the resin's capacity for the primary impurity that is removed by the process step.

4.5.1.4 Resin Cleaning, Reuse, and End-of-Life Validation

Chromatography columns are used for multiple cycles, and it is essential to demonstrate that the cleaning procedures after each cycle are adequate to ensure minimal risk of an increase in carryover of tightly bound product or other impurities from run to run. Cleaning after each cycle extends the life of chromatographic resins. There have been instances reported where viruses undetectable after the first cycle can elute in a subsequent cycle with the product if inadequate sanitization steps are performed after each cycle [98].

Using scale-down models during process development, important factors such as the type and concentration of cleaning solutions, flow rate, and contact time, among others, should be evaluated to ensure adequate cleaning. Prior to developing the purification process, care must be taken to ensure that the chromatographic resins and equipment are compatible with the cleaning regimens in place [98].

Scale-down models are useful for determining the number of times a given column can be cycled to define the useful or functional life of the resin [101–103]. Using representative load material, scale-down models of columns are cycled several times and product pools are periodically collected for various analyses. The useful life of resins should then be confirmed at production scale through periodic testing and monitoring. A comprehensive approach toward determining useful life of resins has been described where a validation program was established to determine the point at which a column might show a measurable deterioration in performance [104]. This program, which included both small-scale and large-scale data, supported the reuse of three Sepharose Fast Flow ion-exchange resins from Pharmacia for at least several hundred cycles [104].

Resin lifetime studies using scale-down models should include an evaluation of column integrity, column cleaning, carryover, chromatograms, product recovery, product purity profile, and impurity clearance (DNA, HCP, viruses), among others. Several tests may be employed to compare pre- and postuse column integrity and attributes of the resin. These include measurements of small-ion capacity, total protein capacity, pressure-flow curves, total organic carbon to test for leachables and extractables, etc. [104]. These tests can also be used to evaluate any loss in chemical functionality of resins as a result of exposure to storage and regeneration solutions. Samples of resins are incubated in cleaning/regeneration solutions for several weeks and the aforementioned tests are performed. Column integrity can be monitored by periodic measurements of HETP and asymmetry factors. Chromatograms from scale-down cycling studies can be compared qualitatively to each other to ensure there are no differences with continued use. In some cases, semiquantitative to quantitative methods have been used to compare chromatograms by comparing certain parameters such as peak apex, peak width, and beginning and end of peak collection [104]. Product recovery over the life of the resin must be monitored to ensure that there are no deleterious trends. Product pools from the cycling studies should be periodically tested for impurities such as HCP, DNA, and protein A (if applicable), among others, to ensure that there is no deterioration in column performance with use [102].

Resins generated from the laboratory-scale cycling studies can be used to pack smaller-scale columns to conduct end-of-life virus validation studies [4,101]. These studies would evaluate the ability of the maximally cycled resin to remove the model viruses compared to unused resin. Another important parameter to monitor is carryover of product and impurities between runs. This is typically determined by conducting periodic mock or blank runs during a cycling study. Mock runs are typical runs without any product loaded on the column. The elution pool from mock runs is analyzed for product and impurity by various analytical methods. The amount of carryover is estimated as a percentage of the amount of product typically eluted from the column. Sufficient data should be gathered prior to setting limits for concurrent testing of production columns.

4.5.1.5 Hold Times for Cell Culture Harvest Samples

Scale-down models are valuable tools in validating process hold times for relatively impure feed streams such as cell culture harvest pools. Any manufacturing process would require that product pools be held for a defined period of time to allow for flexibility in processing. Therefore, it is important that appropriate hold times for the various product pools at different steps in the process be validated. These studies typically involve holding product pools from large-scale manufacturing in smaller containers of similar materials of construction for extended periods of time. Samples are taken at specified times and analyzed by appropriate assays. Changes in purity, activity, and potency of the molecule are monitored. These studies are relatively straightforward when analytical tools are available for in-process pools from a purification process. For impure process streams such as cell culture harvest (or in some cases, product pools after the first purification step), analytical tools are not available to discern differences in product quality upon holding the pools. In such instances, the harvest pools are held for various times and then purified over the subsequent steps using the appropriate scale-down model systems. These samples can be analyzed for changes such as aggregation, modification, and product heterogeneity, among others.

4.5.1.6 Selection of Control Ranges for Cell Culture Processes

Bioreactors are also subject to process variability, and it is important to ensure that the ranges of critical parameters are validated. This would require one to demonstrate that within the operating ranges there is no impact on product quality. Several parameters can affect the performance of bioreactor processes. These include temperature, pH, levels of dissolved O_2 and CO_2, impeller speed in bioreactor, and seed density, among others [105]. Concentration of various media components can also have an impact on cell growth and product quality, and optimal ranges may need to be investigated. The focus of bioreactor process development is usually optimization of parameters such as cell density, product titers, cellular productivity, and various metabolic parameters. Generating product quality end points would necessitate the use of scale-down purification steps to create sufficient product for characterization. Furthermore, these scale-down models could support cell culture robustness studies to evaluate whether manipulating any of the upstream parameters within control ranges has an impact on the purity and potency of the product. It is possible to define linking variables, i.e., output variables of a process step that would have an impact on the performance of a downstream step [106]. Data generated from these scale-down runs are compared to predetermined acceptance criteria and used to validate operating ranges.

4.5.2 Commercial Processes

Scale-down models are especially useful for conducting various routine support functions for commercial processes. These applications include evaluating changes in raw materials, troubleshooting manufacturing deviations, and developing and supporting changes for process improvements to enhance product purity or yield with an overall impact on process economics.

4.5.2.1 Qualify Secondary Vendors for Raw Materials

Manufacturers of important raw materials used in either the cell culture or downstream process often make changes to the manufacturing process for that particular raw material. In other instances, manufacturers may choose to discontinue manufacture of a certain component and alternate suppliers need to be qualified. Other examples of raw material changes would include eliminating the use of animal-derived components in cell culture media or in purification process raw materials to reduce the risk of introducing adventitious viruses or transmissible spongiform encephalopathy (TSE) agents. Therefore, one would need to qualify secondary vendors to assure themselves of uninterrupted supply of raw materials. Furthermore, it is required to demonstrate that the change to the raw material, raw material manufacturing process, or vendor does not have a deleterious impact on product quality. Scale-down models can be used to generate multiple lots of active substance for extensive characterization to confirm that the change had no negative impact. Once the scale-down models provide assurance of comparable performance, the data can be confirmed at manufacturing scale. The amount of data required to establish equivalence depends on the nature of the change and where it is used in the process. For example, if the raw material is used in the final formulation of active substance, one or multiple lots of active drug substance (or drug product) may be required to be held on short-term and long-term stability, which is a more stringent requirement than would be necessary for a minor change upstream.

4.5.2.2 Evaluate Changes in Purification of Raw Materials

When a chromatographic resin manufacturer makes minor or major modifications to their manufacturing processes, the impact of the changes on the performance of the resin should be evaluated. Alternatively, a resin in a commercial process could be considered for replacement by a similar resin having the same functionality. As an example, protein A resin may be offered from the same supplier with ligands derived from both native as well as recombinant sources. Changing from one resin type to the other could affect the resin capacity, protein A leaching, and product purity profile. Equivalence of the step performance to the commercial process should be demonstrated using scale-down models prior to introduction at manufacturing scale. As mentioned previously, the scale-down data can then be confirmed at manufacturing scale.

4.5.2.3 Evaluate Lot-to-Lot Variability of Raw Materials and Troubleshoot Process Deviations

Robustness studies using scale-down models provide information on the effect of variability of operating parameters on the performance of a step. Sometimes the effect of variability of certain parameters in some raw materials (e.g., ligand density of resins) on step performance is also studied. However, it is not possible to test the lot-to-lot variability of all the raw materials encountered in a commercial process. A process in commercial manufacturing uses various raw material lots, and these could have a significant impact on process performance and product purity. In such cases, with the same raw materials used in commercial manufacturing, several laboratory-scale experiments can be performed using scale-down models to understand the cause of shifts in process performance.

Scale-down models are also useful tools in troubleshooting process deviations. During commercial manufacturing, minor changes in process parameters can sometimes lead to altered chromatographic profiles or changes in other output parameters such as yield. These deviations trigger investigations to determine the root cause. Scale-down models using load material from large-scale manufacturing are often useful in determining the cause for deviations since several runs can be performed with limited load material and multiple parameters can be varied to test any given hypothesis. Results from these studies may also determine the impact of the deviation on product quality and whether a batch or multiple batches would be released or rejected.

4.6 SUMMARY

A complete process validation package is a major component of any regulatory filing. Process validation studies are performed either at full scale or using scale-down models. Scale-down models are laboratory-scale systems designed to model a full-scale unit operation used for developing a purification process, which are subsequently scaled up to production scale. Alternatively, they are used prospectively as useful tools designed to mimic large-scale unit operations.

Prior to conducting any process validation studies, it is very important to ensure that the scale-down model system appropriately reflects the performance of the unit operation at full scale. Several parameters need to be considered in designing a scale-down model. These parameters are unique to any given unit operation. It is important to identify the critical parameters, scaling principles, and the appropriate end points for each unit operation prior to designing the scale-down model that would be relevant for comparing the two scales of operation.

For process validations that are used to support product licensure applications for therapeutic proteins, the evaluation of the performance of the small-scale system must be conducted according to cGMP validation guidelines. A qualification protocol that describes the qualification studies to be conducted must be written and should include preapproved acceptance criteria for important performance parameters. The data from the critical process parameters from the scale-down process should be compared, both qualitatively and quantitatively, to the full-scale processes. Qualitative comparisons may be used for evaluation of data from complex analytical methods. For quantitative variables, statistical analyses may be used to more rigorously compare performance at two scales.

Scale-down models have several applications. They have been used to evaluate removal of impurities such as nucleic acids, host cell proteins, viruses, and media additives, among others. Scale-down models are effective tools to determine useful life of chromatographic resins and to evaluate process robustness. For licensed processes, scale-down models play an important role in supporting process changes and in manufacturing investigations.

ACKNOWLEDGMENTS

The authors would like to thank members of the Purification Process Development group at Wyeth BioPharma, who participated in some of the studies described herein.

REFERENCES

1. Center for Biologics Evaluation and Research, FDA, Guideline on General Principles of Process Validation, 1987.

2. Center for Biologics Evaluation and Research, FDA, Points to Consider in the Manufacture and Testing of Monoclonal Antibody Products for Human Use, 1997.

3. Center for Biologics Evaluation and Research, FDA, Guidance for Industry for the Submission of Chemistry, Manufacturing and Controls for a Therapeutic Recombinant DNA-derived Product or Monoclonal Antibody Product for *In Vivo* Use, 1996.

4. International Conference on Harmonization, Viral Safety of Biotechnology Products Derived from Cell Lines of Human or Animal Origin, ICH Viral Safety Document, 1998.

5. Sofer, G. and Little, L.E., Validation: Ensuring the accuracy of scaled-down chromatography models, *BioPharm*, 9, 51–54, 1996.

6. Ghose, S. and Chase, H., Expanded bed chromatography of proteins in small diameter columns. I. Scale-down and validation, *Bioseparation*, 9, 21–28, 2000.

7. Yamamoto, S., Okamoto, A., and Watler, P., Effect of adsorbent properties on zone spreading in expanded bed chromatography, *Bioseparation*, 10, 1–6, 2001.

8. Imamoglu, S., Simulated moving bed chromatography (SMB) for application in bioseparation, *Adv. Biochem. Eng. Biotechnol.*, 76, 211–231, 2002.

9. Smith, T.M., Wilson, E., Scott, R.G., Misczak, J.W., Bodek, J.M., and Zabriskie, D.W., Establishment of operating ranges in a purification process of a monoclonal antibody, in *Validation of Biopharmaceutical Manufacturing Processes*, ACS Symposium Series, Kelley, B.D. and Ramelmier, R.A., Eds., 1998, pp. 80–92.

10. Yamamoto, S., Nakanishi, K., and Maatsuno, R., *Ion Exchange Chromatography of Proteins*, Marcel Dekker, New York, 1988.

11. European Medicines Evaluation Agency, Revised CPMP guideline on virus validation studies, *CPMP*, 268, 95, 1995.

12. Gagnon, P. and Grund, E., Large-scale process development for hydrophobic interaction chromatography. IV. Controlling selectivity, *BioPharm*, 9, 54–64, 1996.

13. Barry, A. and Chojnacki, R., Biotechnology product validation. VIII. Chromatography media and column qualification, *BioPharm*, 7, 43–47, 1994.

14. Sofer, G. and Hagel, L., *Handbook of Process Chromatography: A Guide to Optimization, Scale-Up, and Validation*, Academic Press, New York, 1997.

15. Hjorth, R., Expanded-bed adsorption in industrial bioprocessing: recent developments, *Trends Biotechnol.*, 15, 230–235, 1997.

16. Dasari, G., Prince, I., and Hearn, M.T.W., High performance liquid chromatography of amino acids, peptides and proteins. CXXIV. Physical characterization of fluidized bed behavior of chromatographic packing materials, *J. Chromatogr.*, 631, 115–124, 1993.

17. Thommes, J., Halfar, M., Lenz, S., and Kula, M.-R., Purification of monoclonal antibodies from whole hybridoma fermentation broth by fluidized bed adsorption, *Biotechnol. Bioeng.*, 45, 205–211, 1995.

18. Nilsson, J., Jonasson, P., Samuelsson, E., Stahl, S., and Uhlen, M., Integrated production of human insulin and its C-peptide, *J. Biotechnol.*, 48, 241–250, 1996.

19. Wrotnowski, C., Neose targets complex carbohydrate products, *Genet. Eng. News*, 22, 2002.

20. Bornstein, P. and Balian, G., The specific nonenzymatic cleavage of bovine ribonuclease with hydroxylamine, *J. Biol. Chem.*, 245, 4854–4856, 1970.

21. Antorini, M., Breme, U., Caccia, P., Grassi, C., Lebrun, S., Orsini, G., Taylor, G., Valsasina, B., Marengo, E., Todeschini, R., Andersson, C., Gellerfors, P., and Gustafsson, J., Hydroxyl-amine-induced cleavage of the asparginyl-glycine motif in the production of recombinant proteins: the case of insulin-like growth factor I, *Prot. Exp. Purif.*, 11, 135–147, 1997.

22. Bornstein, P. and Balian, G., Cleavage at Asn-Gly bonds with hydroxylamine, *Methods Enzymol.*, 47, 132–145, 1977.

23. Ladisch, M. and Kohlmann, K., Recombinant human insulin, *Biotechnol. Prog.*, 8, 469–478, 1992.

24. Veronese, F. and Harris, J.M., Introduction and overview of peptide and protein pegylation, *Adv. Drug Delivery Rev.*, 54, 453–456, 2002.

25. Roberts, M.J., Bentley, M.D., and Harris, J.M., Chemistry for peptide and protein pegylation, *Adv. Drug Delivery Rev.*, 54, 459–446, 2002.

26. Glatz, C.E., Precipitation, in *Separation Processes in Biotechnology*, Asenjo, J.A., Ed., Marcel Dekker, New York, 1990, pp. 329–356.

27. Ladish, M.R., Precipitation, crystallization, and extraction, in *Bioseparations Engineering: Principles, Practice, and Economics*, Ladish, M.R., Ed., Wiley-Interscience, New York, 2001, pp. 116–151.

28. Rothstein, F., Differential precipitation of proteins: science and technology, in *Protein Purification Process Engineering*, Harrison, R.G., Ed., Marcel Dekker, New York, 1990, pp. 115–208.

29. Stryker, M.H., Bertolini, M.J., and Hao, Y.-L., Blood fractionation: proteins, in *Advances in Biotechnological Processes*, Vol. 4, Mizrahi, A. and van Wezel, A.L., Eds., Alan R. Liss, New York, 1985, pp. 275–336.

30. Foster, P.R. and Watt, J.G., The CSVM fractionation process, in *Methods of Plasma Protein Fractionation*, Curling, J.M., Ed., Academic Press, London, 1980, pp. 17–31.

31. Chang, C.E., Continuous fractionation of human plasma proteins by precipitation from the suspension of the recycling stream, *Biotechnol. Bioeng.*, 31, 841–846, 1988.

32. Bos, O.J.M., Sunye, D.G.J., Nieuweboer, C.E.F., van Engelenburg, F.A.C., Schuitemaker, H., and Over, J., Virus validation of pH 4-treated human immunoglobulin products produced by the Cohn fractionation process, *Biologicals*, 26, 267–276, 1998.

33. Tatterson, G.B., Process translation, in *Scaleup and Design of Industrial Mixing Processes*, Tatterson, G.B., Ed., McGraw Hill, New York, 1994, pp. 203–266.

34. Bell, D.J. and Dunnill, P., Shear disruption of soya protein precipitate particles and the effect of aging in a stirred tank, *Biotechnol. Bioeng.*, 24, 1271–1285, 1982.

35. Byrne, E.P., Fitzpatrick, J.J., Pampel, L.W., and Titchener-Hooker, N.J., Influence of shear on particle size and fractal dimension of whey protein precipitates: implications for scale-up and centrifugal clarification efficiency, *Chem. Eng. Sci.*, 57, 3767–3779, 2002.

36. U.S. Food and Drug Administration, Guide to Inspections of Viral Clearance Processes for Plasma Derivatives (FDA Web site), http://www.fda.gov/ora/inspect_ref/igs/viralcl.html.

37. Willkommen, H., Experimental experience with virus validation studies, *Dev. Biol. Stand.*, 88, 317–331, 1996.

38. Biescas, H., Gensana, M., Fernandez, J., Ristol, P., Massot, M., Watson, E., and Vericat, F., Characterization and viral safety validation study of a pasteurized therapeutic concentrate of antithrombin III obtained through affinity chromatography, *Haematologica*, 83, 305–311, 1998.

39. Chandra, S., Cavanaugh, J.E., Lin, C.M., Pierre-Jerome, C., Yerram, N., Weeks, R., Flanigan, E., and Feldman, F., Virus reduction in the preparation of intravenous immune globulin: *in vitro* experiments, *Transfusion*, 39, 249–257, 1999.

40. Neal, G., Christie, J., Keshavarz-Moore, E., and Shamlou, P.A., Ultra scale down approach for the prediction of full-scale recovery of ovine polyclonal immunoglobulins used in the manufacture of snake venom-specific Fab fragment, *Biotechnol. Bioeng.*, 81, 149–157, 2003.

41. Boychyn, M., Doyle, W., Bulmer, M., More, J., and Hoare, M., Laboratory scaledown of protein purification processes involving fractional precipitation and centrifugal recovery, *Biotechnol. Bioeng.*, 69, 1–10, 2000.

42. Alonso, W.R., Trukawinski, S., Savage, M., Tenold, R.A., and Hammond, D.J., Viral inactivation of intramuscular immune serum globulins, *Biologicals*, 28, 5–15, 2000.

43. Johnston, A., MacGregor, A., Borovec, S., Hattarki, M., Stuckly, K., Anderson, D., Goss, N.H., Oates, A., and Uren, E., Inactivation and clearance of viruses during the manufacture of high purity Factor IX, *Biologicals*, 28, 129–136, 2000.

44. Dichtelmuller, H., Rudnick, D., Breuer, B., and Ganshirt, K.H., Validation of virus inactivation and removal for the manufacturing procedure of two immunoglobulins and a 5% serum protein solution treated with beta-propiolactone, *Biologicals*, 21, 259–268, 1993.

45. Josic, D., Schulz, P., Biesert, L., Hoffer, L., Schwinn, H., Kordis-Krapez, M., and Strancar, A., Issues in the development of medical products based on human plasma, *J. Chrom. B*, 694, 253–269, 1997.

46. Minor, P., Meeting on the acceptance criteria for virus validation studies, *Biologicals*, 23, 107–110, 1995.

47. Meltzer, T.H. and Jornitz, M.W., *Filtration in the Biopharmaceutical Industry*, Marcel Dekker, New York, 1998.

48. Zeman, L.J. and Zydney, A.L., *Microfiltration and Ultrafiltration: Principles and Applications*, Marcel Dekker, New York, 1996.

49. Mir, L., Michaels, S.L., Goel, V., and Kaiser, R., Crossflow microfiltration: applications, design, and cost, in *Membrane Handbook*, Ho, W.S.W. and Sirkar, K.K., Eds., Van Nostrand Reinhold, New York, 1992, pp. 571–594.

50. Goel, V., Accomazzo, M.A., DiLeo, A.J., Meier, P., Pitt, A., Pluskal, M., and Kaiser, R., Dead-end microfiltration: applications, design, and cost, in *Membrane Handbook*, Ho, W.S.W. and Sirkar, K.K., Eds., Van Nostrand Reinhold, New York, 1992, pp. 506–569.

51. Li, H., Fane, A.G., and Coster, H.G.L., Vigneswaran: an assessment of depolarization models of crossflow microfiltration by direct observation through the membrane, *J. Membrane Sci.*, 172, 135–147, 2000.

52. Wolber, P., Dosmer, M., and Banks, J., Cell harvesting scale-up: parallel-leaf cross-flow microfiltration methods, *BioPharm Manuf.*, 1, 38–45, 1988.

53. van Reis, R., Leonard, L.C., Hsu, C.C., and Builder, S.E., Industrial scale harvest of proteins from mammalian cell culture by tangential flow filtration, *Biotechnol. Bioeng.*, 36, 413–422, 1991.

54. van Reis, R., Gadam, S., Frautschy, L.N., Orlando, S.E., Goodrich, E.M., Saksena, S., Kuriyel, R., Simpson, C.M., Pearl, S., and Zydney, A.L., High performance tangential flow filtration, *Biotechnol. Bioeng.*, 56, 71–82, 1997.

55. Cheryan, M., *Ultrafiltration Handbook*, Technomic Publishing, Basel, 1986.

56. van Reis, R. and Zydney, A.L., Protein ultrafiltration, in *Encyclopedia of Bioprocess Technology: Fermentation, Biocatalysis, and Bioseparation*, Flickinger, M.C., Ed., John Wiley & Sons, New York, 1999, pp. 2197–2214.

57. van Reis, R., Goodrich, E.M., Yson, C.L., Frautschy, L.N., Whiteley, R., and Zydney, A.L., Constant C_{wall} ultrafiltration process control, *J. Membrane Sci.*, 130, 123–140, 1997.

58. Brose, D., Dosmar, M., Cates, S., and Hutchison, F., Studies on the scale-up of crossflow filtration devices, *PDA J. Pharm. Sci. Technol.*, 50, 252–260, 1996.

59. van Reis, R., Goodrich, E.M., Yson, C.L., Frautschy, L.N., Dzengeleski, S., and Lutz, H., Linear scale ultrafiltration, *Biotechnol. Bioeng.*, 55, 737–746, 1997.

60. Meireles, M., Aimar, P., and Sanchez, V., Albumin denaturation during ultrafiltration: effects of operating conditions and consequences on membrane fouling, *Biotechnol. Bioeng.*, 38, 528–534, 1991.

61. Maa, Y.F. and Hsu, C.C., Protein denaturation by combined effect of shear and air–liquid interface, *Biotechnol. Bioeng.*, 54, 503–512, 1997.

62. Kim, K.J., Chen, V., and Fane, A.G., Some factors determining protein aggregation during ultrafiltration, *Biotechnol. Bioeng.*, 42, 260–265, 1993.

63. Frampton, G.A., Evaluating the performance of industrial centrifuges, *Chem. Eng. Prog.*, August, 402–412, 1963.

64. Kempken, R., Preissmann, A., and Berthold, W., Assessment of a disc stack centrifuge for use in mammalian cell separation, *Biotechnol. Bioeng.*, 46, 132–138, 1995.

65. Mannweiler, K. and Hoare, M., The scale down of an industrial disc stack centrifuge, *Bioproc. Eng.*, 8, 19–25, 1992.

66. Ambler, C.M., The evaluation of centrifuge performance, *Chem. Eng. Prog.*, 48, 150–158, 1952.

67. Ambler, C.M., The theory of scaling up laboratory data for the sedimentation type centrifuge, *J. Biochem. Microbiol. Tech. Eng.*, 1, 185–205, 1959.

68. Maybury, J.P., Hoare, M., and Dunnil, P., The use of laboratory centrifugation studies to predict performance of industrial machines: studies of shear-insensitive and shear sensitive materials, *Biotechnol. Bioeng.*, 67, 265–273, 2000.

69. Trowbridge, M.E., Problems in the scaling-up of centrifugal separation equipment, *Chem. Eng.*, August, A73–A87, 1962.

70. Maybury, J.P., Mannweiler, K., Titchener-Hooker, N.J., Hoare, M., and Dunnil, P., The performance of a scaled down industrial disc stack centrifuge with a reduced feed material requirement, *Bioproc. Eng.*, 18, 191–199, 1998.

71. Sofer, G., Virus inactivation in the 1990's — and into the 21st century. IIIa. Plasma and plasma products (heat and solvent/detergent treatments), *BioPharm*, 15, 28–42, 2002.

72. Sofer, G., Virus inactivation in the 1990's — and into the 21st century. IIIb. Plasma and plasma products (treatments other than heat or solvent/detergent), *BioPharm*, 15, 42–49, 2002.

73. Sofer, G., Virus inactivation in the 1990's — and into the 21st century. IV. Culture media, biotechnology products, and vaccines, *BioPharm Int.*, 16, 50–57, 2003.

74. Fisher, G., Hoots, W.K., and Abrams, C., Viral reduction techniques: types and purpose, *Transfus. Med. Rev.*, 15 (Suppl. 1), 27–39, 2001.

75. Roberts, P., Virus safety of plasma products, *Rev. Med. Virol.*, 6, 25–38, 1996.

76. Charm, S.E., Landau, S., Williams, B., Horowitz, B., Prince, A.M., and Pascual, D., High-temperature short-time heat inactivation of HIV and other viruses in human blood plasma, *Vox Sang*, 62, 12–20, 1992.

77. Walter, J.K., Nothelfer, F., and Werz, W., Validation of viral safety for pharmaceutical proteins, in *Bioseparation and Bioprocessing*, Vol. 1, Subramanian, G., Ed., Wiley-VCH, Weinheim, 1998, pp. 465–496.

78. Chandra, S., Groener, A., and Feldman, F., Effectiveness of alternative treatments for reducing potential viral contaminants from plasma-derived products, *Thrombosis Res.*, 105, 391–400, 2002.

79. Tatterson, G.B., Basic processing concepts, in *Scaleup and Design of Industrial Mixing Processes*, Tatterson, G.B., Ed., McGraw-Hill, New York, 1994, pp. 1–52.

80. Committee for Proprietary Medicinal Products, European Medicines Evaluation Agency: Note of Guidance on Plasma-Derived Medicinal Products, CMPM/BWP/269/95, rev 3, London, European Agency for the Evaluation of Medicinal Products, 2001.

81. Roberts, P.L. and Dunkerley, C., Effect of manufacturing process parameters on virus inactivation by solvent-detergent treatment in a high-purity factor IX concentrate, *Vox Sang*, 84, 170–175, 2003.

82. Seitz, H., Blumel, J., Schmidt, I., Willkommen, H., and Lower, J., Comparable virus inactivation by bovine or vegetable derived Tween 80 during solvent/detergent treatment, *Biologicals*, 30, 197–205, 2002.

83. Morfeld, F., Schutz, R., Josic, D., and Schwinn, H., Manufacturing and down scaling process for a virus-inactivated pooled human plasma, *Pharm. Ind.*, 58, 433–435, 1996.

84. Blumel, J., Schmidt, I., Willkommen, H., and Lower, J., Inactivation of parvovirus B19 during pasteurization of human serum albumin, *Transfusion*, 42, 1011–1018, 2002.

85. Adcock, W.L., MacGregor, A., Davies, J.R., Hattarki, M., Anderson, D.A., and Goss, N.H., Chromatographic removal and heat inactivation of hepatitis A virus during manufacture of human albumin, *Biotechnol. Appl. Biochem.*, 28, 85–94, 1998.

86. Lieber, M.M., Benveniste, R.E., Livingston, D.M., and Todaro, G.J., Mammalian cells in cell culture frequently release type C viruses, *Science*, 182, 56–59, 1973.

87. Levy, J., Lee, H., Kawahata, R., and Spitler, L., Purification of monoclonal antibodies from mouse ascites eliminates contaminating infectious mouse type C viruses and nucleic acids, *Clin. Exp. Immunol.*, 56, 114–120, 1984.

88. Levy, R.V., Phillips, M.W., and Lutz, H., Filtration and removal of viruses from biopharmaceuticals, in *Filtration in the Biopharmaceutical Industry*, Meltzer, T.H. and Jornitz, M.W., Eds., Marcel Dekker, New York, 1998, pp. 619–646.

89. Kelley, B.D. and Petrone, J.T., Virus removal by tangential flow filtration for protein therapeutics, in *Membrane Separations in Biotechnology*, Wang, W.K., Ed., Marcel Dekker, New York, 2001, pp. 351–396.

90. Huang, P.Y. and Peterson, J., Scaleup and virus clearance studies on viral filtration in monoclonal antibody manufacture, in *Membrane Separations in Biotechnology*, Wang, W.K., Ed., Marcel Dekker, New York, 2001, pp. 327–350.

91. Saksena, S. and Zydney, A.L., Effect of solution pH and ionic strength on the separation of albumin from immunoglobulins by selective filtration, *Biotechnol. Bioeng.*, 43, 960–968, 1994.

92. Bil'dyukevich, A.V., Ostrovskii, E.G., and Kaputskii, F.N., Ultra-filtration of model solutions of high-molecular-weight compounds. Influence of the ionic strength on the ultrafiltration of protein solutions, *Colloid J. USSR*, 51, 300–303, 1989.

93. van Holten, R.W., Quinton, G.J., and Oulundsen, G.E., Viral Clearance Process, U.S. Patent 6,096,872, 2000.

94. Box, G.E.P., Hunter, W.G., and Hunter, J.S., *Statistics for Experimenters*, John Wiley & Sons, New York, 1978, pp. 31–38 and 73.

95. Seely, R.J., Munyakazi, L., Haury, J., Simmerman, H., Rushing, W.H., and Curry, T.F., Demonstrating the consistency of small datasets, *BioPharm Int.*, 16, 36–58, 2003.

96. Morrica, A., Nardini, C., Falbo, A., Bailey, A.C., and Bucci, E., Manufacturing process of anti-thrombin III concentrate: viral safety studies and effect of column re-use on viral clearance, *Biologicals*, 31, 165–173, 2003.

97. Leonard, M.W., Sefton, L., Costigan, R., Shi, L., Hubbard, B., Bonam, D., Kelley, B.D., Foster, B., and Charlebois, T., Validation of recombinant coagulation Factor IX purification process for removal of host cell DNA, in *Validation of Biopharmaceutical Manufacturing Processes*, ACS Symposium Series, Kelley, B.D. and Ramelmier, R.A., Eds., 1998, pp. 55–68.

98. Adner, N. and Sofer, G., Biotechnology product validation. III. Chromatography cleaning validation, *BioPharm*, 7, 44–48, 1994.

99. Shi, L., Kelley, B.D., Bonam, D., and Hubbard, B., Experimental design for validation of chromatographic process limits, Bio-Pharm meeting, San Francisco, 1997.

100. Kelley, B.D., Establishing process robustness using designed experiments, in *Biopharmaceutical Process Validation*, Sofer, G. and Zabriskie, D., Eds., Marcel Dekker, New York, 2000, pp. 29–59.

101. Breece, T., Gilkerson, E., and Schmelzer, C., Validation of large-scale chromatographic process. I. Case study of Neuleze capture on Macroprep High-S, *BioPharm*, 15, 16–20, 2002.

102. O'Leary, R.M., Feuerhelm, D., Peers, D., Xu, Y., and Blank, G., Determining the useful lifetime of chromatographic resins. Prospective small-scale studies, *BioPharm*, 14, 10–18, 2001.

103. Nigam, S., Ruezinsky, G., and Dugger, J., Reuse validation of an anion exchange chromatography step for purification of clinical grade ciliary neurotropic factor, in *Validation of Biopharmaceutical Manufacturing Processes*, ACS Symposium Series, Kelley, B.D. and Ramelmeier, R.A., Eds., 1998, pp. 125–143.

104. Seely, R., Wright, H., Fry, H., Rudge, S., and Slaff, G., Biotechnology product validation. VII. Validation of chromatography resin useful life, *BioPharm*, 7, 41–48, 1994.

105. Moran, E.B., McGowan, S.T., McGuire, J.M., Frankland, J.E., Oyebade, I.A., Waller, W., Archer, L.C., Morris, L.O., Pandya, J., Nathan, S.R., Smith, L., Cadette, M.L., and Michalowski, J.T., A systematic approach to the validation of process control parameters for monoclonal antibody production in fed-batch culture of a murine myeloma, *Biotechnol. Bioeng.*, 69, 242–255, 2000.

106. Gardner, A.R. and Smith, T.M., Identification and establishment of operating ranges of critical process variables, in *Biopharmaceutical Process Validation*, Sofer, G. and Zabriskie, D., Eds., Marcel Dekker, New York, 2000, pp. 61–76.

5

Adventitious Agents: Concerns and Testing for Biopharmaceuticals

RAY NIMS, ESTHER PRESENTE, GAIL SOFER,
CAROLYN PHILLIPS, AND AUDREY CHANG

CONTENTS

5.1 INTRODUCTION

Adventitious agents are those that are not inherent in the production of biopharmaceuticals. Microbial adventitious agents include viruses, bacteria, fungi, and mycoplasma. Transmissible spongiform encephalopathy (TSE) agents are also potential adventitious agents. Raw materials may contain adventitious agents. Adventitious agents can be introduced during establishment of cell lines, cell culture/fermentation, capture and downstream processing steps, formulation/filling, and even during drug delivery. Therapeutic biotechnology products have an excellent safety record. However, the potential introduction of adventitious agents must continually be evaluated. The testing that is performed for this purpose is addressed in regulatory documents that include ICH guidelines, U.S. Points to Consider, and European, U.S., and Japanese Pharmacopoeia (EP, USP, and JP) documents. In some cases, 9 CFR (U.S. Code of Federal Regulations) and 21 CFR 211 and 610 are applicable. Table 5.1 lists some of the regulatory documents that describe testing requirements.

Since biopharmaceuticals encompass many types of products, there is considerable variability in risks from adventitious agents. In all cases, however, the use of Good Manufacturing Practices (GMPs) (e.g., environmental controls, control of raw materials and personnel flow, and cleaning), suitable safety testing programs, and process validation (including viral and sometimes mycoplasma clearance evaluation) helps to ensure patient confidence in biopharmaceuticals. Some products have minimal inherent risk associated with the introduction of adventitious agents (e.g., recombinant products produced in bacteria). Other types of products, such as those used for cell or gene therapy, are often at the other end of the spectrum and may be associated with greater risk due to their inability to tolerate rigorous processing

TABLE 5.1   Regulatory Documents That Apply to Testing for Adventitious Agents

Guideline on Quality of Biotechnological/Biological Products: Derivation and Characterization of Cell Substrates Used in the Production of Biotechnological/Biological Products (ICH Q5D, 1997), Geneva, Switzerland: International Conference on Harmonization, 1997

Points to Consider in the Characterization of Cell Lines Used to Produce Biologicals (FDA/CBER, 1993), Rockville, MD: Food and Drug Administration, Center for Biologics Evaluation and Research, 1993

Points to Consider in the Manufacture and Testing of Monoclonal Antibody Products for Human Use (FDA/CBER, 1997), Rockville, MD: Food and Drug Administration, Center for Biologics Evaluation and Research, 1997

Guideline on Viral Safety Evaluation of Biotechnology Products Derived from Cell Lines of Human or Animal Origin (ICH 5A, 1997), Geneva, Switzerland: International Conference on Harmonization, 1997

Guidance for Industry: Guidance for Human Somatic Cell Therapy and Gene Therapy (FDA/CBER, 1998), Rockville, MD: Food and Drug Administration, Center for Biologics Evaluation and Research, 1998

Minimising the Risk of Transmitting Animal Spongiform Encephalopathy Agents via Human and Veterinary Medicinal Products (CPMP, 2001), London, England: Committee for Proprietary Medicinal Products, 2001

Draft Guidance for Industry: Preventative Measures to Reduce the Possible Risk of Transmission of Creutzfeldt-Jakob Disease (CJD) and Variant Creutzfeldt-Jakob Disease (vCJD) by Human Cells, Tissues, and Cellular Tissue-Based Products (HCT/Ps) (FDA/CBER, 2002), Rockville, MD: Food and Drug Administration, Center for Biologics Evaluation and Research, 2002

Organization for Economic Cooperation and Development Principles on Good Laboratory Practices, 1998: ENV/MC/CHEM(98)17

Japan Ministry of Health and Welfare, Ordinance No. 21, 1997; Japan Pharmaceutical Affairs Bureau, Ministry of Health and Welfare, Pharmaceutical GLP Guideline, 1995 (lyakuhin GLP kaisetsu), 157–169

conditions. Greater potential risks are often associated with the use of human cells and animal-derived raw materials. Of particular concern are materials derived from bovine and porcine sources. When viable cells are a component of the product (as in *ex vivo* transduction), there may not be sufficient time to perform the required safety testing. In such cases, product may be released prior to completion of relevant tests for adventitious agents, although this testing is still mandated in order to demonstrate that the processes are being performed under adequate controls to maintain patient safety. A risk/benefit analysis determines whether the use of these products is warranted.

In this chapter, we present a description of specific adventitious agents and discuss prevention and control of risks arising from various stages of production. Throughout the chapter, we point out risks associated with various sources.

5.2 VIRUSES

Newly detected viral agents continue to be a source of concern to the general public. Examples include the West Nile virus, monkey pox, and the viruses that cause SARS. Demonstrating freedom from adventitious viral agents enhances confidence in biopharmaceuticals, and it is a regulatory requirement for biologics. This requirement applies for both licensed products and those destined for clinical trials. Viruses are classified by whether they are lipid-enveloped or not, and by size, shape, and resistance to inactivation by physicochemical treatments. A safety testing program for adventitious viral agents requires different assays (Table 5.2). These may include general viral screening assays such as the 14- and 28-day *in vitro* adventitious virus screens and the *in vivo* adventitious viral screen, as well as assays that are designed to detect specific viral agents of concern, such as the *in vitro* bovine and *in vitro* porcine viral assays, the 21-day *in vitro* murine minute virus (MMV) detection assay, and gel endpoint and quantitative polymerase chain reaction® (PCR) assays for specific viral entities.

TABLE 5.2 Assay Methodologies Employed for Viral Detection

Viral Detection Assay	Specificity	DetectionSystem	Duration	End Points
In vitro adventitious virus screen	Broad virus screen	Indicator cell lines	14 or 28 days	Cytopathic effect, hemadsorption, hemagglutination
In vivo virus screen	Broad virus screen	Suckling, adult mice, guinea pigs, hens' eggs	28 days	Survival, egg viability
In vitro bovine virus screen	Bovine viruses	Indicator cells	14 or 21 days	Cytopathic effect, hemadsorption, immunofluorescence
In vitro porcine virus screen	Porcine viruses	Indicator cells	14 or 21 days	Cytopathic effect, hemadsorption, immunofluorescence
In vitro MMV screen	MMV	324K cells	21 days	Cytopathic effect, hemagglutination
PCR	Specific viruses	RNA or DNA	1–2 days	Gel visualization of amplicons
Quantitative PCR	Specific viruses	RNA or DNA	1–2 days	PCR cycle time

5.2.1   Raw Materials

Typically, adventitious viral safety testing of raw materials is performed using the appropriate specific viral detection assay. Bovine-sourced materials (e.g., fetal bovine serum, collagen) are therefore most appropriately evaluated using the 9 CFR-compliant *in vitro* bovine virus detection assay. Additionally, PCR assays for the bovine viruses of most concern (especially bovine viral diarrhea virus [BVDV]) may be performed on such materials. During testing, it is not uncommon for bovine serum samples to display positive results for BVDV, especially the noncytopathic variant. Recently, bovine polyoma virus (BPyV) has become of some concern, especially in the European Union. Bovine serum samples test positive for this virus by PCR at a relatively high incidence, although it is not clear whether the PCR results are indicative of the presence of infectious virus. Detection of infectious BPyV requires the use of an indicator cell line for amplification, with a PCR end point for detection. Similarly, porcine-derived materials, such as trypsin, are evaluated using a 9 CFR-compliant *in vitro* porcine virus detection assay, and such testing may be augmented with PCR assays as necessary.

5.2.2   Cell Banks

Master (MCB) and working (WCB) cell banks are evaluated using both the specific viral assays and the more general viral screening assays, depending on the level of assurance the manufacturer has on the raw materials used. At a minimum, these cell banks are evaluated using the *in vitro* and *in vivo* virus screening assays. It is quite uncommon for viruses to be detected in the cell banks produced in the biologics industry, suggesting that the various controls stipulated in the Good Manufacturing Practice requirements have had the desired effects on quality. This is not the case, however, for cell banks that have been used in basic research laboratories. Care must be taken during the testing of cell banks to ensure that selection agents (e.g., methotrexate, hygromicin) that may be present in the growth media used for cell expansion do not cause excessive cytotoxicity to the indicator cells used

in the *in vitro* assays, as such cytotoxicity can confound interpretation of the tests.

5.2.3 Unprocessed Bulk

Manufactured biologics are expected by the Points to Consider
guidelines to be tested for viral safety in a lot-by-lot manner
at the bulk harvest (unpurified bulk) level. This may be
accomplished using *in vitro* and *in vivo* virus screening assays,
methods intended to detect a broad range of viral contaminants. Three indicator cell lines are used in the *in vitro* virus
screen. Primate and human cell lines are always included,
and the third indicator cell line is expected to be a monolayer
cell of the same or similar species as that of the substrate
employed in the manufacturing process. In the *in vivo* virus
screen, a variety of animal species are inoculated (suckling
and adult mice, guinea pigs, and embryonated hens' eggs).
The detection of viral contaminants in manufactured lots is
rare, with greater risk appearing to be associated with certain
types of products. For instance, cellular vaccines, retroviral
vectors, and monoclonal antibody products rarely have been
found to contain viral contaminants. On the other hand, adenoviral vectors, which are E1-deleted and therefore expected
to be replication-defective in most indicator cells used for
testing, may contain small numbers of recombinant adenoviral particles, which are capable of replicating in these indicator cells and of producing in the cells all the hallmarks of
adenoviral infection. Strictly speaking, this recombination
phenomenon is a natural process and not a case of introduction of an adventitious virus during the manufacturing cycle.
However, the outcome is the same, as the recombinant adenovirus is an unwanted contaminant and, in addition, its detection in an adventitious virus evaluation may mask the
presence of other potential viruses.

The greatest risk of introducing adventitious viral contaminants during the manufacture of biologicals appears to
reside with the production of recombinant proteins in systems
employing Chinese hamster ovary (CHO) cells as substrates.
It is not clear whether this is due to a higher potential of

these cells to serve as viral hosts, relative to the substrates used for other types of manufacture, or to the relatively common use of such cells in terms of number of manufactured products. At any rate, several viral contaminants have been detected with some frequency in CHO cell processes: these include MMV, REO virus (REO), and Cache Valley virus.

MMV has previously been detected in a CHO cell process [1], and as a result of this experience, certain of the Points to Consider documents now mandate that this virus be assayed for in bulk harvests of this type. MMV is a murine parvovirus that represents a special challenge in that it is relatively small (~20 nm) and therefore is difficult to remove by filtration and to inactivate by gamma irradiation. It is nonenveloped and thus resistant to chemical and physical inactivation strategies. In addition, the virus is relatively hardy and the potential for survival of the virus outside of cell cultures therefore exists [2]. In fact, the most likely route of introduction of this virus into manufacturing processes would appear to be contamination of environmental surfaces used for raw materials processing and packaging [1]. This virus has also been found as a contaminant in the Syrian hamster embryo cell line, BHK [3,4]. The most common assays for detection of this virus are (1) the cell infectivity assay using 324K cells as the indicator cell, which detects primarily the fibrotropic strain of MMV (MMV[p], prototype strain); (2) PCR (which can detect both the fibrotropic and lymphotropic or MMV[i] strains); and (3) the mouse antibody production (MAP) test, which should be able to detect both strains of MMV [5,6]. The latter test was used by Nicklas et al. [7] to detect MMV in a number of cell lines.

REO has been isolated from CHO cell cultures on a number of occasions. This infection can be insidious since the virus may propagate slowly in the cell substrate, having minimal if any effect on oxygen or base demand, or on the yield of recombinant protein. Members of the family Reoviridae, genus Orthoreovirus, these viruses are spherical, 60–80 nm in diameter, and nonenveloped and possess a double protein capsid shell. The replication and assembly of these double-stranded RNA viruses occur in the cytoplasm of the host cell, where relatively large numbers of viral particles may be found packaged in crystalline arrays (Figure 5.1). It can be difficult to ascertain the animal species of origin of the various REO viruses (types 1, 2, and 3), confounding investigation of product contamination with these agents. Typically, the presence of such viruses in bulk harvest samples has been ascribed to nonhomogeneously contaminated bovine serum used during the manufacturing process. The relatively low-level contamination of bovine serum lots may prevent the detection of the virus during quality control testing of the serum. The large amounts of serum incorporated into the culture medium during the manufacturing process, coupled with the relatively long culture times employed, may allow the virus to propagate to the point that the virus is detectable in the bulk harvests. The most common assays for detection of this virus are (1) the cell infectivity assay using L929 or CHO-K1 cells as the indicator cell; (2) PCR (using type-specific primers or primers designed to detect all three types); and (3) immunofluorescence staining using anti-REO antisera.

Another viral contaminant that may be introduced into manufacturing processes primarily through use of nonhomogeneously contaminated bovine serum is Cache Valley virus. A member of the family Bunyaviridae, genus Bunyavirus, Cache Valley virus is spherical, 80–120 nm in diameter, with a lipid envelope containing glycoprotein spikes (Figure 5.2). The single-stranded RNA virus is known to infect livestock, being transmitted through insect vectors. As with the REO viruses, a low-level contamination of bovine serum lots with this virus may lead to an inability to detect the agent during quality control testing of the serum. As with REO virus, the large amounts of serum incorporated into the culture medium during the manufacturing process, coupled with the relatively long culture times employed, may allow this virus to propagate to the point that the virus is detectable in the bulk harvests. In contrast to the case for REO virus, amplification of Cache Valley virus during manufacturing campaigns usually leads to detectable changes in substrate integrity, as well as oxygen and base demand by the cultures as cell death occurs. The virus can infect and rapidly cause cytopathic effect

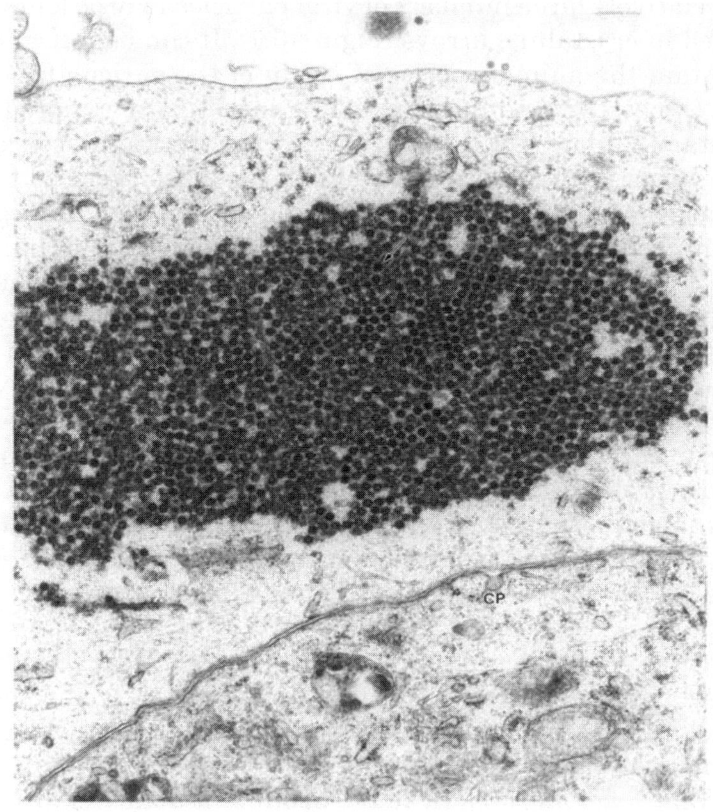

Figure 5.1 REO virus detected in human newborn kidney (324K) cells. 37,000× magnification, showing 65- to 75-nm spherical particles exhibiting crystalline packing pattern near cell nucleus.

in a variety of host cells, including CHO-K1, Vero, MRC-5, and 324K cells. For this reason, the virus is readily detected in *in vitro* viral screens employing these indicator cell lines. Another means of detecting this virus consists of PCR using Cache Valley- or bunyavirus-specific primers.

The three adventitious viral contaminants discussed previously are emphasized since the authors are aware of more than one instance for each virus of detection of the agent in unprocessed bulk harvest samples collected from CHO cell

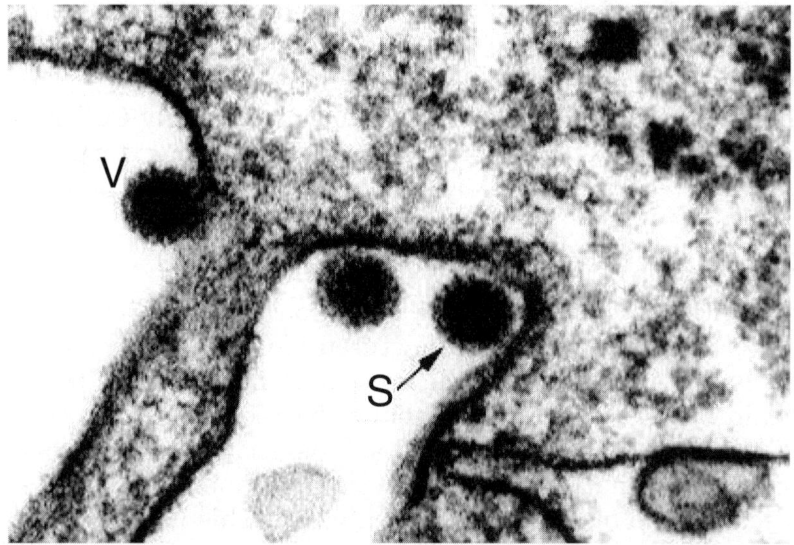

Figure 5.2　Cache Valley virus detected in African green monkey (Vero) cells. 100,000× magnification, showing 80- to 100-nm enveloped particles (V) with external spikes (S) budding from the membrane.

manufacturing processes. As mentioned previously, in the cases of REO and Cache Valley virus, it would appear that the relatively large volumes of fetal bovine serum used in culture medium during scale-up of the production cell substrate may be the origin of the contamination. A low-level nonhomogeneous contamination of a large production lot of fetal bovine serum may be undetectable using the state-of-the-art methods, for which the sampled volumes are relatively small (~200 ml of serum in the case of the 9 CFR bovine virus screen, <1 ml of serum in the case of a gel end point or quantitative PCR assay). One approach to lowering the potential risk associated with these particular viral contaminants would appear to be gamma irradiation of the fetal bovine serum prior to use in manufacturing processes.

At least two additional findings of adventitious viral contaminants in CHO cell systems have been reported. One described the presence of epizootic hemorrhagic disease virus (family Reoviridae, genus Orbivirus) [8] in a genetically engineered CHO cell substrate used for biologic production. The other reported the isolation of a calicivirus, family Caliciviridae, genus Calicivirus, from CHO cells exhibiting cytopathology [9].

5.2.4 Summary of Viral Safety Issues

As mentioned previously, the detection of an adventitious viral contaminant in a manufactured biological for the most part is quite rare and for the most part has been limited to certain types of products. It should be recognized, however, that a negative result in a viral safety assay does not necessarily mean that adventitious viral contaminants are not present in the biological being evaluated. This is due to limitations in the sensitivity of the various viral detection assays and to the fact that only a relatively small volume of each biological is actually sampled for testing. A negative outcome from such testing means that no adventitious viral entities were detected but does not guarantee that there are absolutely none present. In addition to subjecting raw materials, cell substrates, and bulk harvest samples to viral safety testing, viral clearance evaluation studies are therefore performed as a means to ensure patient safety. This testing is done in a proactive manner by spiking known amounts of model viruses into a scaled-down model that is validated to represent manufacturing scale. By performing viral clearance evaluation studies with model viruses selected to encompass a wide range of characteristics, confidence in final product safety is enhanced. These studies are generally performed prior to phase 1 clinical studies and, again, prior to pivotal clinical studies once the process is finalized. In addition, clearance studies involving specific viral entities may be performed in response to the detection, during routine lot release testing, of a viral contaminant. Changes in raw materials, manufacturing control parameters, and unit operations with viral clearance capability require reevaluation of viral safety. If changes have the potential to modify viral safety, clearance studies are repeated. The ICH guideline Q5A (Table 5.1) provides information on viral safety evaluation of biotechnology products derived from cell lines of human or animal origin.

5.3 BIOBURDEN: BACTERIA AND FUNGI

Bacteria and fungi that contaminate a biopharmaceutical raw material, cell bank, cell culture, purification process, or product are likely to grow rapidly. Even when inactivated, these microorganisms pose a safety concern since toxins (e.g., exo- and endotoxins) may remain. A new contaminant or an increase of a specific contaminant upstream may challenge the remainder of the manufacturing process, rendering a final product that is unsuitable for use. Process clearance spiking studies are not normally performed for bioburden, since the actual personnel, environment, and water at the manufacturing site are the most likely sources of contamination. Routine testing and environmental monitoring are required to ensure that a process and product meet requisite microbial safety specifications.

5.3.1 Assays

Sterility assays are imperfect and provide only a statistical probability of nonsterility. For aseptic processes such as the sterility assay or the aseptic fill of a final drug container, a sterility assurance level (SAL) of 10^{-3} is expected. Just imagine that you are the patient that gets that one-in-a-thousand vial! It has been stated [10] that "the concept of what sterile means has now become a matter of degree, i.e., there is a certain probability of sterility for each unit of product being sterilized." In some cases, bioburden testing, rather than sterility testing, is performed. Bioburden testing is intended and appropriate for nonsterile products. Bioburden testing is a type of microbial limits test. It can be quantitative and qualitative, providing a total aerobic microbial count and total yeast and molds count. It may also be used to qualitatively detect the presence of objectionable organisms. Examples of objectionable organisms are described in compendia and include *Pseudomonas aeruginosa*, salmonella species, *Escherichia coli*, *Staphylococcus aureus*, clostridium species, and mycobacteria. Sterility testing can be thought of as a very stringent form of a microbial limits determination, in which no growth of microorganisms is permitted.

Bioburden is sometimes used for testing unprocessed bulk and typically used for setting in-process manufacturing specifications. This is allowed in the FDA's Points to Consider on therapeutic monoclonal antibodies. Unless a sponsor has a sufficient database based on in-house experience, however, setting an acceptable limit for bioburden is problematic. Sterility testing is performed for master and working cell banks, for cells at the limit of *in vitro* cell age (also known as end of production cells), and for unprocessed bulk. During the manufacturing process, in-process alert and action bioburden limits enhance confidence in the safety of the product. Sterility testing of final product is required, and purified bulk is also tested. PDA has petitioned the FDA to discontinue the regulatory requirements for purified (i.e., final) bulk sterility testing. Terminally sterilized product that is sterilized on a cycle not validated as overkill would most probably require bioburden testing of the bulk prior to fill and terminal sterilization in order to ensure that the appropriate cycle SAL for the product is achieved. Overkill cycles are very robust cycles and generally do not require this consideration.

5.3.2 Cell Banks and Unprocessed Bulk

Testing at the cell banking stage is of the utmost importance for minimizing risks from adventitious agents. Testing of cell banks is described by ICH Q5D (Derivation and Characterization of Cell Substrates), which specifies that 1% of the total number but not less than two containers of each MCB and WCB are tested for the presence of bioburden. It does not make sense to move ahead with a bank that has any detectable bioburden, and sterility assays are employed. The ICH Q5D guideline refers the reader to the European, Japanese, and U.S. Pharmacopoeias (EP, JP, USP). However, USP <71> describes a referee test for a pharmacopoeial article purporting to be sterile. Neither EP 2.6 nor JP 54 refers to cell bank testing. The U.S. FDA's Points to Consider in the Characterization of Cell Lines addresses cell bank and unprocessed bulk testing and refers to 21 CFR 610.12; however, 21 CFR 610.12 does not specifically address cell bank or unprocessed bulk testing. Compliance with these methods is thus somewhat problematic, since the specific methods are not designed for testing at cell bank and unprocessed bulk stages. For example, cell banks are established by hand-filling, which is not performed under conditions that can be validated from a microbiological perspective since the number of vials is too small to perform meaningful media fills.

There are two issues that are critical in the design of the sterility testing program for these early stages, namely stasis testing and pooling strategies. As of January 2004, USP and EP refer to stasis testing as the validation test. Bacteriostasis and fungistasis testing provide confidence in the test results by demonstrating absence of growth inhibition by the test article. The requirements for stasis testing at these stages is not explicitly defined in ICH Q5D, but it is expected to be demonstrated that components of the test article are evaluated for inhibitory activity [11]. The validation test (i.e., bacteriostasis and fungistasis) is necessary to ensure the scientific integrity of subsequent sterility testing for a specific test article.

Pooling strategies should take into account the sensitivity of the sterility or bioburden assay. Dilution by pooling is a source of false negatives and can lead to combining "good" and "bad" materials. When cell culture duration is extended, the same issues should be addressed. Was there contamination early or late? How can pooling be justified so that testing results are not compromised?

5.3.3 In-Process/Raw Materials

Raw materials have introduced microorganisms into manufacturing suites. All materials used in microbiologically controlled processes should be tested for microbial quality prior to use. Chromatographic resins, for example, generally have a microorganism specification, but that specification is a numerical limit and does not include speciation. Clearly, if any spore-forming organisms are present, an entire product batch may be compromised. Surprisingly, cleaning and sanitization reagents have also contained resistant microorganisms that have caused contamination.

In-process bioburden specifications are difficult to set. No sponsor wants a failed batch due to a low level of microorganisms during downstream processing, but how can a reasonable level be established? As with unprocessed bulk, the only way to set a limit is to gather a history of manufacturing. This history must include environmental monitoring trends to demonstrate the efficacy of the microbiological control practices applied in a production process. However, when a new facility or new process is established, there may be insufficient experience and data to support realistic limits. Setting limits that are too narrow can lead to out-of-specification batches. On the other hand, setting limits that are too broad is a regulatory issue in the making. Once limits are set, they must be evaluated on a periodic basis in order to ensure that they remain a meaningful and effective monitoring tool.

The use of process analytical technologies (PAT) is being encouraged by the FDA [12]. Briefly, the concept is that rapid in-line, off-line, and at-line evaluation can enhance process control. There are new microbiological tools that are suitable for PAT. Most pick up metabolizing microorganisms and can eliminate the cost of continuing to process at risk. This technology is also suitable for many types of biotechnological final products such as cell and gene therapies and combination products with viable components.

5.3.4 Final Product

Final product sterility testing is addressed in many publications, including regulatory documents. However, for the small volume biotechnology product, final product testing can be problematic. Having to give up two vials of a 10-vial production lot is not easy. And as previously noted for cell banking, the filling is often manual. Media fills, involving a larger number of vials, have been recommended by the EU for clinical studies [13]. Regulatory agencies have recognized that products such as cell therapies do not lend themselves to traditional sterility testing and have encouraged the use of rapid microbiological methods to release product, but this must be followed up with the traditional, required sterility assays.

5.3.5 The Positives and Negatives

A negative sterility assay is not a guarantee that there are no viable organisms. There may remain injured microorganisms that do not demonstrate reproductive growth and are, therefore, not detected by the specified assays. In some cases, such organisms may survive and be able to recover in a suitable host. Furthermore, it is impossible to test enough units to ensure a 100% probability of sterility. Additionally, care must be taken to ensure the test article does not cause inhibition of microbial growth in the assay and lead to false negatives.

Even more problematic are false positives. Deciding to repeat a sterility test can be a regulatory minefield and a production and business nightmare. Common sources of false positives include equipment, supplies, materials, test media, technique, personnel, and the environment in which the sterility assays are performed. Barrier isolators employed for performance of sterility assays have been shown to provide a higher level of confidence. Isolation technology has virtually eliminated human-borne contamination and provides better control over environmental contamination. It has been observed by some that isolators reduced sterility test false positives to almost zero, and the industry-wide failure rate is estimated to be 0.01% to 0.001% [14].

5.4 MYCOPLASMA

Mycoplasmas lack a cell wall and are bound by a single plasma membrane. They are considered the smallest self-replicating prokaryote. There are close to 100 known species of mycoplasma, but eight species constitute over 95% of the identified contaminants [15,16].

Sources of contamination include cell culture media components, serum, cells, viral stocks, and laboratory personnel. The presence of mycoplasma is not always obvious, but an infection may persist for an extended period of time. It has been estimated that between 5 and 35% of cell cultures worldwide are contaminated with at least one species of mycoplasma [17].

Most mycoplasmas are parasites, exhibiting host and tissue specificities. Mycoplasmas affect cell growth properties. They inhibit cell metabolism, disrupt nucleic acid synthesis, produce chromosomal aberrations, produce proteases, phosphatases, and nucleases, change the antigenicity of cell membranes, mimic viral infections, and affect the yield of product. In humans, they can cause atypical pneumonia and are considered to be cofactors for some human diseases.

In a few cases, where there has been contamination of product by mycoplasma, regulatory agencies have required sponsors to perform mycoplasma clearance studies.

5.4.1 Test Methods

Test methods are specified in the regulatory guidelines. The ICH guideline Q5D addresses testing of cell banks for mycoplasma and states that agar and broth media procedures and the indicator cell culture procedure should be performed. Testing from a single container is generally adequate. The FDA's 1993 Points to Consider on Cell Line Characterization recommends testing for both agar-cultivable and non-agar-cultivable mycoplasma for mammalian cells. For insect cells, both mycoplasma and spiroplasma testing are performed. Tests are performed on virus seed and MCB, cell substrate, and each WCB used for manufacture of product.

Whereas much progress has been made in harmonizing sterility tests, specific requirements for mycoplasma testing are still different for different regions of the world. For example, although it is clearly good science to perform inhibition studies, the EP is the only regulatory document that specifies it as a requirement. Recommended positive controls may also differ in regard to mycoplasma concentration and species. In all cases, care must be taken to ensure that mycoplasmas are not inactivated by further processing prior to testing. As noted in the FDA's 1993 Points to Consider on Cell Line Characterization, each lot of product harvest concentrate should be tested prior to clarification, filtration, purification, and inactivation. Prior to testing, the product harvest concentrate sample should be stored between 2 and 8°C for 24 hr or less or at –60°C or lower for 24 hr or more.

For cell therapies and other products that undergo minimal processing, mycoplasma contamination of final product is a potential risk. These products must often be delivered within a matter of days, and the mycoplasma infectivity tests cannot be completed in time for product release. The use of PCR mycoplasma assays that can be performed in 1 day enhances the safety of such products. In a 2003 draft guidance for reviewers, FDA has noted that PCR-based mycoplasma assays are acceptable during development for product release, provided the PCR test has adequate sensitivity and specificity [18]. PCR is also ideally suited for screening cell lines and raw materials susceptible to mycoplasma contamination. Additional considerations for the use of PCR as an alternative method include circumstances (limited volumes, limited time, and interference with indicator cell assay) in which the standard PTC testing may not be feasible. Comparisons of the PCR assay with the standard procedures are promising, and there are several publications that correlate PCR results with those produced by the more traditional methods [17,19–21].

5.5 TRANSMISSIBLE SPONGIFORM ENCEPHALOPATHIES

Addressing regulatory requirements for prevention of transmissible spongiform encephalopathy (TSE) agents has become a big concern of biopharmaceutical manufacturers. The infectious agents are prion proteins, and they are extraordinarily resistant to inactivation methods. Although the infectious agent can be removed by filtration and chromatography, the reuse of filters, resins, and other contact surfaces is problematic. For biotechnological products, bovine spongiform encephalopathy (BSE) is generally the greatest concern. BSE was first identified in 1986, and 1 million cattle have been infected. It is likely spread by feed containing tissue from infected cattle. The infection becomes localized in high-risk tissues, such as brain, spinal cord, central nervous system, and ileum. In 2003, there were 129 human cases (vCJD), which are believed to be caused by consumption of contaminated beef. Sourcing of raw materials, such as fetal calf serum used in cell culture, is essential. Bovine materials can be obtained from countries not shown to have BSE. However, there is always a concern that BSE will be found in countries previously thought to be free of this agent. Some regulatory authorities have gone so far as to forbid the marketing of products using bovine materials sourced from countries where other TSEs, such as elk wasting disease, are found unless the sponsor has done TSE clearance studies. As noted in a European note for guidance, the risk of transmission of TSEs is reduced by controlling the source of animals, the nature of animal tissue used in manufacture, and production processes used for preparation of the animal-derived product [22]. The CPMP now requires that working viral seeds or working cell banks be rebanked if there are any unknown potential risks associated with BSE in the current banks [23].

Clearance studies with spikes of TSE agents can be performed. These studies, however, can take more than 1 year to complete. Testing for TSE agents is by far the most difficult of the agents discussed in this chapter. Currently, the only reliable method capable of detecting one infectious unit employs animal models, most commonly the hamster 263K PrPSc (prion protein scrapie) strain. This strain has been demonstrated to be a model for human PrPsCJD (prion protein scrapie Creutzfeldt-Jakob disease), human PrPvCJD (prion protein variant Creutzfeldt-Jakob), and sheep PrPSc [24]. There are ongoing efforts in the development of amplification methods suitable for detection of one infectious unit, but at this time they are not available. Western blots are commonly used to screen a process to determine where clearance occurs, and then, if necessary, those steps that are shown to be capable of removing scrapie agents are evaluated with the animal models [25].

5.6 SUMMARY

For biotechnological products, absolute freedom from adventitious agents cannot be guaranteed. Often, the sensitivity and precision of infectivity assays are poor. In other cases, when the assay sensitivity is adequate, the time for performance of the assay may limit its utility in releasing product. Highly sensitive assays, such as PCR, are often very specific and can only be used to detect known agents. In spite of these limitations, there have not been incidences of transmittal to humans of infectious agents from purified biotechnology products. The multipronged approach used by today's biopharmaceutical sponsors mitigates potential unknown risks. Equipment design and maintenance, water and air quality, and personnel flow are key elements used to reduce risks from adventitious agents. Qualification and suitable storage of cell banks, testing of incoming raw materials, and stringent sanitization processes eliminate many risks. Compliance with Good Manufacturing Practices is also essential. A robust process that removes real or unknown risks further enhances product safety. Clearance studies using spikes with agents or model agents that represent potential risks are critical when assay sensitivity is insufficient or when routine testing is not feasible (e.g., viral and TSE clearance studies). In-process bioburden assays minimize the risk of contamination by bacteria and fungi. Final product testing for bacteria and fungi, and in some cases their byproducts such as endotoxins, further enhance the safety of biotherapeutics. Table 5.3 summarizes some of the assays and testing stages.

In the near future, we hope that more assays will be harmonized and that virus stocks can be standardized. We anticipate the use of more sensitive, in-line technologies to further minimize the risks from adventitious agents. We continually find new agents as detection technology is improved. And while this may lead to concerns from sponsors, it also

TABLE 5.3 Summary of Testing for Adventitious Agents to Mitigate Risk

Adventitious Agent	Test	Testing Stages
Bacteria and fungi	Sterility and bioburden assays	Cell banks; cells at limit of *in vitro* cell age; unprocessed bulk; in-process testing; final product
Mycoplasma	Mycoplasma assays	Cell banks; cells at limit of *in vitro* cell age; unprocessed bulk
TSE	Sourcing of raw materials[a]	Clearance studies[a]
Adventitious viruses	*In vitro* and *in vivo* assays; specific assays for infectivity and viral nucleic acid	Cell banks; cells at limit of *in vitro* cell age; unprocessed bulk; clearance studies

[a] Currently, the only assay of sufficient sensitivity to detect one infectious prion is the animal bioassay.

enables the development of better tools for control throughout a manufacturing process. As noted by Dr. Kathryn Zoon [26], "For biotech, it's [PAT] definitely applicable. It could be used for online monitoring of adventitious agents found in biotech therapeutics."

REFERENCES

1. Garnick, R.L., Experience with viral contamination in cell culture, in *Viral Safety and Evaluation of Viral Clearance from Biopharmaceutical Products*, Brown, F. and Lubiniecki, A.S., Eds., *Dev. Biol. Stand.*, 88, 49–56, 1996.

2. Jacoby, R.O., Ball-Goodrich, L.J., Besselsen, D.G., McKisic, M.D., Riley, L.K., and Smith, A.L., Rodent parvovirus infections, *Lab. Anim. Sci.*, 46, 370–380, 1996.

3. Nettleton, P.F. and Rweyemamu, M.M., The association of calf serum with the contamination of BHK21 clone 13 suspension cells by a parvovirus serologically related to the Minute Virus of Mice (MVM), *Arch. Virol.*, 64, 359–374, 1980.

4. Zoletto, R., Parvovirus serologically related to the minute virus of mice (MVM) as contaminant of BHK 21 cl. 13 suspension cells, *Dev. Biol. Stand.*, 60, 179–183, 1985.

5. de Souza, M. and Smith, A.L., Comparison of isolation in cell culture with conventional and modified mouse antibody production tests for detection of murine viruses, *J. Clin. Microbiol.*, 27, 185–187, 1989.

6. Parker, J.C., Cross, S.S., Collins, M.J., Jr., and Rowe, W.P., Minute virus of mice. I. Procedures for quantitation and detection, *J. Natl. Cancer Inst.*, 45, 297–303, 1970.

7. Nicklas, W., Kraft, V., and Meyer, B., Contamination of transplantable tumors, cell lines, and monoclonal antibodies with rodent viruses, *Lab. Anim. Sci.*, 43, 296–300, 1993.

8. Rabenau, H., Ohlinger, V., Anderson, J., Selb, B., Cinatl, J., Wolf, W., Frost, J., Mellor, P., and Doerr, H.W., Contamination of genetically engineered CHO-cells by epizootic haemorrhagic disease virus (EHDV), *Biologicals*, 21, 207–214, 1993.

9. Oehmig, A., Buttner, M., Weiland, F., Werz, W., Bergemann, K., and Pfaff, E., Identification of a calicivirus isolate of unknown origin, *J. Gen. Virol.*, 84, 2837–2845, 2003.

10. Berube, R. and Oxborrow, G.S., Methods of testing sanitizers and bacteriostatic substances, in *Disinfection, Sterilization and Preservation*, 4th ed., Block, S., Ed., Lea & Febiger, Philadelphia, 1991, 1058–1068.

11. Sofer, G. and Phillips, C., Sterility testing for master cell banks, working cell banks, and unprocessed bulk, *BioPharm*, 14, 36–38, 2001.

12. Guidance for Industry PAT — A Framework for Innovative Pharmaceutical Manufacturing and Quality Assurance, Draft Guidance, U.S. FDA, August 2003 (http://www.fda.gov/cder/guidance/5815dft.htm).

13. Manufacture of Investigational Medicinal Products, GMP Annex13, EU, July 2003.

14. Akers, J., Oral presentation at BioReliance Workshop: Sterility Testing from Theory to Practice, Boston, January 2002. Available from BioReliance Corp., 14920 Broschart Road, Rockville, MD 20850.

15. McGarrity, G.J. and Katani, H., Cell culture mycoplasmas, in *Pathogenesis of Mycoplasma Diseases. The Mycoplasmas*, Vol. IV, Razin, S. and Barile, M.F., Eds., 1985, pp. 353–390.

16. Bolske, G., Survey of mycoplasma infections in cell cultures and a comparison of detection methods, *Zentbl. Bakteriol. Mikrobiol. Hyg. Ser. A*, 269, 331–340, 1988.

17. Uphoff, C.C. and Drexler, H.G., Comparative PCR analysis for detection of mycoplasma infections in continuous cell lines, *In Vitro Cell Dev. Biol. Anim.*, 38, 79–85, 2002.

18. U.S. FDA, Draft Guidance for Reviewers, Instructions and Template for CMC Reviewers of Human Somatic Cell Therapy Investigational New Drug Applications (INDs), August 2003.

19. Garner, C.M., Hubbold, L.M., and Chakraborti, P.R., Mycoplasma detection in cell cultures: a comparison of four methods, *Br. J. Biomed. Sci.*, 57, 295–301, 2000.

20. Uphoff, C.C. and Drexler, H.G., Detection of mycoplasma in leukemia-lymphoma cell lines using polymerase chain reaction, *Leukemia*, 16, 289–293, 2002.

21. Tang, J., Hu, M., Lee, S., and Roblin, R., A polymerase chain reaction based method for detecting Mycoplasma/Acholeplasma contaminants in cell culture, *J. Microbiol. Meth.*, 39, 121–126, 2000.

22. Committee for Proprietary Medicinal Products/Committee for Veterinary Medicinal Products, Note for Guidance on Minimising the Risk of Transmitting Animal Spongiform Encephalopathy Agents via Human and Veterinary Medicinal Products, Revision 2, London, December 2002 (EMEA/410/01 Rev. 2).

23 Committee for Proprietary Medicinal Products/Committee for Veterinary Medicinal Products, position paper on reestablishment of working seeds and working cell banks using TSE compliant materials, London, September 2002 (EMEA/22314/02).

24. Stenland, C.J., Lee, D.C., Brown, P., Petteway, S.R., Jr., and Rubenstein, R., Partitioning of human and sheep forms of the pathogenic prion protein during the purification of therapeutic proteins from human plasma, *Transfusion*, 42, 1497–1500, 2002.

25. Lee, D.C., Stenland, C.J., Miller, J.L., Cai, K., Ford, E.K., Gilligan, K.J., Hartwell, R.C., Terry, J.C., Rubenstein, R., Fournel, M., and Petteway, S.R., Jr., A direct relationship between the partitioning of the pathogenic prion protein and transmissible spongiform encephalopathy infectivity during the purification of plasma proteins, *Transfusion*, 41, 449–455, 2001.

26. Zoon, K., oral presentation, Plasma Protein Therapeutics Association Conference, Virginia, June 2003.

6

Life Span Studies for Chromatography and Filtration Media

ANURAG S. RATHORE AND GAIL SOFER

CONTENTS

6.1 INTRODUCTION

Chromatography and filtration media often dominate the cost of raw materials for the whole process [1]. As such, from a process economics point of view, it is important to be able to recycle the media to an appropriate number of cycles before replacing it with new media. The optimal number of cycles for a media that should be targeted varies from product to product and company to company and depends on several considerations, which include media cost, approach toward and timing of the various process validation activities, cost of a batch of product, number of batches to be run every year, etc. The cost of the media varies in a wide spectrum, e.g., $6500/l for rProtein A Sepharose Fast Flow® (Amersham Biosciences) to $400/l for High S Macroprep® (BioRad). Similar variation is also seen in the various kinds of filtration media that are on the market today.

Establishing the useful life span of the media, however, remains a critical issue for sponsors producing biological and biotechnological therapeutic and diagnostic products. The primary objective is quite simply the ability to consistently produce intermediates and final products that meet the defined quality and safety attributes. Achieving this goal is complicated by our limited understanding of the surface chemistry of the media and the interactions that take place between the media and the various feed components, such as host cell proteins, nucleic acids, lipids, viruses, and process additives. Once immobilized at the media surface, some impurities may become stabilized. Feed components are washed off to varying extents during cleaning and sanitization cycles. However, after completion of a chromatography or filtration step, a portion of these impurities can remain bound to the media and be slowly removed upon extended storage or even be carried over to the next production lot. Newer and more sensitive detection methods and techniques, such as PCR, can enhance our ability to understand the mechanism and nature of fouling of the media and, thus, aid in developing cleaning, sanitization, and storage procedures that preserve the function and integrity of the media and extend its life span. Nevertheless, validation of media life span requires demonstration at scale of the targeted number of reuses. These studies are often time-consuming and expensive, but they provide confidence in the continued production of consistently pure and safe biotherapeutics and reliable diagnostics.

Regulators have stated that validation of the purification process should also include justification of the working conditions such as column loading capacity, column regeneration and sanitization, and length of use of the columns [2]. Therefore, studies designed to estimate media life span have slowly

become a part of the "process development" of a biopharmaceutical commercial process. In January 2002, Dr. Andrew
Chang of CBER presented a collection of the FDA's findings
related to chromatography [3]. In a review letter, a sponsor
was told to "please provide validation data to demonstrate
there is no negative impact of extended use of the...matrix to
150 production cycles on efficacy of cleaning and regeneration
of the...column. Please provide data that show complete
removal of viral contamination prior to reuse of the system."
In some postapproval inspections, comments included the
following:

> Storage times in between runs for all of the purification
> columns have not been validated for entire life cycle of
> column. Cleaning validation study was conducted only for
> up to 5 uses of the column, which could be used in the
> purification of up to 46 lots per laboratory scale study.
> Cleaning validation including LAL and bioburden studies
> of the...purification columns were only validated for up
> to 5 uses. In addition, the cleaning validation of these
> columns did not include removal of process-related impu-
> rities. However, columns can be used for following number
> of purification runs/years.... Storage in buffer not tested
> for attrition.

The FDA's Therapeutic Compliance Program Guide,
which serves as a guide for investigators, states, "There
should be an estimated life span for each column type, i.e.,
number of cycles. Laboratory studies are useful even necessary to establish life span of columns. There are situations
where concurrent validation at the manufacturing scale may
be more appropriate. Continued use may be based upon routine monitoring against predetermined criteria" [4]. At a
PDA/FDA conference on process validation in 2000, Dr. Barry
Cherney presented CBER's current expectations on determining resin life span [5]. He noted that the 1997 FDA Points to
Consider in the Manufacture and Testing of Monoclonal
Antibody Products for Human Use states that limits must
be prospectively set [6]. The ICH Guideline on Viral
Safety states, "Over time and after repeated use, the ability
of chromatography columns and other devices used in the

purification scheme to clear virus may vary" [7]. European regulatory authorities have also expressed concern over consistency of chromatographic performance. In one CPMP (Committee for Proprietary Medicinal Products) position statement, it was noted that elimination of host cell proteins, in most cases, makes use of chromatographic columns for which the selectivity and yield of the procedures depend not only on the quality of the material but also on the way the columns are used and reused, storage conditions, sanitization, and life span [8]. Similar observations have also been made on filtration steps. One FDA Form 483 noted, "There is no integrity testing of back up filter when the primary nitrogen filter fails integrity test. There may be a lag time of up to…production batches before testing." It is not a big surprise that the issue of chromatography and filtration media life span continues to be discussed at conferences and questioned by regulatory authorities for licensure and during inspections.

In this chapter, we will discuss the various factors that influence life span of chromatography and filtration media and also the key operating and performance parameters that are utilized to monitor integrity of the media. Finally, we will review the different approaches that different companies have taken to successfully validate media life span.

6.2 FACTORS THAT INFLUENCE CHROMATOGRAPHY MEDIA LIFE SPAN

In the following, we discuss the different factors that are listed in Table 6.1 that influence chromatography media life span.

6.2.1 Position of Step in Purification Process

The positioning of a chromatographic step in a process has a profound influence on the expected life span due to the relative purity of the feed stream, which is much higher in the later stages of the process. For example, in the process of purifying albumin from plasma, the ion exchange media in the first step in which product binds is used for 600 cycles, whereas the second ion exchanger is used for 1200 cycles [9].

TABLE 6.1 Factors That Influence Life Span of a Chromatography Column

- Position of step in purification process (capture, purification, or polishing)
- Nature of feed stream (amount and type of the various impurities)
- Mode of chromatography (bind-elute or flow-through)
- Type of chromatography media (physical and chemical stability)
- Maintenance (efficacy of cleaning, sanitization, and storage procedures)
- Column packing and attrition (packing method and physical stability of media)
- System components (design of column and supporting instrumentation)
- Quality of raw materials (nature of impurities in raw materials)
- Economics (cost of batch of media vs. validation costs)

In general, the early chromatographic steps have to face not only feed streams containing a variety of impurities that interact with the column media, but also relatively aggressive cleaning and sanitization protocols that are required to maintain the integrity of the column for the next reuse. The decision to place a chromatographic step earlier or later in a process is totally dependent on the process under consideration, and the optimal solution is frequently a result of compromise between counteracting considerations. For example, placing an affinity chromatography step later in the process will allow more reuses of the column media. However, due to the higher selectivity of affinity chromatography, using this column for capture of the product might reduce the number of steps required for purification. Finding an optimal solution in such cases requires performing small-scale studies to compare the different options.

6.2.2 Nature of the Feed Stream

The nature of the feed stream is also a critical factor in determining media life span. Chromatographic separations performed early in the process are often complicated by the presence of a variety of components in the feed material, including host cell impurities (host cell proteins, endotoxin,

TABLE 6.2 A CIP Protocol for a Feed Stream from Cell Culture

Feed stream:	Hybridoma cell culture
Chromatography media:	STREAMLINE® rProtein A
CIP protocol:	1. 1.0 mM NaOH and 2 M NaCl in 20% ethanol, 2 hours, 100 cm/h
	2. 5% sodium lauroylsarcosinate, 20 mM EDTA, and 0.1 M NaCl in 20 mM NaH$_2$PO$_4$, pH 7.0, 1.5 h
	3. 50 mM acetic acid in 20% ethanol

nucleic acids, lipids, viruses), process-related impurities (raw materials, additives), and the various product-related impurities [10]. Due to the requirement of more stringent cleaning for such steps, maximizing media life span requires carefully planned development of cleaning and sanitization steps early in process development. For example, in expanded bed adsorption techniques, whole broths are often applied directly from cell culture. A cleaning-in-place (CIP) protocol for such a step is shown in Table 6.2. It is obvious that this cleaning protocol is quite stringent, but it is compatible with the media, which was used for five cycles with an expectation that more could be obtained. Product recovery, purity, and breakthrough capacity remained constant over these life span studies [11].

Many feed streams contain colored substances that bind strongly to chromatographic media. This is particularly noticeable with *E. coli* feed streams from inclusion bodies and in plasma fractionation. Visual inspection in such cases can cause concern. Cleaning validation studies, however, can be utilized to demonstrate that these columns continue to perform consistently with no loss of capacity and no change in product purity, impurity profiles, and other performance attributes.

6.2.3 Mode of Chromatography

The mode of chromatography, bind-elute versus flow-through, also plays an important role in determining the life span of the column. In contrast to the more commonly used bind-elute mode, flow-through mode is often used with the objective to bind other host cell impurities (most commonly host cell proteins or DNA), while letting the product of interest flow through the chromatography column. It is recommended to keep the mode of chromatography in mind while deciding on the acceptance criteria for media life span.

6.2.4   Type of Chromatography Media

When a chromatography column is scaled up and its diameter increases, the wall support contribution to bed stability starts decreasing. For column diameters greater than 25–30 cm, the lack of wall support may become an issue and could cause redistribution of packing particles and settling of the bed [12]. This often results in formation of high-porosity regions at the column inlet and maldistribution of flow across the column. This phenomenon is more prominent for nonrigid gel materials and is often reversible within limits but almost always with a marked hysteresis. The issue of physical stability of the column bed becomes particularly significant at large scale as the column is put to more reuses during commercial manufacturing, and hence the physical stability of the media must be taken into account for robust column design.

Considerations of chemical stability of the packing material include any factors that may result in deterioration of the column performance over a period of use. It may be the leaching of ligands into the mobile phase as often experienced with affinity chromatography, destruction of the matrix in the mobile phases used for column operation, regeneration or storage (e.g., silica packings at high pH), or irreversible binding at the packing surface. These factors directly impact the column life span.

6.2.5   Column Maintenance

Good column maintenance is essential for maximizing media life span. This consists of three primary steps: cleaning, sanitizing, and storage, which have a very significant impact on column life span. Column life spans are diminished when inadequate cleaning protocols are employed. Unsuitable protocols allow a continual buildup of contaminants, often leading to reduced flow rates and clogged columns. The optimal cleaning protocol depends on several factors including compatibility of the media with cleaning solutions, nature of substances that must be removed, contact time, and temperature. A practical approach should be taken. For example, in the evaluation of cleaning calf thymus DNA from an anion exchanger, it was found that 1 M NaOH containing 1 M NaCl was effective in removing all residual DNA, as measured by the Threshold System. However, with a monoclonal antibody sample containing a high level of DNA, the DNA was not removed even with 2 M NaOH or 3 M NaCl [13]. A DNase treatment did remove the residual DNA; however, this is not an inexpensive approach for manufacturing, since the addition of DNase requires validation of its removal. A practical approach is to evaluate consistent capacity and flow properties, protein product purity, and DNA impurity levels. If no changes are observed, then the use of 1 M NaOH with 1 M NaCl should be sufficient for cleaning. Affinity media with proteinaceous ligands are usually the most difficult to clean. In the purification of Factor VIII with an immobilized monoclonal antibody column, for example, special care is taken to protect the expensive column. The feed stream and all buffers and cleaning solutions are prefiltered, and the column is kept isolated by sterile filters [14]. At the other extreme, there are many ion exchangers, hydrophobic interactions, and gel filtration media that tolerate cleaning with up to 2 M NaOH and provide life spans of up to 1200 cycles or more [15]. Data on compatibility of the chromatography media with a variety of cleaning agents is generally available from vendors. However, this often serves just as a starting point, and each user must consider what is optimum for their particular application.

Sanitization of chromatography columns is required to ensure consistent performance. Microorganisms can leave behind endotoxins, enterotoxins, and other potentially harmful substances, which may be quite difficult to remove. For example, negatively charged endotoxins bind strongly to anion exchangers [10]. Routine monitoring for bioburden and endotoxin levels is part of a quality assurance program that ensures consistent performance of packed chromatography columns.

Storage is another critical parameter to be considered as part of the development studies. Proper storage is essential to ensure expected media life spans. Storage solutions, temperature, and air quality may all have an impact on a firm's ability to reuse a column. When a column is stored for a considerable time period — for example, when campaigning in a multiproduct facility — it is advisable to periodically check the column for cleanliness and suitability for reuse. Storage solutions often have an excellent cleaning capability. There are many stories in the industry of extensively cleaned columns that, after storage, have "nucleotide-like" and other substances in the rinse. As a result of this phenomenon, it is necessary to establish criteria for complete removal of storage solutions.

Other factors related to maintenance that can enhance media life span include proper gowning, air quality monitoring, and humidity control [16]. Minimizing worker contact with the media once it is sanitized is recommended. Air quality in the purification suite is usually Class 10,000. In cold rooms, humidity control is critical, since high humidity is more likely to allow the growth of spore-forming organisms. Water quality, too, should be defined. WFI is usually used for cleaning and rinsing packed columns. In some cases, however, this is not necessary — for example, in the first purification step of an *E. coli*-derived feed stream.

6.2.6 Column Packing and Attrition

Column packing and attrition also influence media life span. The considerations mentioned during the discussion on "physical stability" of the media in Section 6.2.4 apply here as well. When in spite of rigorous cleaning and sanitizing routines a deterioration in the chromatographic profile is seen, product purity changes, backpressure increases, or flow decreases, most firms remove the media from the packed column and clean it out of place with stirring. This often restores performance, but the user must requalify the column after packing, and in most cases some media is lost. New column designs that allow for automated unpacking and repacking may reduce the attrition, but newer, rigid media are sometimes more brittle and repacking may result in more fracturing of the particles. Hence, physical stability of the media should be taken into consideration while deciding on the life span at large scale.

6.2.7　System Components

System components can have a significant influence on the media life span. It is always necessary to consider not only media compatibility with cleaning and sanitizing agents, but the column hardware and system compatibility as well. If the cleaning solution causes leaching from components, e.g., O-rings, then the cleaning problem is only exacerbated, and batch failures may occur. In-line filters can also be problematic and should be taken out of line during cleaning and sanitization. At least one firm learned this the hard way when a filter remained in line during sanitization with NaOH. Since it was not known what might leach out of the filter, the entire column contents had to be replaced.

6.2.8　Quality of Raw Materials

Another consideration is the use of consistent, high-quality raw materials. Although the feed stream is often expected to be variable, especially with cell culture, raw material quality can be controlled. Raw material quality can have a major impact on media life span. For example, if laboratory-grade acetone is used as a test molecule to measure HETP, the impurities in the acetone can start to accumulate. Stories are told in the industry about cleaning agents that have been found to contain microorganisms; therefore, if detergents or similar agents are used in cleaning or sanitizing columns, a firm should ensure their quality. Buffers and salts have sometimes been found to contain high levels of undefined impurities [17]. These can also accumulate and lead to a reduction in column life spans. Loss in performance of hydroxyapatite columns due to presence of metals, such as iron, in raw materials is well known.

6.3 EXPERIMENTAL APPROACHES TO DETERMINE AND VALIDATE CHROMATOGRAPHY MEDIA LIFE SPAN

Determination of media life span can be done via concurrent validation or prospective validation [18], and these approaches are outlined in Figure 6.1 and Figure 6.2 [19], respectively. Validation of media life span, however, has to be performed at manufacturing scale. The most common approach is to use small-scale data for "guidance" followed by "confirmation" and "validation" at full scale (Strategy 2) as it reduces the risk of "failure" at full scale and the resulting loss of batches if life span is solely determined at large scale.

While designing the experiments, it is essential to recognize that each feed stream and each process are unique. Expiry dates established for identical media used for similar end products from similar feed streams may be used to estimate media life span. This may, for example, be considered if a firm is producing several monoclonal antibodies from the same basic source and same culture conditions. If these data are to be used for a license application, however, one should discuss this early with the appropriate regulatory authorities to ensure they accept the concept and the data.

6.3.1 Small-Scale Models

A small-scale model of the chromatography step is required to be generated and then qualified before life span studies can be performed at small scale. The percentage of scale-down from manufacturing may be quite variable and depends on several factors including the scale of the final unit operation. As long as the scale-down is verified to represent full scale, the degree of scale-down is not significant. In some cases, a scale-down of 2000-fold or more is acceptable. With very expensive feed streams or those that are hard to obtain plus

- STRATEGY 1: CONCURRENT VALIDATION
  - Perform cycling studies at large scale
  - Evaluate column performance every n^{th} run
  - Perform blank run every $n^{th} + 1$
  - Material made in the last n cycles is quarantined until criteria are met for the final run
- Advantages:
  - No small-scale studies required
  - Entire dataset is pertinent as obtained at full scale
- Disadvantages:
  - Evaluation at full scale is more cumbersome and expensive
  - At any point, "n" lots are at risk

Figure 6.1 Concurrent validation strategy for determination and validation of column life span: performing studies only at manufacturing scale.

- STRATEGY 2: PROSPECTIVE VALIDATION
  - Perform cycling studies at small scale
  - Evaluate column performance every n^{th} run
  - Perform blank run every $n^{th} + 1$
  - Once lifetime known at small scale, validate at full scale with appropriate safety factor
- Advantages:
  - Most work done at small scale (less expensive and faster)
  - With appropriate safety factor, no material at risk
  - Only suitable approach for evaluating clearance of hazardous impurities
- Disadvantages:
  - Small-scale dataset serves only as a guide and the full-scale validation is still required
  - Safety factor is critical as lifetime at small scale does not guarantee performance at full scale

Figure 6.2 Prospective validation strategy for determination and validation of column life span: performing studies at both small and manufacturing scales.

very expensive affinity chromatography media, this level of scale-down is not uncommon.

TABLE 6.3 Steps for Designing Small-Scale
Chromatography Models

- Create an effective cleaning procedure
- Use manufacturing feed stream
- Simulate manufacturing-scale chromatography system
- Maintain bed height and linear flow rates (contact time)
- Apply proportional sample load and maintenance solutions

In this section, we will briefly review some of the guidelines that should be considered while generating a scale-down model for performing life span studies. These are listed in Table 6.3. The topic of "scale-down modeling" is discussed in much more detail in Chapter 4.

First, a procedure needs to be identified or created that can be used for effective cleaning of the chromatography column. A recently published study highlighted the importance of having optimal cleaning and sanitization procedures [20]. The study was performed using DEAE-Sepharose CL-6B anion-exchange media used in purification of prothrombin-complex concentrate from cryoprecipitate-depleted human plasma. The authors used a recycling procedure that includes two NaCl washes: one before and one after hydroxide washes. They found that although the majority of the material is removed during the first NaCl wash, the second wash removes material that has been solubilized by the NaOH. The cleaning and storage procedures that resulted from this investigation were found to significantly reduce carryover on the column and could be expected to have a positive effect on column life span.

Second, experiments should be performed using manufacturing feed stream or a feed stream that is representative of manufacturing scale. Prior to implementation of this work, the cell culture or fermentation conditions, including additives, should be well defined.

Third, attempts should be made to mimic the manufacturing-scale chromatography system as much as possible or account for the deviations by using similar or appropriate components (e.g., identical chemicals in contact with product where possible) and configurations (e.g., distance from column outlet to monitor should be appropriately scaled). Inevitable differences may occur due to differences in flow cell path lengths and diameters, tubing diameter, availability of similar wetted materials, etc. Where deviations occur, however, they should be noted. The preferred approach is to compare the scaled-down model to the manufacturing scale in terms of the various performance criteria, which depend on the objective of the column. These performance criteria are discussed in more detail in the next section. If significant differences exist between the two scales, a careful determination of the impact of these differences should be made and, if necessary, the small-scale model should be redesigned. In any case, having a qualified scaled-down model "prior" to performing small-scale cycling studies is necessary, and using a scaled-down model that is flawed would only lead to unreliable life span study results and a waste of time and resources. In cases where satisfactory scale-down cannot be performed, Strategy 1 outlined in Figure 6.1 can be used for determining column life span, provided life span studies do not require virus clearance evaluation or clearance of other hazardous substances.

Fourth, for most cases it is recommended to maintain bed height and linear flow velocity when scaling down. The ICH guideline on viral safety states that the validity of the scaling down should be demonstrated and that column bed height should be shown to be representative of commercial-scale manufacturing [21]. However, it is often possible to scale down without maintaining the bed height, as long as residence time is maintained [22]. And in some cases, it is simply not realistic to maintain the bed height. For example, in several cases firms have scaled down immobilized Protein A columns without maintaining bed height. In at least one case, the scaled-down column had a bed height that was reduced twofold from full scale. If linear flow rate cannot be maintained, retention time must be kept constant by changing the bed height. As with any such deviations from a guideline such as those produced by ICH, it is advisable to discuss the plan with regulators prior to implementation.

TABLE 6.4 Comparison of Performance of Small-Scale Model
with Full-Scale Manufacturing Column

Scale	Cycle #	Yield, %	CHOP[a], ppm	DNA, ppm	Protein A, ppm
Small scale	1	88.7	75	<0.006	<7.8
	51	88.3	34	0.01	<7.8
Manufacturing scale	1	84.6	116	<0.07	<7.8
	50	81.1	72	<0.03	<7.8

[a] Chinese hamster ovary proteins (host-cell proteins).
Source: Adapted from O'Leary, R.M., Feuerheim, D., Peers, D., Xu, Y., and Blank, G.S., *Biopharm*, 14, 10–18, 2001. With permission.

Fifth, apply proportional sample load to chromatography media volume. Where possible, apply the worst-case parameters to provide a safety margin. For adsorption techniques, total protein should be kept within the established specifications for manufacturing (usually expressed as grams total protein per liter of chromatography media). For gel filtration techniques, it is critical that the percentage of sample volume relative to column volume be kept within established production specifications, preferably toward the upper limit. Sample concentration should also be constant. Maintain constant ratios of wash, elution, regeneration, cleaning, and equilibration volumes relative to chromatography media volume. Buffers should be made according to manufacturing SOPs.

Table 6.4 presents an example of a successful scale-down of a cation-exchange chromatography step and its use for measuring column life span [18]. It is observed that at both scales the step yields are comparable and the key functions of the column step, i.e., reduce Chinese hamster ovary proteins (CHOP) and DNA and clear Protein A, are met at both the scales.

6.3.2 Parameters to Measure

Since the purpose of small-scale cycling studies is to determine or demonstrate life span for a chromatography column, a variety of functional, chemical, and physical parameters can

TABLE 6.5 Commonly Measured Parameters for Small-Scale Models

- Chromatographic profile and related parameters
- Product yield and purity
- Clearance of impurities
- Column qualification measurements (HETP and Asymmetry)
- Pressure/flow
- Media particle properties
- Product carryover (blank runs)
- End-of-life testing

be measured to ensure that the media will perform over the targeted number of reuses. The logical approach is to pick parameters that would be expected to affect the ability of the column in achieving its objective. In the following, we list and discuss some of these operating and performance parameters that have been used in the industry to successfully determine column life span. It is expected that the reader will take these as suggestions and pick those that make the most sense to the application under consideration.

Table 6.5 lists some of the operating and performance parameters that are commonly used to monitor column integrity during cycling studies. These are discussed in more detail in the following text.

6.3.2.1 Chromatographic Profile

This is the simplest observation one can make to observe changes in performance. Often, however, production chromatograms look like mountain slopes and changes are hard to decipher. Experiences collected in process development and transferred to production will enable the observer to judge the quality of the chromatogram and assess whether it reflects a change in performance.

Since comparison of the chromatogram is qualitative, several attributes have been used to quantitate this analysis. These include pool volume, absorbance, and conductivity at start of pool collection, absorbance and conductivity at end of pool collection, number of column volumes (CVs) from gradient start to start of pool collection, A280 and conductivity at peak maximum, peak area for collection, number of CVs from gradient start to peak maximum, and number of CVs from gradient start to end of pool collection. As is evident, the objective of all these parameters is to be able to spot any trends or deviations in the chromatographic profile with increasing number of cycles. Care should be taken in drawing conclusions, however, since changes in retention are often influenced by variability in the feed stream. This is particularly true for cell culture, even more so for continuous cultures. Figure 6.3 shows a plot of conductivity of the column eluent at start collect, peak maximum, and stop collect versus number of cycles. It is seen that the data are indicative of a consistent chromatographic profile over the 250 cycles that were investigated.

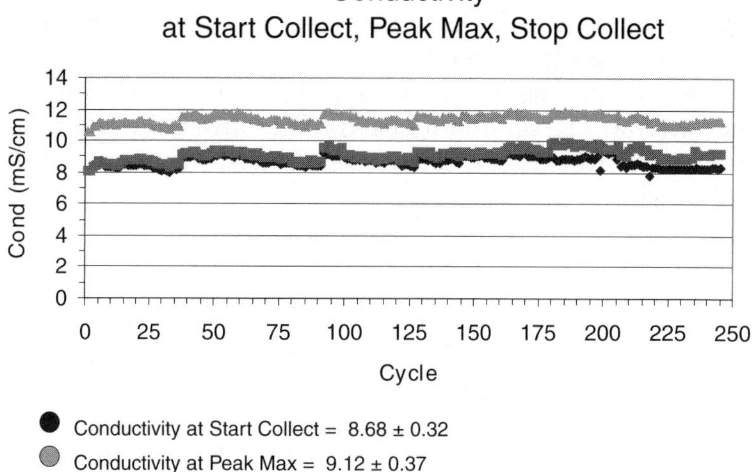

Figure 6.3 Conductivity at start collect, peak maximum, and end collect for an ion-exchange column as a function of the number of reuses (CM Sepharose High Performance® media, 2.6 cm diameter, 18 cm bed height). Data kindly provided by Karen Dane and Jim Seely, Amgen, Inc.

6.3.2.2 Product Yield and Purity

For most applications, quality of the final product is a key performance criterion for a chromatographic step. Product yield is also important to ensure consistent performance over column life span. Evaluation of both purity and impurity profiles by multiple orthogonal methods (e.g., IEC HPLC, SDS-PAGE) measures the ability of the media to remove specific impurities relevant to this step in the process. In some cases, it may also be necessary to perform a biological assay. These determinations can be performed at an appropriate interval, depending on the targeted media life span.

6.3.2.3 Clearance of Impurities

In most cases, chromatographic steps are used not only to separate product-related impurities, but also to provide clearance for host cell impurities (e.g., host cell proteins, endotoxin, nucleic acids, lipids, viruses) and process-related impurities (e.g., raw materials, additives). For example, DNA and bovine IgG may need to be removed from cell culture products, and endotoxin and DNA from *E. coli* products. It is essential to assess removal of these specific impurities over media life span. If, for example, a given step is designed to remove DNA and deamidated forms of a protein product, then the relevant assays should be performed to confirm consistent removal of these impurities to the specified level. This is particularly important for specific impurities that require spiking studies or those whose presence in the final product adversely affects its safety, potency, or efficacy.

One area of particular concern for cell culture products is the ability of the chromatographic media to remove viruses after repeated usage. Since viral clearance testing is quite costly, this work requires some special considerations. It is not realistic to test every few runs. For example, one firm tested the ability of Protein A Sepharose Fast Flow to remove viruses in the first, eleventh, and thirty-fourth cycles. Work performed in the plasma fractionation industry indicates no loss of ability to remove viruses after more than 400 cycles [23]. More recently, Brorson et al. have shown that retroviral clearance was not impacted for 100 cycles beyond the point that an immobilized Protein A media quality deteriorated [24].

6.3.2.4 Column Qualification Measurements

Periodic determinations (at an appropriate interval) of HETP and asymmetry (A_s) can be useful in pointing to any deterioration in column integrity with reuse. These measurements are particularly important for gel filtration steps but may not always be relevant, e.g., in "on-off" step gradient separations commonly found early in a purification process

6.3.2.5 Pressure/Flow

A buildup of impurities can result in an increase in pressure or decrease in flow. Changes in pressure or flow can also indicate compression or breakdown of the media, or clogging of column screens, nets, or in-line filters. Pressure at certain process points can thus be a useful indicator of the physical stability of the media and can easily be monitored for each cycle. Figure 6.4 shows a plot of pressure drop across an ion-exchanger column at the end of the loading step versus number of column reuses. It is seen that the pressure drop slowly increases from an average of 40 psi to 45 psi after 450 reuses, indicating a slight buildup over time.

6.3.2.6 Chromatography Media Properties

Various physicochemical attributes of the media particles can be used to characterize fouling of the chromatography column during reuse. Some of these attributes are typically listed in the certificate of analysis provided by the media manufacturer. Criteria often evaluated during ion exchange reuse studies include small-ion capacity, total protein capacity, particle-size distribution, flow-versus-pressure curves, and total organic carbon (TOC) removed by extreme cleaning solutions [15]. A comparison of results obtained from media at the end of life span to the corresponding values for fresh media can yield an insight into the mechanism of media fouling, e.g.,

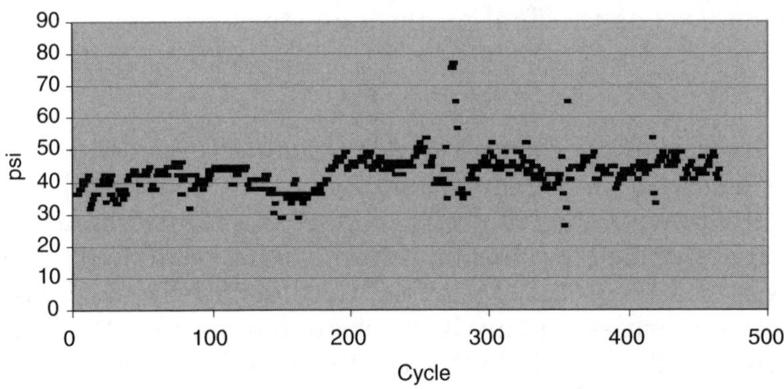

Figure 6.4 Pressure drop across the column at the end of the loading step for an ion-exchange column as a function of the number of reuses (S Sepharose Fast Flow® media, 2.6 cm diameter, 25 cm bed height). Data kindly provided by Dana Becker, David Dripps, and Jim Seely, Amgen, Inc.

buildup in column pressure along with a reduction in mean particle diameter indicates breaking of media particles due to shear experienced during column repacking.

6.3.2.7 Blank Runs

Performing blank runs periodically (at an appropriate interval) is commonly used to evaluate efficacy of cleaning and potential of product carryover. In a blank run, the column is operated following the normal procedure except that the load is substituted with water or buffer. When gradient elution is used, the elution pool is collected in the same portion of the gradient where the product is typically pooled and is analyzed for any product-related or other impurity. Analytical techniques often utilized for this purpose include product-related assays (if they have the required sensitivity), SDS-PAGE, silver stain, TOC, and total protein assays. The target must be set appropriately, based on the quality of the feed material and function of the column, i.e., the target can be higher for a capture column that is being loaded with the crude cell broth and can be more stringent for a polishing column that is being used as the final purification step.

6.3.2.8 End of Media Lifespan Testing

This is typically performed to demonstrate that media that has surpassed the targeted number of reuses can still successfully provide the required clearance of specific impurities and the specified product or intermediate purity. In some cases, it can be useful to use feed that has been spiked with the key impurities that are being cleared in the step. Performing this study may help reduce the risk in implementing column life spans determined at small scale to manufacturing scale.

An example of measurable parameters of column performance over time is shown in Table 6.6. Drevin et al. observed a decrease in retention volume, bed height, and peak height during 300 analytical separations. These decreases were attributed to protein clogging of the top filter [25]. Optimization of the washing procedure and column configuration improved column performance. This example illustrates the value of small-scale studies that allow for improvements to be made prior to scaling up for full-scale manufacturing and further extending media life span.

TABLE 6.6 Changes in Performance over 300 Cycles

Run No.	Bed Height, cm	Cl⁻ Capacity, mmol	Retention Vol, ml			
			Peak I	Peak II	Peak III	Peak IV
1	10.2	3.53 ± 0.08	48.87	74.04	84.69	100.74
150	9.5	3.53 ± 0.08	47.19	72.81	82.89	99.48
250	8.9	No data	46.98	71.70	82.62	99.27
300	8.9	3.54 ± 0.07	47.91	73.14	84.00	99.12

Source: Adapted from Reference 25.

A recently published study showed the utility of performing combined reuse and characterization studies for a cation-exchange column, Macroprep High-S, used as the capture step in the manufacturing process for Neuleze, a nerve growth factor [26]. The effect of multiple parameters on the percent yield and clearance of impurities, such as host cell proteins, DNA, and a cell culture media component, was evaluated. Various fermentation lots, equilibration pH, elution pH, and absorbance at start of collection were investigated. This was achieved via a DOE (design of experiment) consisting of 42 experiments, and it was concluded that the media could be reused for 42 cycles. Approaches such as DOE can lead to a considerable savings in time and resources that are required to perform these studies.

6.3.3   Concurrent Validation at Pilot or Full Scale

In addition to the model columns that allow for large numbers of cycles to be run, analyses must be performed on production columns to determine media life span. This is typically done during preparation of consistency batches and concurrently in production. The operating and performance parameters that should be monitored at full scale are similar to the ones mentioned in Section 6.3.2 and are typically chosen based on the results from small-scale studies. Most firms routinely monitor both bioburden and endotoxin. These determinations are more a reflection of compliance with GMPs than media life span, but they remain useful to establish that good hygiene routines are being followed over the life span of the packed column and are usually necessary in the event a column is unpacked, cleaned, and repacked. Small-scale end-of-life-span testing can be performed using media from a manufacturing column that has reached the targeted life span. This type of study may provide an additional safety margin.

Table 6.7 shows representative data from a very large-scale manufacturing facility producing Phase III clinical material on three ion exchange columns. The process was fully validated at the time these data were collected, and a comprehensive monitoring program was in place to justify

TABLE 6.7 Data from Monitoring of Ion-Exchange Chromatography Columns in a Large-Scale Manufacturing Facility

452 L S-Sepharose Fast-Flow Column

No. Cycles Prior to Chromatogram	41	300
Cumulative Cycle No.	41	341
Most recent HETP	0.04 cm	0.04 cm
Yield (%)	79	86
Start	1.51	1.55
Peak	2.25	2.3
End	2.78	2.81
Width	1.27	1.25

378 L Q-Sepharose Fast-Flow Column

No. Cycles Prior to Chromatogram	26	208
Cumulative Cycle No.	26	234
Most Recent HETP	0.05 cm	0.02 cm
Yield (%)	82	80
Start	2.26	2.59
Peak	2.97	3.14
End	3.46	3.65
Width	1.20	1.06

452 L CM-Sepharose Fast-Flow Column

No. Cycles Prior to Chromatogram	25	208
Cumulative Cycle No.	25	233
Most Recent HETP	0.04 cm	0.04 cm
Yield (%)	70	74
Start	3.00	2.85
Peak	3.16	2.99
End	3.52	3.49
Width	0.52	0.64

Note: Data kindly provided by Holly Hutchins and Robert Seely, Amgen, Inc.

continued reuse. Media replacement was based on 1 year's use (potentially 1000 cycles) and not based on the number of cycles. Two runs are shown in the table for each of the three ion exchange columns used in manufacturing. Two chromatograms from each column were selected —one from the early part of the campaign and a later one. Peak profile and position were evaluated. Column yield from each run was also noted along with an estimate of the number of cycles prior to the selected chromatograms. HETP tests were performed on the columns every fifth batch, and the most recent HETP value for each of the column cycles is shown in the tables. Although there is some variability, for example, in the yield for the S Sepharose Fast Flow column, the preestablished specifications for yield and retention position were met.

6.4 EXPERIMENTAL APPROACHES TO DETERMINE AND VALIDATE FILTRATION MEDIA LIFE SPAN

The key concepts that form the underlying basis for determination and validation of life span for chromatography media also apply for filtration media. Hence, this section will focus on aspects that are unique to filtration. The commonly used approach is to use small-scale data for "guidance" followed by "confirmation" and "validation" at full scale. While this discussion is more focused on tangential flow filtration (TFF) applications, some aspects apply to depth flow (DF) filtration applications as well.

6.4.1 Small-Scale Models

Table 6.8 reviews guidelines that could be useful when creating a scale-down model for a filtration step. Once again, this discussion focuses on the issue of media life span. A more detailed discussion is provided in Chapter 4.

First, an effective cleaning and sanitization procedure is identified. It is common to try the vendor-recommended procedures, as they are supported with data from the required leachables/extractables studies. Cleaning/sanitizing solutions

TABLE 6.8   Design of Small-Scale Filtration
Models

- Create an effective cleaning procedure
- Use manufacturing feed stream
- Simulate manufacturing-scale filtration system
- Use identical operating conditions

tend to be reactive and corrosive, and hence care must be taken to operate within the concentrations, temperatures, contact times, and other conditions that are covered by the vendor's package. If, for some reason, a new solution has to be used or conditions outside those recommended by the vendor have to be used, one has to plan for performing the appropriate leachables/extractables studies. These studies, however, tend to be time-consuming and expensive. The issue of extractables from product contact surfaces was recently reviewed [27].

Second, experiments should be performed using feed material that is manufactured at full scale. This is particularly true for process streams in the upstream portion of the process, since unit operations such as centrifugation and homogenization are difficult if not impossible to mimic at lab scale. As a result, the feed material in the laboratory may not be representative of full scale in terms of the amount of host cell impurities and other constituents. These impurities, such as endotoxin and DNA, have a significant impact on the life span of a filter. Thus, it is best to use feed material generated at full scale or representative of pilot scale.

Third, an attempt should be made to have an accurate scale-down system. Step recovery for ultrafiltration/diafiltration at lab scale is often marred by considerable losses due to high system holdup volume relative to the final pool volume. While it may not be possible to achieve the exact recovery that could be obtained at pilot or manufacturing scale, care must be taken to minimize the differences in performance of the step across the two scales. This can be achieved by ensuring that the system design reflects the manufacturing scale. Further, it is important that the membrane material and the design format of the cassette be identical to that used at manufacturing scale.

Fourth, it is common to keep membrane area per unit amount of product the same while scaling down, i.e., operate at identical protein loading as compared to the large scale. It is recommended to make buffers using the appropriate SOPs and keeping the other operating conditions such as pH, ionic strength, temperature, transmembrane pressure (TMP), and cross-flow rate identical to large scale.

6.4.2 Parameters to Measure

Table 6.9 lists some of the operating and performance parameters that are commonly used to monitor filter integrity during cycling studies. These are discussed in more detail in the following text. Once again, the parameters that are chosen for monitoring and their specifications or control ranges depend on the intended application.

6.4.2.1 Normalized Water Permeability (NWP)

Percent recovery of NWP is perhaps the most commonly used performance parameter for monitoring the integrity of a UF/DF (ultrafiltration/diafiltration) membrane and should be performed after every reuse in the life span study. This parameter measures the permeability of the membrane using water and allows for a comparison of the integrity of the membrane pre- and postuse. Percent recovery of NWP typically declines with number of uses since every time the membrane is used,

TABLE 6.9 Commonly Measured
Parameters for Small-Scale Models

- Normalized water permeability (NWP)
- Product yield and purity
- Clearance of impurities
- Filter integrity measurements
- TMP vs. flux curves
- Filter analysis
- Product carryover (blank runs)

product or other species in the feed material can bind to the pores of the membrane, causing decay in the permeability. It is very common to use NWP criteria for determining the number of cycles a membrane should be used, e.g., 75–125% of original NWP. While the filter vendors provide the criteria for a particular membrane product, it is recommended that cycling studies be performed by the user, and a variety of performance criteria should be monitored. The data should then be evaluated to determine the appropriate NWP criteria for the specific application under consideration.

6.4.2.2 Product Yield and Purity

Just as for chromatographic separations, product yield and purity should be monitored at an appropriate interval during the life span study. This is to ensure that product degradation is not induced due to repeated use of the membrane. This is particularly important if one is using particularly reactive cleaning solutions, such as bleach. Minute amounts of carry-over of the bleach in the system can result in a significant increase in product-related impurities in the final pool.

6.4.2.3 Clearance of Impurities

Filtration steps are often used for clearance of host cell-related as well as process-related impurities. This clearance of the appropriate impurities should be monitored during reuse studies at an appropriate interval to demonstrate that the "efficacy" of the step in performing the clearance is not marred by reuse.

6.4.2.4 Filter Integrity Measurements

These measurements are used to identify problems such as macroscopic holes in the membrane, cracks in the seals, or improperly seated modules, which can lead to product leakage or unsatisfactory clearance of impurities [28]. A common way to do this is via an air diffusion test. When air is applied to the retentate side at a controlled pressure, it diffuses through water in the pores at a predictable rate. However, in the presence of any defects, the air flows through at a significantly higher rate and, thus, fails the test value. Such measurements could easily be performed after every reuse.

Besides air diffusion, several other tests are also employed to evaluate membrane integrity. These include bubble point determination and pressure hold–decay test [29–31]. It is recommended that the reader evaluate the applicability of these different tests to the application under consideration and then pick the appropriate integrity testing method. A more detailed discussion on the various approaches is presented in Chapter 7.

6.4.2.5 Transmembrane Pressure (TMP) versus Flux Curves

TMP is the average applied pressure from the feed to the filtrate side of the membrane. As TMP increases, the flux across the membrane typically increases such that the slope of the curve keeps decreasing with increasing TMP. These curves serve as a good indicator of the performance of a filtration step and are commonly used as a qualitative measurement. A carryover of product or impurities often results in decay of the TMP–flux curve. Measurements at an appropriate interval can be useful in deciding an appropriate life span for a membrane. It is recommended that these curves be obtained at three different cross-flow rates that span the range of manufacturer recommendations [27].

6.4.2.6 Filter Analysis

With the advent of new and more sensitive spectroscopic methods such as Fourier transform infrared Raman (FTIR) spectroscopy, it is possible to analyze the filter surface and quantify the buildup of protein or absence of such. This kind of analysis, at least at the end of intended filter life span, can be done in consultation with the filter vendor and can be useful in characterization of filter fouling.

6.4.2.7 Blank Runs

Performing blank runs periodically (at an appropriate interval) is commonly used to evaluate efficacy of cleaning and potential of product carryover. In the case of the blank run, filtration is performed using load material that does not contain any product, and the resulting pool is analyzed for any product-related or other impurity. Just as for chromatographic separations, analytical techniques often utilized for this purpose include HPLC assays, SDS-PAGE, and total organic carbon analysis.

6.4.3 Concurrent Validation at Pilot or Full Scale

Once the life span studies have been performed at small scale, a target for number of reuses is set. Next, full-scale runs are performed to determine filter life span. This can be done during preparation of consistency batches and concurrently in production [32,33]. Appropriate operating and performance parameters are monitored at full scale. As mentioned previously, blank runs should be performed at an appropriate interval at full scale to show absence of any carryover.

6.5 CONCLUSIONS

In this chapter, we have discussed the various factors that influence useful life span of chromatography and filtration media and also the key operating and performance parameters that are utilized to monitor integrity of the media. It is clear that determining life span of chromatography and filtration media requires several approaches and evaluation of multiple parameters. The key output of this effort is in the form of a validation report that presents the results from qualification of the scale-down model and data from the small-scale and large-scale studies in a concise tabular form for evaluation by regulatory authorities.

It is always advantageous to build in a safety margin by performing an excess number of runs at small scale before implementing the targeted life span at manufacturing scale. Figure 6.5 shows a plot of the cost of chromatography media,

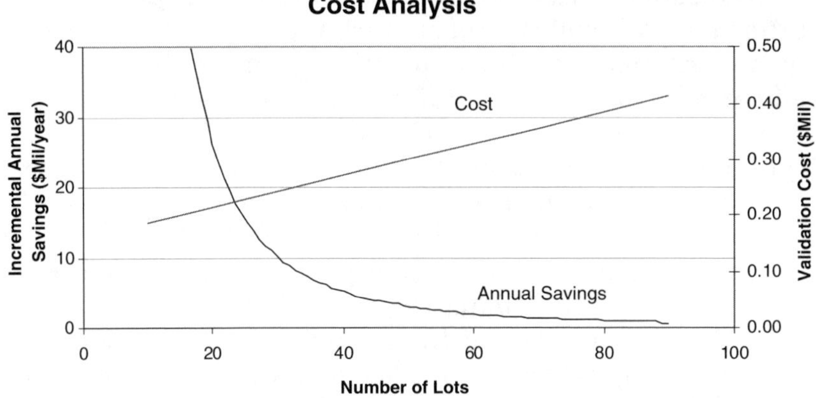

Number of Lots	Incremental Annual Savings ($M/year)		ValidationCost ($M)	
10	$	112.67	$	0.19
30	$	14.86	$	0.24
50	$	2.97	$	0.30
70	$	1.27	$	0.36
90	$	0.71	$	0.41

Figure 6.5   Cost analysis for an Amgen product — cost of media, validation cost, and net savings as a function of number of reuses. Data provided by Traci Taggart, Amgen, Inc.

cost of validation, and net savings as a function of the number of reuses for an Amgen product [34]. It is seen that while the cost of new media decreases with increasing number of media reuses, the cost of validating media life span increases. Thus, the number of reuses targeted is a function of the application under consideration and various factors such as cost of chromatography or filtration media, number of batches to be run every year, gap between different campaigns when the media will be needed to be stored, resources available to the project, etc. It is not uncommon for the same company to perform different sets of activities for different products.

Indications of deterioration in chromatography and filtration media include loss of product purity, recovery, or capacity and changes in the impurities' profile. More specific indications involve monitoring of changes in retention time/volume, pressure–flow curves, HETP, and A_s for chromatography media, and testing of the NWP and filter integrity for filters. Use of blank runs to evaluate carryover is currently the *de facto* standard for either kind of media.

In this chapter, we have attempted to present the current approach toward determination and validation of media life span. However, in view of the dynamism that results from tightening regulatory standards and different successful approaches that companies take, it is essential to continue to challenge and evolve one's approach and stay abreast of further developments.

ACKNOWLEDGMENTS

The authors would like to acknowledge Jim Seely and Robert Seely, Amgen Inc., Colorado, for their helpful comments.

REFERENCES

1. Rathore, A.S., Levine, H., Latham, P., Curling, J., and Kaltenbrunner, O., Costing issues in production of biopharmaceuticals, *Biopharm*, January 2004.

2. European Commission, The Rules Governing Medicinal Products in the European Union, Vol. III, Addendum 3, Guidelines on the quality, safety and efficacy of medicinal products for human use, Production and Quality Control of Medicinal Products Derived by Recombinant DNA Technology, III/3477/92, pp. 47–56.

3. Chang, A., oral presentation, Chromatography: FDA Regulator's Experience WCBP, Washington, D.C., January 2002.

4. U.S. FDA, Compliance Program, Chapter 41, Inspection of Licensed Therapeutic Products, March 1999.

5. Cherney, B., CBER's Expectations on Determining Resin Lifespan, FDA/PDA Process Validation Meeting, Washington, D.C., 2000.

6. U.S. FDA, Points to Consider in the Manufacture and Testing of Monoclonal Antibody Products for Human Use, U.S. Dept. of Health and Human Services, FDA, CBER, February 1997.

7. Viral Safety Evaluation of Biotechnology Products Derived from Cell Lines of Human or Animal Origin, ICH, 1997.

8. EMEA, CPMP Position Statement on DNA and Host Cell Proteins (HCP) Impurities, Routine Testing Versus Validation Studies, CPMP/BWP/382/97, http://www.eudra.org/emea.html.

9. Data from South African Blood Transfusion Center, Durban.

10. Rathore, A.S., Sobacke, S.E., Kocot, T.J., Morgan, D.R., Dufield, R.L., and Mozier, N.M., Analysis for residual host cell proteins and DNA in process streams of a recombinant protein product expressed in E. coli cells, *J. Pharm. Biomed. Anal.*, 32, 1199–1211, 2003.

11. Data File: Expanded Bed Adsorption, Uppsala, Sweden, 1996.

12. Rathore, A.S. and Velayudhan, A., An overview of scale-up in preparative chromatography, in *Scale-up and Optimization in Preparative Chromatography*, Rathore, A.S. and Velayudhan, A., Eds., Marcel Dekker, New York, 2002, pp. 1–32.

13. Dasarathy, Y., A validatable cleaning-in-place protocol for total DNA clearance from an anion exchange resin, *BioPharm*, 9, 41–44, 1996.

14. Feldman, F., Chandra, S., Hrinda, M.E., and Schreiber, A.B., Quality assurance in production of plasma proteins, in *Quality Assurance in Transfusion Medicine*, Vol. 2, CRC Press, Boca Raton, FL, 1993, pp. 259–284.

15. Seely, R.J., Wight, H.D., Fry, H.H., Rudge, S.R., and Slaff, G.F., Validation of chromatography resin useful life, *BioPharm*, 7, 41–48, 1994.

16. Sofer, G. and Hagel, L., *Handbook of Process Chromatography*, Academic Press, London, 1997.

17. Gagnon, P., *Purification Tools for Monoclonal Antibodies*, Validated Biosystems, Inc., Tucson, AZ, 1996.

18. O'Leary, R.M., Feuerheim, D., Peers, D., Xu, Y., and Blank, G.S., Determining the useful lifespan of chromatography resins, *Bio-Pharm*, 14, 10–18, 2001.

19. Rathore, A.S., Explore an Approach to Process Validation for an Acceptable Validation Package, Course on Process Validation, Barnett International, Philadelphia, PA, January 2003.

20. Turton, J. and Moola, Z., Storing an ion-exchange chromatography gel in dilute alkali during recycling improves cleaning, *BioPharm*, April, 24–30, 2002.

21. ICH, Quality of Biotechnological Products: Viral Safety Evaluation of Biotechnology Products Derived from Cell Lines of Human or Animal Origin, International Conference on Harmonization Step 4, March 1997.

22. Yamamoto, S., Nomura, M., and Sano, Y., Resolution of proteins in linear gradient elution ion exchange and hydrophobic interaction chromatography, *J. Chromatogr.*, 409, 101–110, 1987.

23. Andersson, L., Connor, S.E., Lindquist, L.-O., and Watson, E.A., A Validation Study for the Removal/Inactivation of Viruses during a Chromatographic Process for Albumin and IgG, oral presentation, International Society of Blood Transfusion, Japan, March 1996.

24. Brorson, K., Identification of Chromatography Performance Quality Attributes to Assure the Retrovirus Clearance of Multiply Cycled Resins, poster presentation, prep 2000.

25. Drevin, I., Larsson, L., and Johansson, B.-L., Column performance of Q-Sepharose HP in analytical- and preparative-scale chromatography, *J. Chromatogr.*, 477, 337–344, 1989.

26. Breece, T.N., Gilkerson, E., and Schmelzer, C., Validation of large-scale chromatographic processes, *BioPharm*, July, 35–42, 2002.

27. Bennan, J., Bing, F., Boone, H., Fernandez, J., Seely, B., van Denise, H., and Miller, D., Evaluation of extractables from product-contact surfaces, *Biopharm Int.*, December, 22–34, 2002.

28. Millipore Technical Brief, Protein Concentration and Diafiltration by Tangential Flow Filtration.

29. Jornitz, M.W., Agalloco, J.P., Akers, J.E., Madsen, R.E., and Meltzer, T.H., Filter integrity testing in liquid applications, revisited, *Pharm. Tech.*, October, 34–50, 2001.

30. Sundaram, S., Brantley, J.D., Howard, G., and Brandwein, H., Considerations in using bubble point type tests as filter integrity tests, *Pharm. Tech.*, September, 90–114, 2000.

31. Trotter, A.M., Meltzer, T.H., Bai, F., and Thoma, L., The effects of bacterial cell loading, *Pharm. Tech.*, March, 72–80, 2000.

32. Morris, G.M., Rozembersky, J., and Schwartz, L., Validation of filtration, in *Biopharmaceutical Process Validation*, Sofer, G. and Zabriskie, D.W., Eds., Marcel Dekker, New York, 2000, pp. 213–233.

33. Parenteral Drug Association Technical Report No. 26, Suppl. Vol. 52, No. S1, Sterilizing Filtration of Liquids, 1998.

34. Taggart, T., Dripps, D., Cameron, M., Kessler, T., Seely, J., and Todd, B., Resin Reuse Validation and Evaluation of Performance over Resin Lifespan, ACS National Meeting, March 2003.

7

Validation of a Filtration Step

JENNIFER CAMPBELL

CONTENTS

7.1 FILTRATION VALIDATION OVERVIEW

Process validation has been defined by the FDA as "establishing documented evidence which provides a high degree of assurance that a specific process will consistently produce a product meeting its predetermined specifications and quality attributes" (FDA, 1987). It is an assurance that a process is robust and reproducible and will consistently produce a product that meets specifications. Validation is born out of Good Manufacturing Practices (GMPs), which require that quality be built into a manufacturing process. The process must exhibit control at each step or unit operation. Sources of variation must be identified, and these variations must be controlled and monitored. Final testing of the product is not sufficient to ensure quality.

Validation is a matter of proving a claim regarding the performance of a device or unit operation. Filters have functions relating to flow rate, throughput, sterilizability, organism or particle retention, extractable levels, particle shedding, product stability, compatibility, toxicity, nonpyrogenicity, and thermal and pressure tolerance. The manufacturer is best equipped to assess some of these functions, and most manufacturers document claims of sterilizability, lack of toxicity and nonpyrogenicity, maintenance of integrity under pressure, extractable levels, particle shedding, organism retention, and air and liquid flow rates as a function of pressure. The user may accept the validation claims from the filter manufacturer. However, the responsibility for validation rests with the user [1].

If a sterilizing-grade filter is used to sterile filter the product in a process, then the filter must be validated to be sterilizing grade. However, the same filter could be used to filter a process intermediate to remove particulate and reduce bioburden, but it is not intended to sterilize the process intermediate. In this case, the filter does not have to be validated to be sterilizing grade. Instead, it must be validated to remove an adequate amount of particulate and bioburden to ensure optimal performance of the downstream operations. Only the claims made regarding the performance of a filter device must be validated. A method must be developed to validate the claim, and this constitutes validation protocols.

There are three phases to the validation process: installation qualification (IQ), operational qualification (OQ), and performance qualification (PQ). Equipment validation also normally has a design qualification (DQ) or enhanced design review (EDR) as well as defining user requirements and how the design meets these requirements [2]. The IQ confirms that all equipment and components are included, properly installed, and meet the design specifications [3]. Calibration procedures are established for all components and instruments. The OQ verifies that each component in the system functions as specified in the design and that the components operate together as a system as specified. The PQ comprises the manufacturing of the drug product and the cleanability of the system. In the United States, a minimum of three manufacturing runs are required for the PQ. At present, it is a common practice to perform five manufacturing runs in support of a European filing. The following are examples of what the PQ must prove:

- All equipment in contact with the process fluids is chemically compatible and does not contaminate the product.
- System integrity is maintained.
- Passage of product (where appropriate) is sufficient.
- Retention of product (where appropriate) is sufficient.
- Passage of contaminants (where appropriate) is sufficient.
- Retention of contaminants (where appropriate) is sufficient.
- Recovery of the product is sufficient.
- Total process time is in conformance with the design.
- Finished drug product fulfills the product specifications.

- Cleaning solutions remove all residual drug product, cells, and contaminants between processing runs.

As a manufacturing drug moves through the different phases of manufacturing, emphasis on validation increases. Phase I is performed at the laboratory scale. Limited process data exist, and the drug is in clinical testing. At this point, assays may not be well developed and the process is not well defined. The final formulation may not be set. Key concerns are filter membrane selection, chemical compatibility, product and preservative binding, and assay validation. Membrane compatibility screening determines whether filter materials are compatible with the process fluid to be sterilized. Parameters evaluated before and after product exposure are water flow, membrane weight, product bubble point, and membrane visual inspection. Any effects of the filter on the product formulation need to be described, such as adsorption of preservatives, active drug substances, or extractables.

Phase II is typically performed at pilot scale. The process is more defined and assay development is progressing. Further scale-up may be required, and during scale-up, process operating parameters such as differential pressure and flow rate, temperature, and filtration time must be evaluated. Product yield should be evaluated. Integrity testing should be documented.

Phase III is typically performed at large manufacturing scale. Process validation is a requirement, as the product will be released for manufacturing if its BLA is approved. Validation includes product-specific microbial retention testing, physical compatibility testing and product-specific integrity testing (if formulation is set), filter sterilization requirements, and extractables documentation. All assays must be validated and instruments calibrated prior to initiating the process validation. Consideration should be given to the level of sensitivity of assays with respect to the level of control required in the corresponding process step. Software on automated systems must be validated. Per ICH Q7A Section 5.40, "GMP related computerized systems should be validated" [2].

The validation criteria will define the acceptable ranges of critical parameters in the process, such as pressure, flow rate, temperature, and processing time. This chapter will focus on the validation of the critical parameters of filtration unit operations, as well as the cleaning requirements and sampling plan for reuse filters such as tangential flow devices.

7.2 SCALES OF VALIDATION

The process scale at which validation occurs may differ. Certain operations may be validated using scale-down studies. This is advantageous as a cost savings and sometimes as a safety consideration. In the case of viral spiking or microbial challenge studies, scale-down experiments are often performed for safety reasons. When performing scale-down studies, it is important to mimic the process-scale conditions as closely as possible (see Figure 7.1). Despite differences in volumes, the scale-down studies should emulate the holding times, mixing times, and transfer times of the manufacturing-scale process. Maintaining these times reduces differences in product quality between the two scales. If the manufacturing process incorporates an overnight hold step at 4°C, this step must be performed in the scale-down study. However, certain aspects cannot be duplicated. If the manufacturing product is then brought to room temperature by gentle mixing in the suite over several hours, this will be difficult to duplicate in the scale-down study. The smaller volume of product will achieve room temperature more quickly, so it either will be exposed to a shorter warming time or will sit at room temperature for a longer time if mimicking the process-scale time

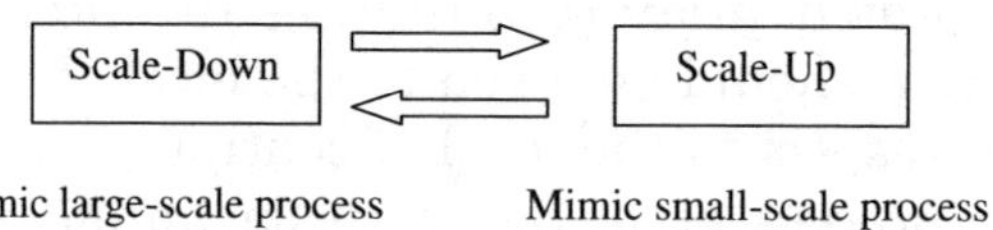

Figure 7.1 Scale-up and scale-down.

frame. In such situations, product degradation must be evaluated. Aspects that do not scale well include heat transfer rates, surface-to-volume ratios, and pumping rates.

Properties that are not affected by the scale of operation can be tested at small scale, such as compatibility, extractables, and cleanliness. Product assays measuring the effect of the filtration on the product can be performed at small scale. Bacterial retention and viral retention testing can be performed at small scale as long as the full-scale process is modeled properly. Full-scale validation should demonstrate that the scale of operation does not alter the product quality or filtration process. The filter validation can be integrated with the process validation [4].

7.3 STERILIZING-GRADE FILTER VALIDATION

Validation of sterilizing filtration focuses on retention of microbes in the feed stream and integrity testing of the filter. Other considerations are chemical compatibility of the feed stream with the filter, grow-through, adsorption, sterilizability, extractables, oxidizables, particle shedding, toxicity, and thermal and hydraulic stress resistance. Most filter manufacturers provide validation guides and services to the user. These will aid the drug manufacturer in the validation of the filter in their specific application. However, validation of the filter for its intended use is the drug manufacturer's responsibility (see Table 7.1). "If any validation task is contracted to a sterilizing filter vendor, it remains the sterile drug product manufacturer's ultimate responsibility to ensure that worst-case formulation and processing parameters are adequately studied, evaluated, and documented" (Human Drug CGMP Notes [Dec. 1995]).

7.3.1 Bacterial Retention

The definition of a sterilizing grade filter is that it retains 10^7 CFU *Brevundimonas diminuta* ATCC® 19146 or appropriate challenge organism per square centimeter of filter surface area [5]. In the biopharmaceutical industry, a filter with a

TABLE 7.1 Responsibilities of the Filter Manufacturer and the Filter User in Sterilizing Filtration Validation

Filter Manufacturer Responsibilities	Filter User Responsibilities
Validate filter manufacturing process	Audit filter vendor and outside labs
Establish specifications for integrity testing, sterilization, pressure, and temperature	Operate within manufacturer's specifications
Validate filter claims	Validate key filter claims and test methods including product compatibility, cleaning, and filter sterilization
Meet regulatory requirements for non-fiber releasing, endotoxin, toxicity, sterilizing-grade performance, and extractables	Validate filtration process Qualify operators

0.2-um pore size rating is typically used as a sterilizing-grade filter [6]. Challenge bacteria must be cultured according to ASTM® standards to ensure organism viability and prevent aggregation of the organism. The manufacturers of sterilizing-grade filters perform this destructive bacterial challenge test and correlate the results of this bacterial challenge with non-destructive integrity tests such as bubble point and diffusion. The drug manufacturer is responsible for performing these nondestructive integrity tests according to the filter manufacturer's instructions.

Some drug products may contain components that are inhibitory to the challenge organism. If this is the case, the bacterial retention challenge using the inhibitory drug product is not valid. Even though the drug product has an inhibitory effect on the challenge organism, it may not have an inhibitory effect on a naturally occurring organism in the feed stream. Two possible solutions to validating retention in this situation are as follows:

- The filter can be equilibrated with the drug product, then flushed to remove the drug product, and challenged with the appropriate organism. The filter is exposed to the drug product to prove that the product does not interact with the filter and change the pore sizes. In this case, the drug product's effects on organism size are not known.
- The inhibitory component can be removed from the feed stream and the challenge is performed with the appropriate challenge organism in the placebo feed stream [6].

7.3.2 Bubble Point Integrity Test

The bubble point test has a direct correlation with bacterial retention, whereas the diffusion test has an indirect correlation with retention. The theory behind the bubble point integrity test is that the pores of the filter membrane retain liquid due to the surface tension of the liquid and the capillary forces of the pores (see Figure 7.2). Smaller pores retain liquid more strongly than larger pores. If pressurized gas is used to displace the liquid from the pores, the largest pores become clear of liquid at a lower gas pressure than the smaller pores. This type of integrity test requires thorough wetting of the filter to be tested. The manufacturer's instructions should be consulted for the wetting volumes and pressures. Gas pressure is then slowly raised on the upstream side of the filter until

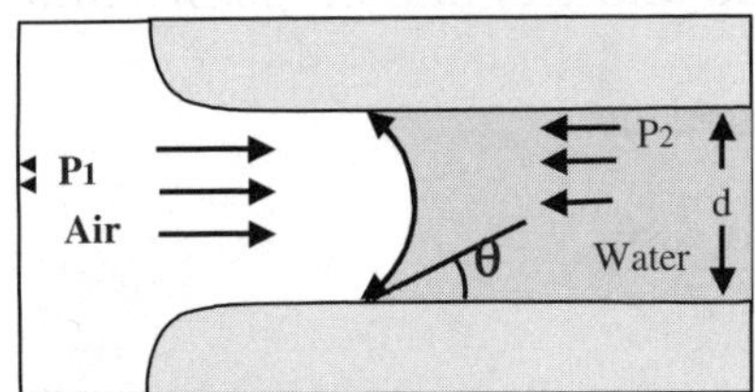

Figure 7.2 Forces within a wetted membrane pore.

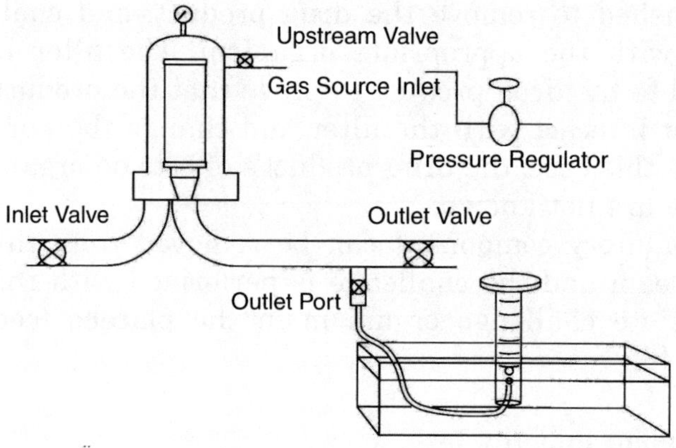

Figure 7.3 Manual integrity testing equipment setup.

liquid is displaced from the largest set of pores, allowing bulk gas flow through the filter. In a manual test, downstream gas flow is monitored by placing the outlet tube in a container of liquid (see Figure 7.3).

Bubble point can be used to determine the pressure at which the largest set of pores allows bulk gas flow. It can also be used to determine the pore size of an unknown filter. There is a direct correlation between the size of the pores and the pressure required to release the liquid wetting the pores [5]. This can be displayed graphically as the relationship between the microbial log reduction value and the bubble point value (see Figure 7.4).

The bubble point is expressed as

$$BP = \frac{4k\gamma\cos\theta}{d}$$

where

k = shape correction factor
γ = surface tension
θ = contact angle
d = pore diameter

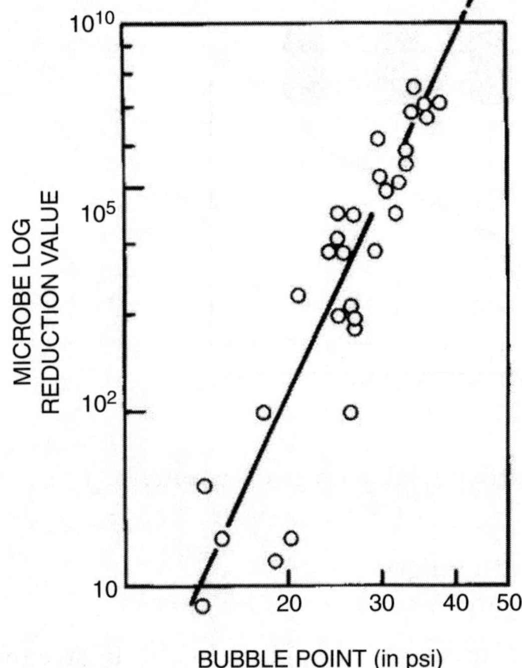

Figure 7.4 Relationship of bubble point values to microbial log reduction.

7.3.3 Diffusion Integrity Test

The diffusion test is based on the diffusivity of gas into the liquid wetting the filter membrane pores. The amount of gas diffusion into the wetting liquid is a factor of the solubility of the gas in the wetting fluid, the path length of the membrane, the membrane porosity, the gas pressure, and the total membrane area.

$$\text{Diffusion} = \frac{K(P_1 - P_2)A\rho}{L}$$

where

$\qquad\qquad K = \text{diffusivity/solubility coefficient}$

$\qquad P_1 - P_2 = \text{pressure difference across the system}$

$\qquad\qquad \rho = \text{membrane porosity}$

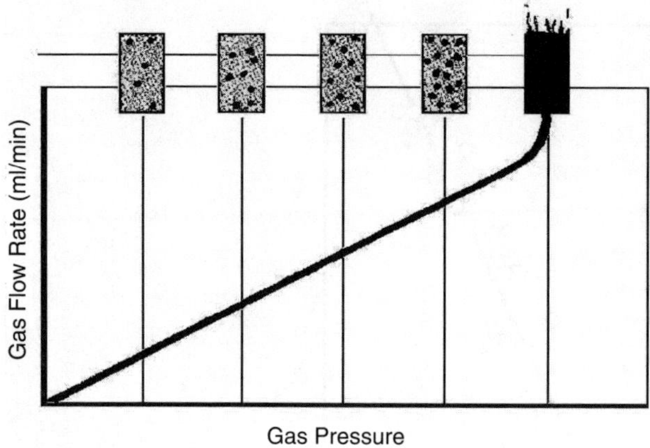

Figure 7.5   Gas pressure in relation to gas flow rate.

L = effective path length
A = membrane area

As increasing gas pressure is applied to the upstream side of the filter, the amount of gas that dissolves in the wetted pores and travels across the membrane increases (see Figure 7.5). Since diffusion is based on the porosity of the membrane and not the pore size, there is no direct correlation between the amount of gas diffusion and the pore size of the membrane. Diffusion values can be similar between membranes of different pore sizes when membranes are tested at differential pressures below their bubble points. Values above the diffusion specification indicate a gross defect in the filter or a faulty connection in the filter housing. Diffusion values should be tracked to monitor trends and outliers with respect to upper and lower quality control limits (see Figure 7.6).

Regardless of the type of integrity test selected, it is preferred by regulatory agencies to test the filter *in situ*, which means not only the filter is tested for integrity, but the housing and connections as well. A postuse integrity test is required by regulatory agencies. Preuse integrity testing is a good practice and is favorably received as part of the validation plan.

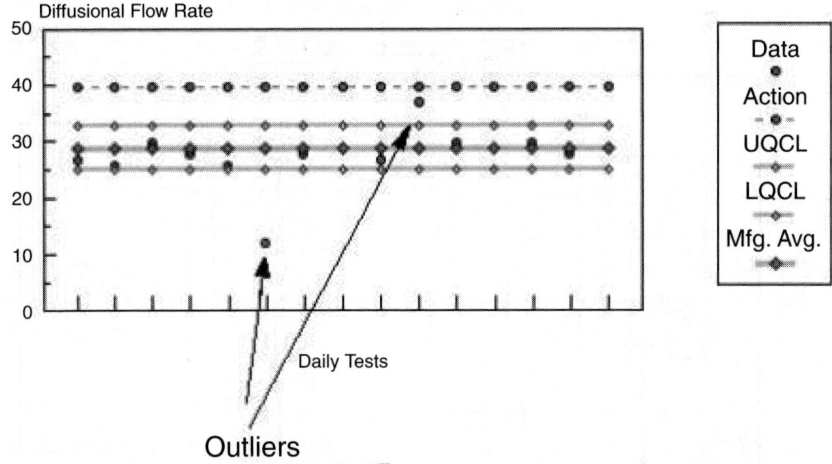

Figure 7.6 Tracking of integrity test values.

7.3.4 Integrity Test Validation

When validating integrity tests, it is crucial to follow the manufacturer's instructions. Wetting fluids, test gases, and test pressures are different between filter types (hydrophilic and hydrophobic) and pore sizes. Using the incorrect test gas (compressed air vs. nitrogen) or wetting fluid (water vs. alcohol mix) will give incorrect test results. Compressed air is more soluble than nitrogen and so results in higher diffusion rates. The most common mistake when performing integrity tests is incomplete wetting of the filter. If all the pores of the membrane are not completely wet out, bulk gas flow will occur at low pressures, causing integrity test failures. Protocols should be in place in the event of an integrity testing failure. Protocols should include checking the sealing of the filter in the housing and all connections in the system. Rewetting can be performed with increased volumes or increased wetting pressure. The decision tree in Figure 7.7 can be used to aid in the troubleshooting of integrity testing procedures.

The FDA requires written procedures detailing the sequence of actions to be taken in the event of an integrity

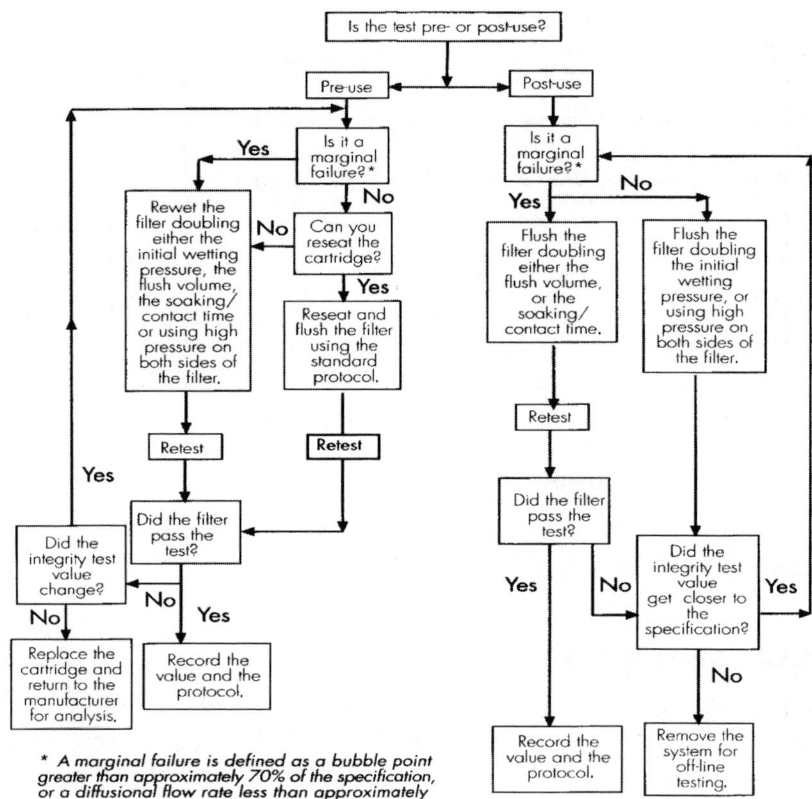

Figure 7.7   Integrity testing troubleshooting decision tree.

testing failure. If additional wetting is to be performed, the wetting volumes and pressures should be specified. If an alcohol wetting or soak is to be performed, the volumes and times, along with the alcohol flushing protocol, must be specified. Some FDA 483 observations are as follows:

- "There is no written procedure describing the actions to be taken if a nitrogen filter fails the integrity test performed according to procedures FL 124 and FL 124A."

- "There is no integrity testing of back up filter when the primary nitrogen filter fails integrity test. There may be a lag time of up to ___ production batches before testing."

7.3.5 Postuse Integrity Testing and Product Bubble Point Test

Per PDA Tech Report No. 26, "it is generally regarded as a CGMP requirement that filters or filter systems routinely be integrity tested both prior to and after use" [7]. Obtaining water-wetted bubble point values after use requires removal of the product from the filter device by flushing. Residual product can change the bubble point value of the membrane since the surface tension of the product is often different from water. Some products are very difficult to remove from the membrane and may require copious amounts of water. This can be time-consuming and costly, especially if pharmaceutical-grade water is being transported in from a separate location. There are several solutions to this problem. One is an alcohol or detergent wetting or soaking of the membrane to remove the residual formulation components, followed by a water flush to remove the alcohol or detergent. If this method is used, the flushing volume to remove the alcohol or detergent must be validated. The compatibility of the filter with the cleaning agent must also be validated [8].

A second solution is to use a lower surface tension reference fluid such as isopropyl alcohol (IPA). The surface tension of IPA is so low compared to water that it is unlikely that residual drug components will affect the IPA bubble point. Filter manufacturers often provide validated specifications for alcohol-wetted bubble points.

Another option is a product bubble point test. The bubble point of the membrane wetted with product is determined, and this value becomes the postuse integrity test specification for the bubble point. Per PDA Tech Report No. 26, "the appropriate product-wetted integrity test limit for a specific product/filter combination can be established by relating product-wetted value to the water-wetted values for the same filters"

[7]. The use of this test avoids flushing of the membrane after the product filtration, saving time and flushing fluid. It is very useful when the product is incompatible or immiscible in water, or surface active components adsorb to the membrane during the filtration. If testing is required mid-process, flushing is not required and product dilution is avoided. When validating the product bubble point, it is important to mimic the process filtration time, because components in the feed stream may adsorb to the membrane over time, changing the bubble point until the point at which the membrane is equilibrated with the product (see Figure 7.8). Because there can be variability between product lots, the product bubble point must be validated using a minimum of three product lots on a minimum of three membrane lots. Each membrane lot is tested with the water bubble point test to show consistency in the membranes. Each membrane is then tested with the product bubble point test to show consistency in the product. If the product tests are inconsistent, it can be assumed that

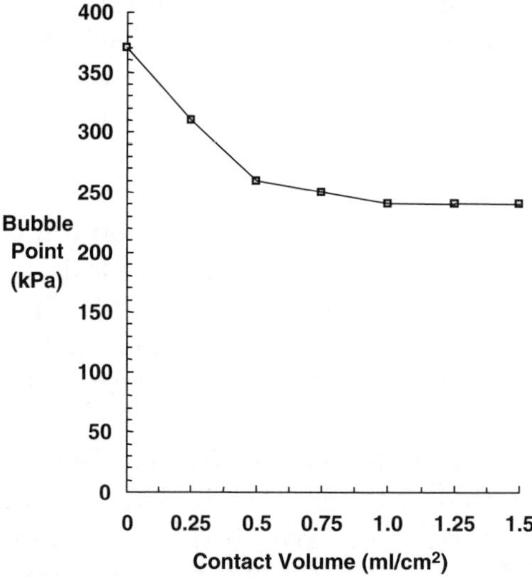

Figure 7.8 Bubble point suppression in relation to product contact volume.

Bubble Point Ratios	% of Samples Tested	Product Examples
0.4 – 0.5	2	Oil based Alcohol based
0.5 – 0.8	38	Surfactant-containing solutions, e.g., Tween
0.8 – 1.0	60	Aqueous solutions Salt solutions Sugar solutions
>1.0	<1	High salt solutions

Figure 7.9 Product bubble point ratios of over 200 sample fluids tested.

the product lots are too variable to validate a product bubble point test, and water flushing is the recommended procedure. The majority of aqueous solutions suppress the water bubble point due to a change in the surface tension of the fluid. Data in Figure 7.9 is based on over 200 solutions tested.

Preliminary testing is conducted on laboratory scale, typically using 47-mm disc filters. It is not possible for the lab to emulate exactly the size filters and conditions that will be used in the process, or the exact conditions. Per PDA Tech Report No. 26, "the scale down study is only the first part of the validation; the second part is obtaining additional ongoing product attribute data" [7]. The product bubble point is then confirmed under normal processing conditions, as part of the PQ, on three consecutive filtration runs. If the PQ results deviate from the laboratory study, then the lab validation is discarded in favor of a revalidation using filter devices in the process stream under normal processing conditions. Acceptable bubble point ratio variability is achieved by CV <5% [8]. See Figure 7.10.

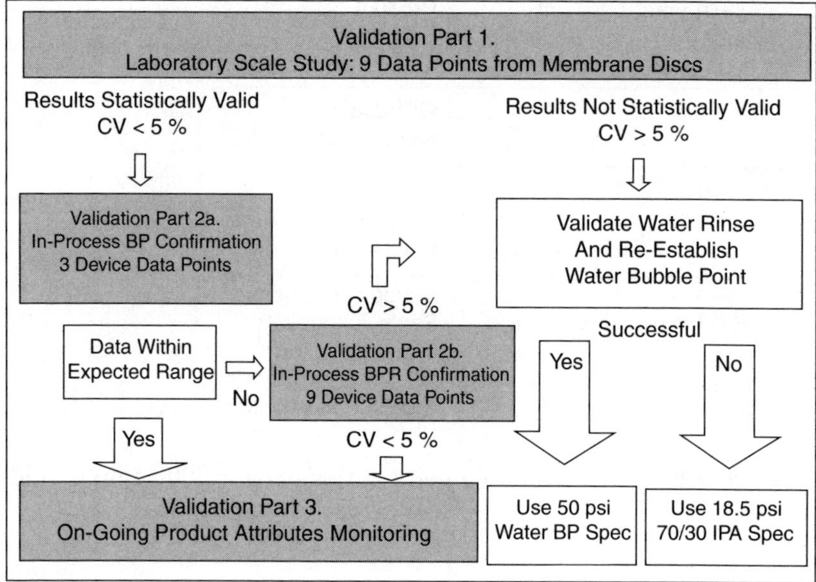

Figure 7.10 Validation of product bubble point testing.

7.3.6 Grow-Through and Endotoxin

The filter must not experience grow-through during the filtration step. If the filter is removing live bacteria, these cells can reproduce and potentially pass through the filter membrane [9]. Filtrations at higher temperatures, but not exceeding 40°C (for *B. diminuta*), represent a worst-case scenario. Grow-through can occur on a filter when liquid flow is ongoing or during static periods when the filter is wet. Even sterilizing-grade filters capable of removing $\geq 10^7$ CFU of *B. diminuta* per square centimeter of membrane area are subject to grow-through over time. This occurs when organisms divide by binary fission, and the smaller daughter cells are able to penetrate the pores of the membrane [1]. For this reason, sterile filtrations should only be performed for as long as validated to produce a sterile filtrate.

At certain stages, a process intermediate may be held for a variety of reasons, such as transport to a different processing location, pooling of multiple batches, or an unseen event delaying the downstream process. A sterilizing-grade filter is commonly used to remove bioburden from process intermediates prior to planned holds. This allows for some flexibility in the manufacturing schedule. The duration of the hold time of the process intermediate must be validated.

Endotoxin limits are confirmed to be <0.5 EU/ml using the Limulus amebocyte lysate (LAL) assay. Validation methods for the LAL assay are available from the FDA [10]. It should be noted that the LAL test is sensitive and fast but only detects endotoxin. Certain buffers may interfere with the LAL assay since it is enzyme based, and this should be accounted for in the assay validation [11]. The rabbit test can also be used to test for endotoxin, as it detects pyrogenic substances.

7.3.7 Adsorption

Filters should neither add anything to the fluid being processed (extractables) nor remove anything from the fluid being processed (adsorption). In reality, trace extractants and adsorption are likely. The purpose of validation, then, is to quantify the effects of extractables and adsorption by empirical study. The purpose of an adsorption (binding) study is to determine whether a given filter adsorbs components from a drug product. Adsorption can cause loss of drug product, conformational changes, and reduced activity and stability. If adsorptive interaction or conformational changes are discovered, the drug manufacturer must determine whether the interaction affects drug safety and efficacy. If it does, that filter is not acceptable for use in the manufacturing process. If it does not, it must be determined whether it is possible to compensate for the effect of the filter (i.e., prequenching the filter membrane with preservative to tie up the binding sites).

Product adsorption is assessed by product assays pre- and postfiltration and may be affected by other factors, such as flow rate, drug concentration, excipient concentrations, pH, ionic strength, and temperature of the solution. For this reason, it is important to conduct adsorption assays on product filled in the actual process. However, laboratory-scale adsorption studies can be useful in understanding adsorption kinetics.

Adsorption studies are most easily performed by scaling down the process volume and flow rate based on the membrane area. Typically, 47-mm filter discs are suitable for laboratory-scale studies. Other process parameters such as temperature and differential pressure should remain constant. Samples are taken from the feed, from sequential fractions, and from the pooled filtrate to analyze for component concentration. From the data, the volume needed for saturation of the filter binding capacity by the formulation product or excipient at manufacturing scale is determined. Table 7.2 shows an example of a preservative binding laboratory study.

The filtrate was assayed for the concentration of two preservatives. See Figure 7.11 for the preservative adsorption profiles of the two preservatives. This laboratory study shows initial adsorption of preservative by the filter and directs focus on the critical first liters of the manufacturing-scale filtration. The manufacturing-scale study should also take into consideration all flexible materials of contact that could result in drug product adsorption (i.e., tubing, plastic containers, stoppers, etc.). Interruptions in processing, such as line stoppage, increase exposure time of the drug product to a potentially adsorptive medium and should be considered in the validation process.

TABLE 7.2 Scale-Down Parameters for Filtration Operation

	Process Scale	Laboratory Scale
Filter area	1000 cm^2	13.8 cm^2
Volume	100 liter	1.38 liter
Flow rate	2 liter/min	30 ml/min
Differential pressure	20 psi	20 psi
Temperature	23°C	23°C

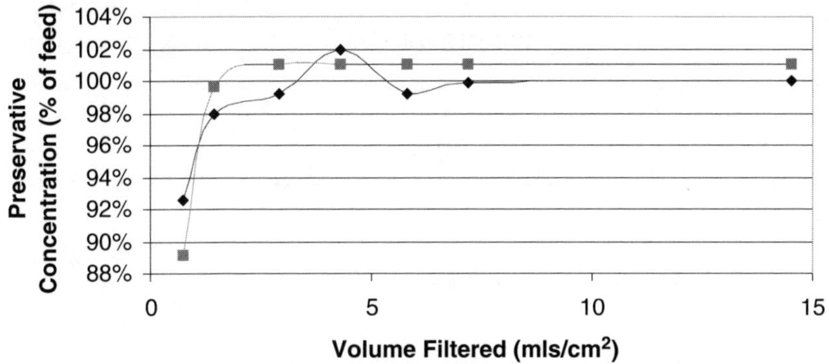

Figure 7.11 Adsorption profiles of preservatives in a drug product.

Adsorption studies are critical for final filling applications. The results of the adsorption studies will determine the initial flush volume of product to discard. Adsorption studies are important but somewhat less critical for batch filtration. Often in these cases, the quantity of material adsorbed to the filter is undetectable when assaying the concentration in the filtered bulk.

7.3.8 Extractables

Filters must be validated to show that they do not add extractables to the drug product being filtered. Extractables are inherent in the filter manufacturing process and are present to some degree in all filter devices. Extractables may include filter materials of construction, wetting agents, surfactants, and particulates [12]. Process variables such as temperature, contact time with solvents, sterilization methods, and flushing procedures all have an impact on extractable levels. Extractable levels will increase with increased contact time, increased temperature, and more rigorous sterilization methods [13,14]. Flushing is intended to remove extractables to an acceptable level (see Figure 7.12). Most filter manufacturers publish data showing the extractable level in specified flush volumes of model solvents. The following question arises: Will

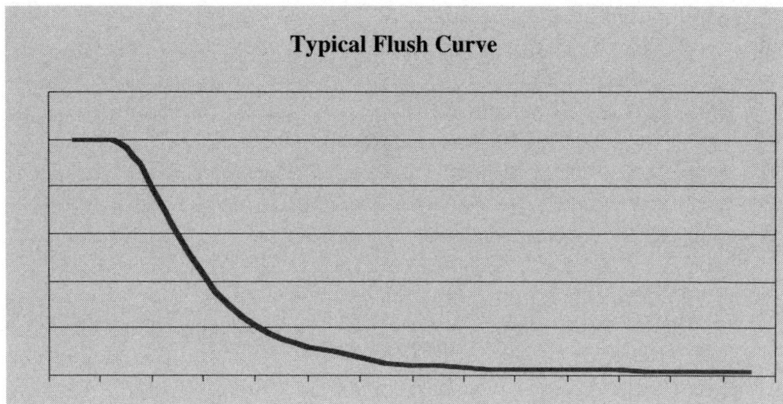

Figure 7.12 Typical filter extractable levels in relation to flush volumes.

the process fluids extract a different extractable level from the filter?

Filter manufacturers ensure that the materials of construction meet USP requirements for Class VI Biological Tests for Plastics [15] and are nontoxic per USP General Mouse Safety Test [16]. However, these tests are performed using model solvents specified in the USP guidelines. The USP also requires that plastics be extracted with a drug product vehicle. If extractions with the drug product vehicle result in extractable types and levels comparable to the manufacturer's claims, then the manufacturer's toxicity studies can be used to assess the impact of extractables on biopharmaceutical product quality and safety [17]. The USP Oxidizable Substances Test is used to determine the minimum required flushing volume prior to use.

The filter manufacturer may provide data on water and model solvent extraction, but it is the responsibility of the drug manufacturer to test for extractables in the drug product formulation. Testing for filter extractables in product is the ultimate goal or ideal for an extractables study, and it is possible in limited cases to do some work in product. However, complex drug product solutions present several issues:

- The extractables must be separated into individual species in order to identify each component [16].
- Typical drug product formulations will contain components at concentrations two to four orders of magnitude higher than the maximum filter extractable level [13]. This can confound even powerful analytical techniques such as RP-HPLC.
- Drug products and filter components are typically organic in nature. Because most drugs contain a much greater concentration of organic material as compared to filters, it is often impossible to develop a practical analytical method to accurately detect and quantify extractables. Therefore, even the most precise analytical equipment employing the most accurate methods often cannot detect filter extractables when using actual drug product.

Extractables may be identified using analytical and toxicological methods. Analytical methods may be qualitative or quantitative. The following assays are commonly used:

- Gravimetric testing quantifies nonvolatile extractables.
- Total organic carbon (TOC) quantifies organics via oxidizable carbon.
- Fourier transform infrared (FTIR) spectroscopy identifies polymeric and oligomeric solutes.
- Reverse-phase high-performance liquid chromatography (RP-HPLC) identifies low-level organic solutes.

Toxicological methods are intended to generate all potential extractables from the filter device and ensure the safety thereof. These methods include the following:

- USP Class VI test
- USP General Mouse Safety test
- Ames mutagenicity test
- Cytotoxicity tests

No single analytical method can provide reliable extractables information for all filters. There are factors that affect the accuracy of each analytical test. NVR analysis can be affected by the purity of the extraction solvent, the accuracy of the balance, and contamination during sample handling. High concentrations of solutes in NaCl, NaOH, and Tween 80 extraction solutions can cause high background levels, which can mask the extractable levels. Water, pH 2.0 HCl, and ethanol extraction solutions give more accurate results due to low levels or an absence of nonvolatile solutes. TOC does not detect inorganic extractables, and interference can result from carbon-containing extraction solutions such as 0.1% Tween 80. High concentrations of chloride ions in 20% NaCl solutions can also cause assay interference. FTIR spectroscopy becomes difficult to interpret as the number of components in the sample increases, and it is also subject to effects from extraction solutions. Solutions of NaCl, pH 2.0 HCL, pH 12.5 NaOH, and Tween 80 may be indistinguishable from controls, and therefore low extractable levels cannot be identified. RP-HPLC may be more robust for use with different extraction solutions, but it has poor sensitivity for polymeric or oligomeric molecules, which compose the majority of filter extractables. In general, water and ethanol exhibit the least amount of interference with analytical methods. TOC and RP-HPLC can be used with acidic and basic extraction solutions [13].

If the drug product contains interfering components, it may be possible to perform the extraction validation using a model solvent. Appropriate solvent streams should be selected, test protocols developed, and analysis performed. The specific model solvent streams tested and the specific analytical methodologies employed should be specific to the filtration device. In most drug formulations, the primary solvent is water. If an organic solvent or surfactant is present that interferes with the analytical assays, a noninterfering organic solvent that is appropriate for the filter device may be substituted. Acids and bases may be replaced by noninterfering agents that achieve the desired pH. A rational systematic approach should be used that simulates the worst-case conditions for a filtration device. The worst-case scenario will be represented by the longest contact time, the maximum process filtration temperature, and the most rigorous sterilization procedure. This approach should detect and quantify extractables and be generic so it can be applied to any filtration device. However, each application should be evaluated on a case-by-case basis [13]. As a process is scaled up, the filtration time often increases. If this is the case, the process validation should reflect the longest anticipated filtration time.

Extractables should be tested both in water and in drug product. Drug product testing should be performed with the drug product and under the exact conditions of the filtration process. A soaking period must be defined by actual process time (worst case). The standard time is typically 24 hours. The use of buffers high in salt, urea, and organics can result in higher levels of filter extractables [17]. If a mixture to be filtered contains multiple components, each component should be considered separately, as well as the mixture of components. The detrimental effect of a compound of low concentration in the mixture may or may not be lessened by its dilution in the mixture, whereas the interaction of two separately innocuous components may have a detrimental effect [16].

If the filter will be steam sterilized or autoclaved for use in the process, this step should be performed during the extractables testing. A worst-case scenario for filter extraction is to wet the filter with the extraction solvent and then autoclave it in the extraction solvent. The prewetting of the filter ensures contact with the boiling extraction solvent. If the filter is autoclaved dry, steam must diffuse into the pores and the extraction strength of the solvent is minimized [16]. Studies on PVDF membrane filters demonstrated that autoclaving resulted in higher extractable levels than steaming [14]. When validating either autoclaving or steaming of a filter, the total anticipated cycle time of the sterilization method, including warm-up and cool-down time, should be used as the time at the maximum sterilizing temperature during the validation study [14]. The extractable components should be identified and classified as toxic or nontoxic. It can be challenging to measure trace levels of filter extractables in the presence of high protein and excipient levels. As with any contaminant, if it cannot be identified, it must be assumed to be the most toxic component. Filter extractable levels should be considered in terms of the batch size. A larger batch size will dilute extractables and produce a lower level in the final formulation.

Sterilizing-grade filters must be non-fiber-releasing as defined in 21CFR 210.3(b)(6). The sterile filtration represents the final operation in the drug manufacturing process, and any contaminants added to the product will not be removed by a subsequent unit operation. The filter must not release any particulate or fibers into the drug product. Fiber shedding claims are validated by flushing the filter with a specified volume of filtered water at a specified upstream pressure and passing the effluent through a disc filter of a specified pore rating. The disc filter is then examined microscopically for the presence of fibers.

7.3.9 Thermal and Hydraulic Stress Resistance

If the filter is to be steam sterilized prior to use, the filter must be validated to maintain integrity after the sterilization process. Steam sterilization is often the harshest step in the lifetime of the filter. Most filter devices are composed of plastic polymers, and these polymers become weaker at steam temperatures, thereby increasing the chance of damage to the device. The preuse integrity test should occur after steam sterilization or autoclaving to show integrity immediately prior to the filtration of the product.

Pleated filter devices are susceptible to flexing of side seams and filter pleats, as well as the bonding points of the filter to the end caps. The hydraulic stress resistance of the filter should be assessed by subjecting the filter to the anticipated pumping impulses it will receive over the process filtration. Many filter manufacturers perform this test by pulsing the filter devices to certain pressures a specified number of times. The pressures are achieved by plugging the filters with suspensions such as bentonite clay. The filters are then integrity tested to prove hydraulic stress resistance. These tests may be performed at different temperatures to document both thermal and hydraulic stress resistance [18]. If hydraulic stress studies are performed on scaled-down devices, it should be noted that the pleat lengths are different between the small-scale device and the cartridge device, and the effects of the stress may be different on the devices.

7.3.10 Other Considerations

If the filter user needs to operate the filter in a manner outside of that tested by the filter manufacturer, the operation must be validated. Examples include an in-line filter on a filling machine where there is no surge tank present. This filter may be subject to pressure surges above the recommended reverse-pressure limitations. The filter should be validated to perform as intended in these operating conditions.

7.4 CLARIFICATION/PREFILTRATION FILTERS

As with sterilizing-grade filters, prefilter manufacturers perform validation testing on their products. Validation performed by the prefilter manufacturer typically includes claims of particle retention efficiency, water flow rates, USP biological safety, hydraulic and thermal stress resistance, 21 CFR toxicity compliance, extractables, oxidizables, and absence of fiber shedding. It is the drug manufacturer's responsibility to review this data, audit the filter manufacturer, and validate the prefilter in their specific process. The user should demonstrate filtrate clarity, drug product consistency, and activity/stability and evaluate product yield, process time, chemical compatibility, adsorption, and extractables with their drug product solution.

7.4.1 Retention Ratings

Prefilters are given both absolute and nominal retention ratings. Absolute retention is defined as 100% removal of all particles at or above the rated pore size. Absolute retention ratings are generally reserved for sterilizing grade membranes, although some filter manufacturers will give absolute ratings for prefilters with retention efficiencies of 99.9% or greater. Prefilters are not validated for absolute retention in the filtration process. Nominal retention is the removal of less than 100% of particles at or above the rated pore size. When validating the particle retention of a prefilter, the retention efficiency value should include a particle size and a percent retention of particles of that size [19].

Normal flow filters must be validated to retain contaminants while allowing the passage of desired molecules. The percent retention efficiency test is used to classify and rate the retention of prefilters. Filter manufacturers perform non-biological retention testing of prefilters with particles of known size. Formerly used test particles such as latex beads, glass beads, and AC fine test dust (ACFTD) have been replaced by a new standard particle contaminant medium test dust (MTD) sold by the National Institute for Standards (NIST) [20]. Filter retention testing is performed by challenging the filter with a solution containing a known number of particles at specific size ranges. Filters are wetted and flushed with clean water at a specified flow rate and temperature and then challenged with particle solutions. Particle counts are recorded at intervals on both the upstream and downstream side of the filter. In the percent retention efficiency calculation, clean water background counts are subtracted from the cartridge effluent counts. Percent retention efficiency may be expressed as a beta ratio, which is the number of feed particles divided by the number of effluent particles [21].

7.4.2 Throughput Testing

Filter capacity or throughput testing must be performed with the drug product solution. Testing procedures should be application-specific and may require different fluid types, particle types and concentration, and flow conditions (constant pressure vs. constant flow, single pass vs. multipass). This testing can be performed at small scale. Acceptable methods include V_{max}^{SM} testing, constant-flow trials, and flow decay trials.

7.4.3 Toxicity and Fiber Shedding

Although integrity testing is not a requirement for prefilters, prefilters used in the final process filter train are subject to the same toxicity requirements as are the sterilizing-grade filters [21]. Although it is preferable to have a fiber-shedding claim for all the filters in the drug manufacturing process, prefilters do not need to have a fiber-shedding claim as long as there is a non-fiber-shedding filter downstream. 21 CFR, part 211.72 states, "If use of a fiber-releasing filter is necessary, an additional non-fiber-releasing filter of 0.22 micron maximum mean porosity (0.45 micron if the manufacturing conditions so dictate) shall subsequently be used to reduce the content of particulates in the injectable drug product." Asbestos was a very common filtration material for over 50 years. Asbestos filters were banned in the mid-1970s because of the toxicity issues associated with asbestos fibers. Per 21 CFR, part 211.72, "Use of an asbestos-containing filter, with or without subsequent use of a specific non-fiber-releasing filter, is permissible only upon submission of proof to the appropriate bureau of the Food and Drug Administration that use of a non-fiber-releasing filter will, or is likely to, compromise the safety or effectiveness of the injectable drug product." Per 21 CFR, part 210.3(b)(6), "All filters composed of asbestos are deemed to be fiber-releasing filters."

7.4.4 Bioburden and Endotoxin

Although the prefilter should not add bioburden or endotoxin to the product, the prefiltration step may not have a claim for bioburden reduction or endotoxin removal. Prefilters should demonstrate nontoxicity per USP Class VI Biological Tests for Plastics and the USP General Mouse Safety Test [15]. Extracts from the filter are tested for endotoxin per the USP Bacterial Endotoxins Test.

7.4.5 Extractables

Extractables are defined as static or dynamic and are reported as milligrams per cartridge. Static extractables are the material extracted from a filter after an 18- to 24-hour static soak at ambient temperature. The soak can be in water or a compatible organic solvent, which is then evaporated to allow for weighing of the extractables [22]. The residue can be analyzed by FTIR. Solvent extraction will typically generate a higher level of extractables than water extraction. Dynamic extractables are the material extracted from a filter under clean water flush conditions. The filter is flushed until the effluent reaches a prespecified resistivity below that of the feed water, and the time to reach this resistivity is related to the dynamic extractables [23]. The USP Oxidizable Substances Test is used to determine the minimum required flushing volume prior to filter use. Reference Section 7.3.8 for more information on extractables testing.

7.4.6   Product Stability

In the case of a clarifying filter, the stability of the product over the filtration time must be assessed. Proteases and other products that may damage the protein are likely to be present in the feed stream. A maximum processing time may be important in maintaining product quality. The product may not be stable at the pH or conductivity of the cell culture solution, and this may warrant a speedy clarification and commencement of purification to preserve the product quality. Nonspecific binding of product or excipients to the filter should be assessed and documented (see Section 7.3.7). Any effects the filter material will have on the drug product solution must be evaluated. Most filter materials will have some nonspecific binding of proteins, the degree of which varies with the type of filter material. Since the degree of binding is also dependent on the drug product and its concentration in the solution to be filtered, testing must be performed with the drug product solution under the actual processing conditions (flow rate, differential pressure, temperature, contact time). A lengthy filtration time can allow for the replication of bacteria present in the feed stream. Filtration time should be validated using the worst-case scenario. If a clarification step will require a certain filtration time, then the process should be validated using that same filtration time. This will demonstrate whether there is a problem with grow-through of bacteria on the filter.

7.4.7 Processing Considerations

The validation of the clarification step should include testing the subsequent operation at the range of outcomes from the filtration step. This allows for establishment of the normal operating ranges for the filtration step and gives enough process knowledge to determine the minimum specification for clarity to ensure a successful subsequent operation. These specifications may be measured in nephelometric turbidity units (NTUs) or the capacity of a downstream filtration step (i.e., V_{max} testing of the clarified filtrate on a sterilizing-grade filter). When clarifying mammalian cell cultures, low operating pressures and low flow rates are required to maintain the cell membrane integrity. Cell lysis results in contamination of the filtrate with cellular debris and proteins. These contaminants may not be adequately removed by subsequent steps that were not intended to clear them. System design can contribute to shear effects resulting in cell lysis. Filtration skids should be designed such that the pumps, valves, instrumentation, and piping do not contribute to shear.

The clarification step may be followed by a unit operation that requires a particulate-free filtrate from the clarifying filter. In the case of a subsequent chromatography step, the clarifying filter must generate a particulate-free filtrate that will not limit the life of the chromatography media. Chromatography media is subject to blinding if the feed stream is not prefiltered to remove cell debris and other particulate. Particulate may also adversely affect the flow distribution within a column, causing channeling, which in turn lowers the binding capacity of the column. Differential pressures will increase across the column if particulate in the feed stream lodges in the interstitial spaces of the media. A range of operating pressures, flow rates, and volumetric loading (volume/membrane area) should be tested to set specifications that meet the criteria for particulate removal. A clarifying filter may give a filtrate of acceptable clarity at a low flow rate and operating pressure, but not at a higher flow rate and pressure. The pressures and flow rates tested should generate a filtrate free of cellular debris. A clarity specification is necessary to ensure the required purity of the feed stream moving forward in the purification process.

If the feed stream is subject to forming colloids or aggregates as the processing time increases, this must be considered in the validation. Also, previously frozen feed streams can present difficulties in filtration. If a feed stream must be frozen and thawed, or held for an extended period of time prior to filtration, the validation of that filtration step must be performed under the same conditions. The duration of the hold time must also be validated. This is an instance where scaling of the process may require revalidation, as the amount of time for a small volume of feed stream to thaw is much less than the thawing time for a large volume. The difference in thawing time could contribute to product quality differences due to the degradation by proteases and other enzymes present in the feed stream.

7.5 VIRAL CLEARANCE FILTERS

7.5.1 Definitions and Regulatory Requirements

In order to understand the regulatory requirements, it is first necessary to define the different categories of virus according to how they contaminate the product, and to define viral clearance.

Viruses can be grouped into three classifications according to how they contaminate the product:

- Endogenous viruses are viruses "whose genome is part of the germ line of the species of origin of the cell line and is covalently integrated into the genome of animal from which the parental cell line was derived....Intentionally introduced, non-integrated viruses...fit in this category" [24]. In plasma-derived products, endogenous viruses are natural contaminants of donor blood. Mammalian cell culture systems are susceptible to endogenous retrovirus-like particle (RVLP) contamination. RVLPs are present in virtually all mammalian cell lines and cannot be screened out of the master cell bank because they integrate their genome into the host cell genome [25].

- Nonendogenous viruses are "viruses from external sources present in the Master Cell Bank" [24].
- Adventitious viruses are "unintentionally introduced contaminant viruses" [24]. Contamination with adventitious virus may occur through the addition of contaminated raw materials or through extraneous contamination.

Viruses can also be categorized according to their relevance as model test viruses:

- Relevant virus is "the identified virus, or of the same species as the virus that is known, or likely to contaminate the cell substrate or any other reagents or materials used in the production process" [24].
- Specific model virus is a "virus which is closely related to the known or suspected virus (same genus or family), having similar physical and chemical properties to those of the observed or suspected virus" [24].
- Nonspecific model virus is "a virus used for characterization of viral clearance of the process when the purpose is to characterize the capacity of the manufacturing process to remove and/or inactivate viruses in general, i.e., to characterize the robustness of the purification process" [24].

Viral clearance can be classified as specific or general:

- Specific virus clearance — "To provide evidence that the production process will effectively inactivate/remove viruses which are either known to contaminate the starting material or which could conceivably do so" [24].
- General virus clearance — "To provide indirect evidence that the production process might inactivate/remove novel or unpredictable virus contamination" [24].

This relates to robustness of the unit operation.

Regulatory guidance for viral clearance promotes a three-tiered approach. First, raw materials are controlled and qualified for use through virus-screening measures. Second, specific steps in the manufacture of the product are included in the process line and validated to clear virus. Third, the final product is screened for the presence of virus [26].

The ICH makes the following recommendations in Topic Q5A [24]:

- Test the process source material.
  Test cell lines, raw materials, media components, etc., for viruses.
- Test the process.
  Assess the capability of the manufacturing process to clear viruses.
- Test the product.
  Test the product at appropriate points in the process for the absence of contaminating infectious viruses.

The overall process targets a product SAL (sterility assurance limit) of 6, meaning that in 10^6 doses, no more than one dose will be contaminated. For biotech products that carry endogenous viruses, RVLPs are found at titers of 10^6–10^9/ml. In order to reduce the titer to 10^{-6}/ml in the final product, industry standard requires a 1–15 log reduction value (LRV) in the process. It is difficult to measure the effectiveness of viral clearance beyond 6 LRV in a particular step due to limits of detection of the assay; therefore, at least two effective steps should be used in the process to achieve 12–15 LRV. These effective steps should be orthogonal, meaning they utilize different viral clearance methods, such as size exclusion and adsorption [27]. If a process relies on one methodology for viral clearance, it is more likely to fail. If two adsorption chromatography steps are used to clear virus, a shift in the pH of the feed stream may reduce the binding capacity of the chromatography media, resulting in breakthrough of virus from both steps. If orthogonal methods are implemented, the adsorption step is coupled with a size exclusion or inactivation step, neither of which will be affected by the pH shift. More recent trends also include testing at process extremes such as flow rate, protein concentration, and pressure.

Commonly accepted practice is to demonstrate 6 LRV for adventitious viruses. This requires at least one effective step. An "effective" step is defined as providing a minimum of 4 LRV and as being scaleable and robust. An "ineffective" step provides an LRV of 1 or less. A "moderately effective" step falls between the two [27]. Robustness refers to two concepts, the first being that the viral clearance step is capable of clearing a wide range of viruses [24], and the second being that the step can withstand perturbations of process variables [28]. Minor changes in the feed stream should not affect the performance of the viral clearance step. Examples of unit operations categorized as robust are pH 3.9, heat inactivation, solvent-detergent, and filtration (15 to 40 nm) [29]. Adsorption-based unit operations are less robust, as adsorption is dependent on process variables such as ionic strength, pH, temperature, and flow rate. A risk analysis is required showing the clearance capability of various steps and the overall process. The risk analysis also evaluates the likelihood of contamination in the final product.

7.5.2 Virus Spiking Studies

Most viral clearance validation studies incorporate a Phase I study. For biotech products, MuLV is the RVLP model virus [24]. For plasma products, a range of model viruses is used, with a full panel of viruses submitted with the BLA. Relevant viruses are those identified viruses of the same species likely to contaminate the cell substrate. Specific models are viruses of the same family as the suspected or identified virus. They are available in high titers, safer than the virus of concern, and practical if the actual virus is not culturable. Relevant and specific model viruses are used to demonstrate the capability of the process to remove viruses present in the master cell bank. Nonspecific models are viruses with different properties than the suspected or identified virus. This category of viruses is used to demonstrate the robustness of the process to remove/inactivate viruses with wide physicochemical

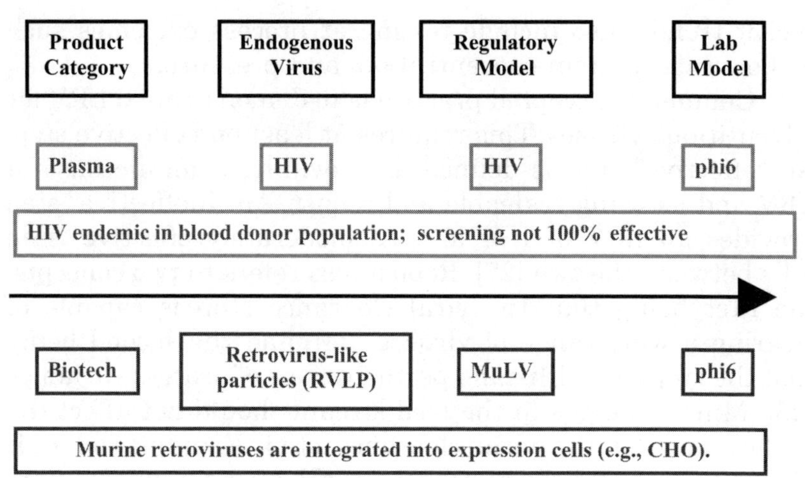

Figure 7.13 Viral contaminants and respective models.

TABLE 7.3 Common Viruses and Their Properties

Virus	Natural Host	Genome	Enveloped	Size (nm)
Vesicular stomatitis virus	Bovine	RNA	Yes	70 × 150
Parainfluenza virus	Various	RNA	Yes	100–200
MuLV	Mouse	RNA	Yes	80–110
Sindbis virus	Human	RNA	Yes	60–70
BVDV	Bovine	RNA	Yes	50–70
Pseudorabies virus	Swine	DNA	Yes	120–200
Poliovirus Sabin	Human	RNA	No	25–30
Encephalomyocarditis virus	Mouse	RNA	No	25–30
Reovirus 3	Various	DNA	No	60–80
SV40	Monkey	DNA	No	40–50
Parvoviruses	Canine/porcine/ murine	DNA	No	18–24

Source: Federal Register/Vol. 61, No. 92/Friday, May 10, 1996/ Notices.

properties (see Figure 7.13) [30]. Table 7.3 lists common viruses and their properties.

Viral clearance validation is performed with viral spiking studies, in which a heavily virus-spiked solution is filtered through a test filter to characterize the retention capability of the filter. It is performed for known endogenous viruses in the Master Cell Bank (MCB) to provide assurance for clearance of such viruses, and for unknown contaminants to characterize the robustness of the removal/inactivation step. Viral clearance validation is performed at small scale for multiple reasons. Viruses are spiked into the feed stream, and thus enormous quantities would be required at the process scale. The required quantities are not practical. The safety of manufacturing personnel is also a concern. The scale-down model should include all critical parameters, maintain relative values, and represent the production procedure. The parameters include the following:

- Same challenge solution (product)
  pH
  Protein concentration of the input/output
  Ionic strength
- Same process parameters
  TMP or flow rate
  Process time
  Temperature
  Relative volume/filter area

A minimum quantity of virus should be used so as not to change the characteristics of the test product. A 0.5–5% v/v ratio of virus suspension to challenge solution is typical.

Virus should be nonaggregated to avoid overstating physical removal. TEMs of the virus prep should reflect monodispersed intact particles with no cellular debris. Hold controls should be included to monitor infectivity of the virus during the process conditions. The product should be evaluated for toxicity to the indicator cells used in the assays. Duplicate studies should be done to provide reproducible results.

The reduction factor is the $\log_{10}$ of the ratio between the total virus load before clearance and the total virus load after clearance.

$$\text{Reduction factor} = \log_{10}[(V_1 \times T_1)/(V_2 \times T_2)]$$

where

V_1 = volume of spiked feed stock that has been used to challenge the clearance step

T_1 = virus concentration of spiked feed stock prior to the clearance step

V_2 = volume of material that has been treated by the clearance step

T_2 = virus concentration of material after the clearance step

The current guidance states that "sufficient sample volumes should be tested to ensure that there is a high probability of detecting virus in the sample if present" [29]. If no virus is detected in the sample, the theoretical virus concentration in the sample must be calculated before the LRV is determined. For samples representing a percentage of the total volume, it is possible that the volume not sampled contains virus. The probability (p) of this is dependent on the total volume of filtrate (V), the sample volume of filtrate (v), and the number of viruses in the total volume (n). The following equation quantifies the probability [24]:

$$p = ((V - v)/V)^n$$

If the sample volume is a very small percentage of the total volume, the probability is expressed as the Poisson distribution:

$$p = e^{-cv}$$

where c = virus concentration. If 95% confidence limits are applied, $p = 0.05$. In solving for c, the equation becomes

$$c = 3/v$$

This value for c is then used as the value for T_2 in the first equation, and the reduction factor is calculated as above [26].

Serial dilutions should be performed when the expected titer of the undiluted sample is outside the statistically significant range. Multiple replicates of the final dilution should be assayed to increase the accuracy and precision of the assay.

Assay methods can be quantitative or qualitative. Quantitative methods include 50% tissue culture infectious dose ($TCID_{50}$) assays where the cell culture is scored as being either infected or not. The titer is measured by the proportion of the culture infected. Another method is to measure the genomic equivalent units (geu) using polymerase chain reaction (PCR). The genome is amplified by PCR until the limit of detection of the assay is reached. The number of cycles to reach the limit of detection is indicative of the amount of genomic material present in the original sample.

Quantitative assays include plaque assays in which one plaque corresponds to a single infectious unit. For negative results, when only a portion is assayed, there is sampling error involved. The amount of virus to achieve a positive result should be calculated using the Poisson distribution and taken into consideration when determining LRV. The FDA recommends 95% confidence limits when calculating LRV. Probability of detection is $p = e^{-cv}$ or $c = \ln(p)/-v$ where c is the concentration, ln is the natural logarithm, p is the percent confidence, and v is the volume of the material assayed.

Example 7.1

100 mL of MuLV with initial titer of $1.5 \times 10^6\,TCID_{50}$/ml suspension is filtered through a viral clearance scale-down device. There is no virus detected in the filtrate. If 4 ml of the filtrate was assayed, the LRV is calculated as follows:

Initial virus load: $1.5 \times 10^6\,TCID_{50}$/ml $\times 100$ ml $= 1.5 \times 10^8\,TCID_{50}$

Final viral load is less than the limit of detection.

For 95% confidence: $c = \ln(0.05)/-4 = 0.75$

Final virus load is less than 100 ml $\times 0.75$ or <75.

LRV is calculated as $\log(1.5) \times 10^8 - \log(75) = 8.2 - 1.9 = 6.3$ LRV >6.3.

The steps of a typical viral spiking study are outlined below. See Figure 7.14 for equipment setup for a viral spiking study.

1. Assemble holders with membrane.
2. Attach holders to manifold.
3. Attach downstream of filter holders to tared collection vessels.
4. Attach air filters to collection vessels and manifold (for venting).
5. Spike product with virus and mix. Note the exact volume.
6. Prefilter challenge material with a 0.1-µm membrane (low protein binding).
7. Remove a sample of the spiked feed to determine the initial virus concentration and a hold control sample.
8. Transfer spiked feed into pressure vessel (in BL2 cabinet).
9. Connect the outlet of the vessel to the manifold.
10. Connect the inlet of the vessel to pressure source via an air filter.
11. Pressurize vessel.
12. Vent manifold.
13. Open two-way valve and vent membrane holder.
14. Start filtration.
15. When desired amount of filtrate has been collected, shut downstream valve off and remove filtrate vessel.
16. Determine the exact filtrate volume.
17. Sample feed and compare to initial to determine if virus inactivation is occurring.
18. Perform a postuse integrity test.

7.5.3 Integrity Testing of Viral Clearance Filters

Viral clearance filters are available in NFF and TFF configurations, all devices being single use, regardless of the configuration. Regardless of the type of device selected, it must be integrity tested. NFF devices can be integrity tested using the diffusion test as described in Section 7.3.3. The user should comply with the manufacturer's recommendations for

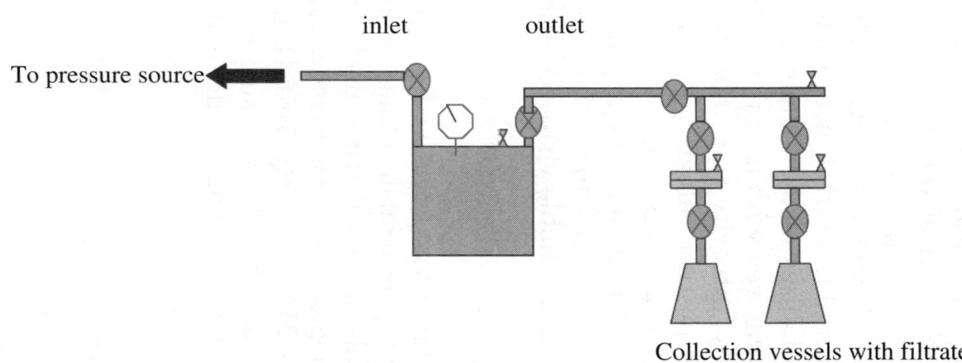

Figure 7.14   Equipment setup for viral spiking study.

the wetting fluid, test gas, and test pressures. The CorrTest™ integrity test of TFF viral clearance membranes is patented by Millipore Corporation. The CorrTest integrity test uses a pair of immiscible fluids, one of which is employed as a wetting fluid and the other as an intrusion fluid. The result is a ratio of two membrane permeabilities measured at preselected operated conditions. The first operating condition is chosen so as to selectively intrude those pores accessible to ϕX-174, a 28-nm bacteriophage, using a two-phase fluid system. The second operating condition, a water permeability measurement, is selected such that all of the membrane pores are intruded. The ratio of the two permeabilities is the amount of flow through the membrane pores accessible to ϕX-174 relative to the total flow and is a direct measure of the intrinsic virus retention capabilities of the membrane. These two components are easily removed with a simple flushing protocol, allowing the CorrTest integrity test to be used both pre- and postprocessing. For postuse integrity testing, the membrane should be cleaned prior to testing to avoid biofoulants interfering with the test. Customer integrity tests are combined with vendor tests on devices and membrane to provide assurance of consistent and reliable virus retention.

7.5.4   Other Considerations

Effluent from the filter must test negative for USP oxidizable substances after the appropriate flush volume. Manufacturers ensure that the materials of construction meet USP requirements for Class VI Biological Tests for Plastics and are non-toxic per USP General Mouse Safety Test [15]. Endotoxin limits are confirmed to be <0.5 EU/ml using the LAL test. Filters must be non-fiber-releasing as defined in 21CFR 210.3(b)(6).

7.6 VALIDATION OF TANGENTIAL FLOW FILTERS

7.6.1 Overview

In a purification process, TFF may be used for multiple steps. Upstream applications for TFF are media depyrogenation, mammalian cell culture perfusion, mammalian and bacterial cell harvest, and bacterial cell lysate clarification. Downstream applications are product concentration, buffer exchange, viral reduction, and small-molecule depyrogenation (see Figure 7.15). Although each of these applications has different performance outcomes, each operation must demonstrate performance consistency through the claimed number of runs, as well as ruggedness of the process over the normal range of operating conditions.

Per PDA Technical Report No. 15, "Studies supporting the selection of TFF systems, membranes, and operating parameters should be performed as part of process development and should be completed before full scale production begins" [31]. The IQ and OQ portions of the validation plan should be completed prior to full-scale production.

The process validation of a microfiltration or ultrafiltration TFF operation involves common elements as well as special considerations. The PQ of a tangential-flow filtration operation involves the claims described in Section 7.1 as well as special considerations, such as the following:

- Passage of product by MF membranes
- Retention of product by UF membranes
- Passage of contaminants in diafiltration process
- Recovery of the product from the system
- Cleaning solutions remove all residual drug product, cells, and contaminants between processing runs

We will discuss the common elements first, followed by the special considerations.

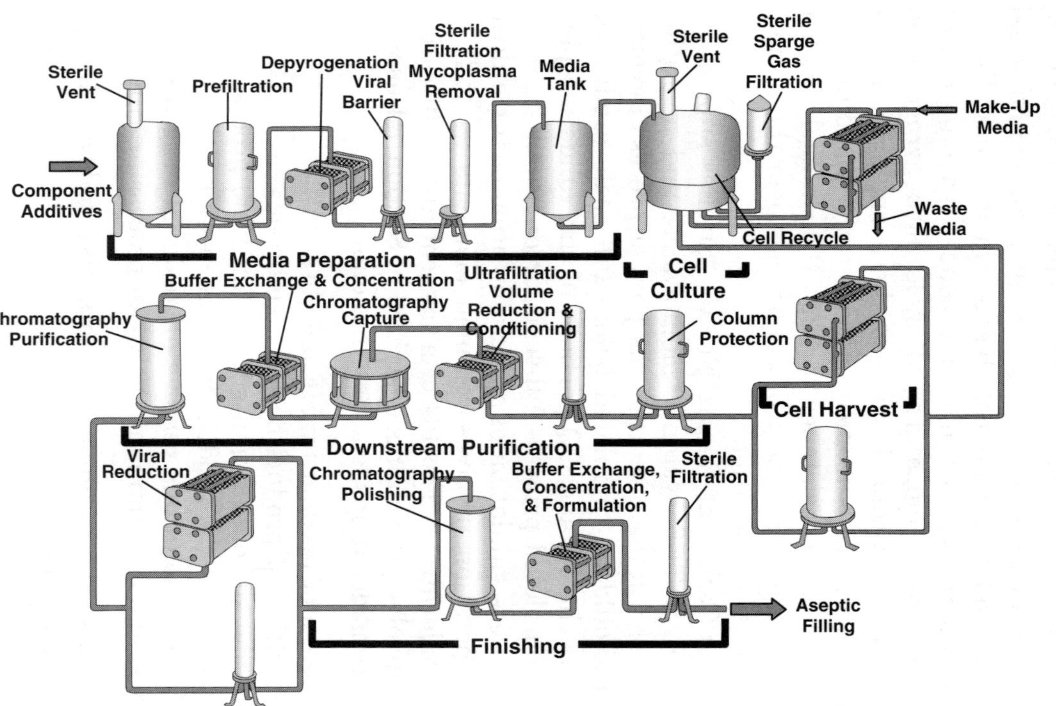

Figure 7.15   General monoclonal antibody manufacturing process.

7.6.2 Process Flux

During process development, experiments should determine the required average flux at the process temperature and pressure. Consistency and reproducibility of process flux should be monitored run to run. A decreasing flux value indicates a difference in this rate of passage, the difference being due to some form of resistance. This resistance is the result of fouling, which is the physical or chemical binding of solutes to the membrane surfaces. In a reuse process, membranes are cleaned in order to remove these foulants and restore process flux. A decreased process flux value indicates inadequate removal of foulants during the cleaning regimen. Figure 7.16 shows a tangential-flow filter with an adsorbed layer of foulants. A decreased flux means that additional processing time is required to meet the concentration and purity specifications of the process intermediate. See Figure 7.17 for an example of trending process flux over multiple process runs.

7.6.3 Pressure Profiles

As well as monitoring process flux, pressure profiles should also be monitored. At a constant feed flow rate, the same solution will generate equivalent pressure profiles. A change in pressure profile at a constant feed flow rate is indicative of a change in fluid viscosity or channel geometry. In a robust

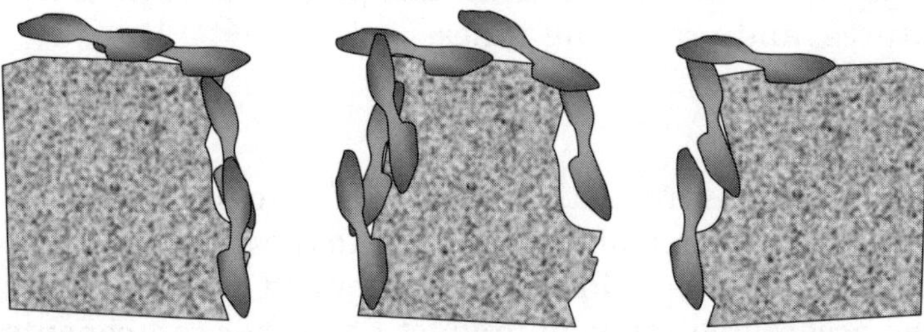

Figure 7.16 Polarization and fouling of a tangential flow filtration membrane.

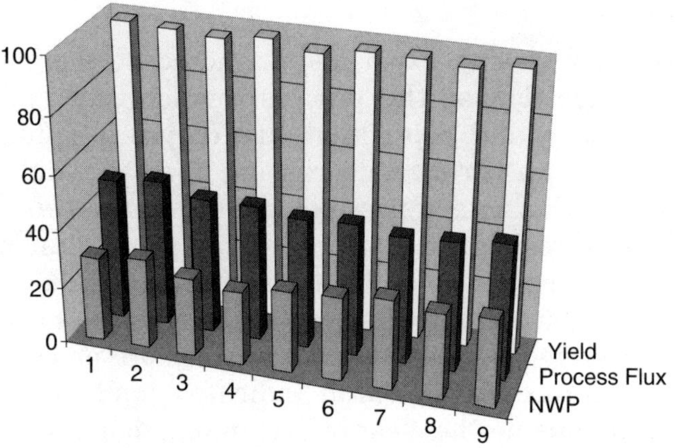

Figure 7.17 Monitoring yield, process flux, and clean water flux over multiple process runs.

process, changes in the feed stream should be minor. Changes in viscosity will be discussed with respect to microfiltration applications, owing to the fact that cell densities may vary in a cell culture clarification. Critical validated parameters such as the transmembrane pressure and cross-flow will be specified in the chemistry manufacturing controls (CMC) section of the BLA. Set points should be established, as well as normal operating ranges (NOR) and maximum operating ranges (MOR). These will specify the minimum and maximum volumes, transmembrane and differential pressures, flow rates, temperatures, and processing times.

7.6.4 Retention

Retention is a measure of the amount of a solute that does not pass through the membrane relative to the amount of that solute in the feed stream. Process development studies should define the acceptable range of product and other components in the feed stock. Retention of the drug product should be consistent throughout the lifetime use of a membrane. For UF applications, retention should be at least 99% to ensure adequate recovery of the drug product. Increased retention can be due to foulants decreasing the pore size of the membrane or to a polarization layer of solutes impeding the passage of other solutes to the membrane surface. Decreased retention can be due to harsh cleaning regimens altering the membrane pores. The molecular weight cutoff of membranes can change with exposure to a chemical that degrades the membrane matrix.

7.6.5 Yield

Product yield should be consistent over membrane reuse. Changes in yield are indicative of changes in product retention. A decreased yield of product in the filtrate of an MF step may be attributed to the polarization layer impeding the passage of product or product loss due to aggregation, denaturation, or precipitation. A decreased yield of retained product in a UF step may be attributed to unwanted passage through the membrane where the molecular weight cutoff has increased or, again, losses due to aggregation, denaturation, or precipitation. Product assays should be developed to ensure that the product is recovered from the system in an active nondenatured and nonaggregated form. A yield of greater than 100% may indicate the unwanted activation of a product by the unit operation [32]. See Figure 7.17 for an example of trending drug product yield over multiple process runs.

7.6.6 Chemical Compatibility

For all applications, the compatibility of the membranes as well as all wetted components of the system must be determined with each process fluid. It is imperative that none of the wetted surfaces, including the filters, corrode, extract, swell, or weaken with exposure to any of the process fluids. Process fluids include the feed stream and flushing, cleaning, sanitizing, and depyrogenating agents. Membrane retention must not change over the course of use of the devices. Membrane selectivity must also not change over the course of use. The lifetime of the expendable device must be determined. The cleaning and sanitization of the membranes must be validated.

7.6.7 Bioburden and Endotoxin

The membrane and the TFF system must not add microbial contamination to the product. This is of particular importance if the TFF unit operation is near the end of the purification process. Sterility requirements and maximum endotoxin levels should be specified. Bioburden and endotoxin reduction must be documented. Both are removed after processing by cleaning with caustic agents, typically 0.5–1.0 N NaOH. Some UF TFF membranes are susceptible to degradation by these cleaning agents. In this case, the membranes can be bypassed when the system is cleaned.

Endotoxin is capable of producing a pyrogenic response in humans at levels of 0.1 ng (1 EU) per kg of body weight. Typical gram-negative bacteria contain 10^{-15} g of LPS; therefore, 0.1 ng or 1 EU of endotoxin may be generated by 10^5 bacterial cells [33]. The acceptable level of endotoxin is dependent on the type of product. Since endotoxin limits are often rated per dose, a product that is administered in large frequent doses, such as a monoclonal antibody, has a lower specification for endotoxin than a product that is administered infrequently in low doses, such as a vaccine. For example, Factor IX has an endotoxin limit of ≤5 EU/dose, which is equivalent to ≤0.1 EU/ml. HIb vaccine has an endotoxin limit of ≤25 EU/dose, or ≤50 EU/ml [33].

The filter device must not add endotoxin to the product that has been filtered. Although a 0.2-μm filter will retain gram-negative bacteria, it may pass the endotoxin released from these bacteria into the filtrate. Endotoxin can be removed from media and buffer solutions by ultrafiltration TFF. Endotoxin can be removed from product by adsorption on charged membranes or chromatography media. The LRV of either method must be validated. The endotoxin removal step should be able to accommodate variability in endotoxin loads due to changes in the cell disruption method. Cell disruption methods are subject to change during process scale-up, and so the load of endotoxin to be removed from the product can vary [34].

Validation methods for the LAL assay are available from the FDA [9]. It should be noted that the LAL test is sensitive and fast but only detects endotoxin. Certain buffers may interfere with the LAL assay since it is enzyme-based, and this should be accounted for in the assay validation [11]. The rabbit test can also be used to test for endotoxin, as it detects pyrogenic substances.

7.6.8 Membrane Qualification

Another consideration in the validation of a TFF process is qualification of the membrane. Three lots of membrane should be tried using three lots of feedstock. It is wise to qualify a second vendor for all materials used in the manufacturing process, with filters being no exception. In case of a supply deficiency from the primary vendor, having qualified a second vendor in advance can avoid lost processing time. When selecting any vendor, important considerations are the vendor reputation for quality, service, and dependability. If the vendor provides validation guides with their devices, it will assist in the validation process.

7.6.9 Other Considerations

Manufacturers ensure that the materials of construction meet USP requirements for Class VI Biological Tests for Plastics and are nontoxic per the USP General Mouse Safety Test [15]. Effluent from the filter must test negative for USP oxidizable substances after the appropriate flush volume. The membrane and the TFF system must not add chemical contamination to the product. This is of particular importance if the TFF unit operation is near the end of the purification process. Users of TFF membranes must also demonstrate that the preservative solution is completely removed from the device by the recommended flushing procedure and that the cleaning and storage solutions are effectively removed by the recommended flushing procedure. The manufacturer's flushing guidelines should be used to establish the appropriate cross-flow and pressures for flushing of the preservative or storage solution. The user may be able to validate the flushing procedure with substantially lower flushing volumes than the manufacturer's recommended volumes, saving on water costs and time. The assay showing clearance of the preservative or storage solution should be easy to use. The validation of an assay that can be run in the purification suite will save processing time, rather than collecting samples and submitting them for QC testing.

7.6.10 Bacterial Cell Harvest and Lysate Clarification

Special considerations surround the validation of a TFF system for microfiltration due to exposure to cells. Whether bacterial, yeast, or mammalian, the cleaning of the TFF system must be adequate to show removal of all cells between runs. The processing of bacterial cell products involves two potential MF steps: a cell-harvesting step, in which the cells are concentrated and the spent media removed, and a lysate clarification step, in which the cell debris is removed from the product. Important considerations in process validation of bacterial cell harvests are the potential for changes in the feed stream. Bacterial cells grow rapidly, and there may be a range of cell concentrations over which the harvest must take place. Also, the pH and viscosity of the feed stream may vary between fermentations. Bacterial cell walls make them relatively insensitive to lysis by shear. The bigger validation issue surrounding bacterial cell harvest is the containment of recombinant organisms and equipment decontamination. If a claim is made that the filtrate from the TFF system should be free of recombinant organisms, then protocols should specify testing of the filtrate for such. The TFF membranes should be integrity tested before and after use.

Bacterial cell lysate clarification presents a challenge in that cell wall debris, organelles, and hundreds of host cell proteins are released upon cell lysis. The large amounts of proteinaceous material present in the bacterial lysate may complicate identification of contaminants. This should be kept in mind during assay development and qualification. The clarification of product from mammalian cells is not as complicated since these cells are capable of secreting products and can be clarified from the product intact. In a lysate clarification, product is being passed through the membrane, and cell debris is retained.

7.6.11 Mammalian Cell Clarification

In mammalian cell separations, the objective is to keep the cells intact, thereby preserving a cleaner feed stream. A marker such as lactate dehydrogenase can be used to measure cell lysis, or alternatively trypan blue can be used to count viable versus nonviable cells. Cell lysis can affect the quality of the product by releasing proteases and other enzymes that may damage or alter the product. Variability in the feed stream quality may be measured further downstream. During the cell separation, the pressures and shear must be kept to a minimum to avoid cell lysis. These are critical parameters for which an optimal range must be validated. A batch process will have a higher cell viability and lower cell count than a perfusion process. In a perfusion process, it is critical to maintain sterility of the perfusion system. Procedures for cleaning and sterilizing the TFF system should be validated, and the cell culture should be monitored over time to ensure that product expression and cell viability are not affected by the membrane.

It is common in the industry to steam MF systems and devices used for vaccine production, although the devices do not have to be sterile. In applications where steaming is not desired, or the devices cannot be steamed, they are often cleaned *in situ* and then removed for steaming of the system. Devices must be cleaned prior to steaming, or the steaming cycle will fix the existing residues onto the membranes.

7.6.12 Protein Concentration and Diafiltration

As a protein is being concentrated in a UF process, a polarization layer builds up on the surface of the membrane. This polarization layer results from the transmembrane pressure driving solutes in the feed stream against the membrane, where they are retained (see Figure 7.16). If this polarization layer becomes excessive, it can impede the passage of small solutes that were intended to pass through the membrane [35]. The polarization layer, in effect, becomes a second layer of resistance to filtration above the membrane itself. This is of concern if it interferes with the intended separation. An optimal transmembrane pressure and cross-flow should be selected that avoid this situation and produce a product of the acceptable purity and yield. A second consideration involves the concentration of contaminants concomitant with the product concentration. If the feed stream contains proteases that become concentrated with the product, the product quality could be affected. Product must be tested for quality as well as yield.

The diafiltration (DF) process must produce a product that meets the specification for a maximum level of the contaminant being removed from the drug product. The DF process should not lead to any changes in the composition of the finished drug product. Stability and solubility of the drug product in the starting buffer and the final DF buffer should be determined during process development at the laboratory scale. In the validation of the DF process, samples should be taken from the starting solution and throughout the DF to show removal of contaminants (see Figure 7.18). Validation of the DF operation should also show that the change in buffer does not cause osmotic effects that alter the permeability of the membrane. Rejection for small-molecular-weight contaminants in a UF process is calculated according to the formula below. The specification for the maximum allowable contaminant concentration in the drug product after the DF step must be measurable by a reproducible and accurate assay. Consideration should be given to the limit of detection of the assays for the contaminants being removed.

$$\% \text{ contaminants remaining} = [e(R - 1)(V_d/V_s)] \times 100$$

where

V_d = diafiltration volume
V_s = system volume
R = retention of contaminant

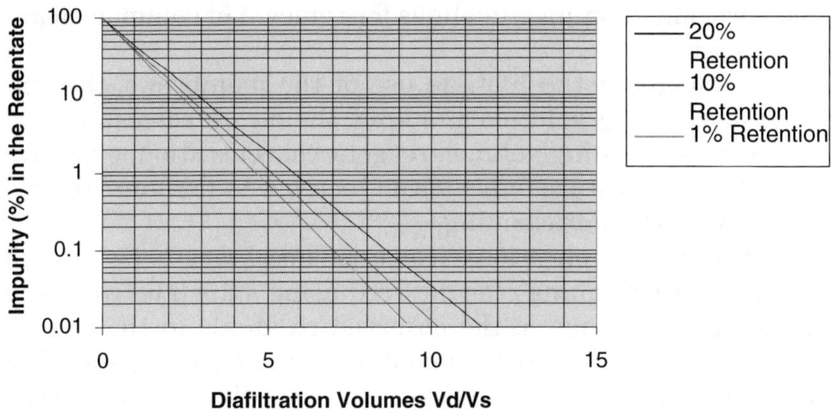

Figure 7.18   Impurity removal in relation to diavolumes at varying impurity retention levels.

7.7   VALIDATION OF A TFF SYSTEM CLEANING PROTOCOL

7.7.1   Cleaning Considerations

Section 211.67(a) of part 21 of CFR states, "Equipment and utensils shall be cleaned, maintained, and sanitized at appropriate intervals to prevent malfunctions or contamination that would alter the safety, identity, strength, quality or purity of the drug product beyond the official or other established requirements."

A cleaning protocol must be developed, documented, and validated. The objectives of a cleaning protocol are multifold. Devices must be cleaned or flushed prior to initial use to remove storage agents and preservatives. After processing the product, cleaning serves to remove residual proteins and contaminants thereby restoring membrane permeability. Proper cleaning enhances the long-term performance of the device and can extend the lifetime of the device. The cleaning protocol should be developed using the filter manufacturer's recommendations for compatible cleaning solutions and contact times and temperatures. Many filter manufacturers also provide flushing guidelines for removal of common cleaning agents.

Throughout the lifetime use of the membrane, the volume of cleaning solution required should be consistent. An increase in cleaning volume, reagent concentration, exposure time, or temperature indicates an increase in foulants, requiring more stringent cleaning.

For some applications, it may be necessary to clean with two separate cleaning reagents, requiring a flush between the cleanings. A change in the observed residuals in the critical flush step also indicates a deviation in the cleaning step. The critical flush is the flush performed immediately prior to the introduction of the product to the TFF system. It is the most important cycle to identify trace contaminants using the TOC method. A typical TFF critical flush volume is 20 l/m^2 membrane area.

If the cleaning agent is water-soluble, it can be flushed with water or aqueous buffer. If it is a multi-ingredient agent, will certain components be harder to remove than others? If the product is not water-soluble, the rinse water will have to be removed prior to introduction of the product. The rinse procedure that removes the cleaning agent must be validated. If the cleaning agent can be measured by pH or conductivity, these can be validated as the assay to demonstrate removal of the cleaning agent from the TFF system. For example, if WFI is being used to rinse 0.5 N NaOH from a system after cleaning, the conductivity or pH of the rinse WFI could be used as the specification for clearance of the cleaning agent. A word of caution regarding the use of pH as an assay to show removal of caustic cleaning agents: A small amount of ions in WFI results in a high pH, even though the solution has a low conductivity. It may be easier to validate removal of cleaning agents using a conductivity assay instead of pH. A solution of very low conductivity can have a high pH. From personal experience, a solution of 0.0025 N NaOH measures approximately pH 10, yet has a conductivity of only approximately 0.7 mS/cm.

A critical flush volume of 20 l/m^2 of membrane area should yield TOC values below a 1.0 ppm level [36]. The toxicity of the cleaning agent usually dictates the specification for residuals, with the level of detection of the assay commonly used. A warning here is that with advancements in technology, assays are continually becoming more sensitive. Setting a residual limit at the level of detection of the assay may prove troublesome if the assay becomes capable of detecting a lower level of residual [37]. Selecting an industry-standard value (such as less than 1 ppm) avoids this complication and will be acceptable for most applications.

7.7.2 Chemical Compatibility

The development of the cleaning protocol requires investigation into the compatibility of the filtration device as well as all the wetted components of the system with the cleaning agents. Because TFF devices are often reused, they are subjected to rigorous cleaning protocols. The cleaning protocol must not have an adverse effect on the membranes or the devices. There are different options available for cleaning the devices and systems, and the selection of these affects the cleaning protocol. If the devices are cleaned *in situ*, the cleaning regimen must be able to effectively clean both. In some cases, it will be advantageous to clean the devices *in situ* and then bypass the devices to clean the system at higher flow rates or with a more concentrated reagent. For system sanitization with 1 N NaOH or sterilization with steam, it may be necessary to bypass the membranes, which may not be compatible with these procedures. If the system is to be steam sterilized, steam temperatures and pressure must not have an adverse effect [38]. Membrane retention must not change over the course of use of the devices. Membrane selectivity must also not change over the course of use. The lifetime of the expendable device must be determined. The cleaning and sanitization of the membranes must be validated.

The system itself must not adulterate the product. "Any substances associated with the operation of equipment, such as lubricants, heating fluids or coolants, should not contact intermediates or APIs so as to alter their quality beyond the official or otherwise established specifications" [2]. Attention must be paid to the surface coatings, the wetted components of the pump, the sealants and lubricants used in the pump, etc. One particular instance involved a system being cleaned with a reagent that was compatible with the devices but not with the internal components of the pump. The pump had rubber-lined rotary lobe heads, which over time were dissolved by the caustic cleaning agents and were trapped in the feed channels of the TFF device. This is an example of an incompatibility not of the devices, but of the system. Large systems will typically have 316L SST piping. With small-scale systems, tubing may be a variety of materials including but not limited to PTFE, silicone, neoprene, and tygon. It is important to ensure the compatibility of the tubing. Chemical degradation of the tubing components can result in these components contaminating the product.

7.7.3 System Design

There are many factors that affect the cleaning of the system. The geometry of the system is very important. See Figure 7.19 for examples of valve design. Piping should be sloped to allow proper drainage, and dead legs should be minimized to facilitate cleaning. Length/diameter ratios of system dead legs should be less than 2 to facilitate cleaning and flushing. All connections should be sanitary. This includes all the piping, valves, instrumentation, and the pump head. The surface finish should be a maximum of 35 Ra to minimize trapping

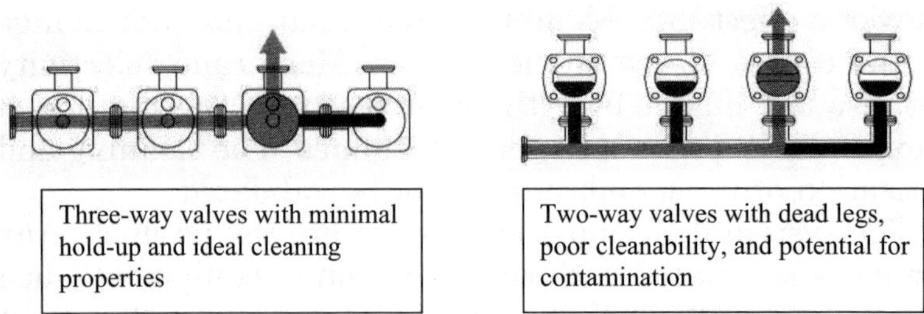

Figure 7.19 Impact of valve design on product holdup and contamination.

of particulate and bioburden. The composition of the metals in the system can affect the cleanability of the system, with 316L (low-carbon) SST being the industry standard for product contact surfaces, owing to its increased corrosion resistance. According to cGMPs, all equipment should be nonporous, nonreactive, nonadditive, and nonadsorptive. As with cleaning any surface, the temperature and concentration of the cleaning agent, as well as the flow rate and exposure time, affect the cleaning.

Different pump heads have different levels of cleanability. Peristaltic pumps are the most sanitary, since the product does not come in contact with the pump. The flexible tubing is changed between uses. Rotary lobe, centrifugal, and gear pumps are sanitary but require cleaning between uses. The necessary cleaning flow rates for the particular pump head should be validated. The pump manufacturer should be consulted for optimal cleaning flow rates.

7.7.4 Cleaning Specifications

When developing SOPs for cleaning, factors to consider include the maximum length of time that the equipment can sit in between processing and cleaning. Oftentimes, the focus is on the product and speeding it along in the downstream process, and equipment is left to sit before cleaning while operators concentrate on the next unit operation. If residuals are allowed to dry on the equipment surfaces, a cleaning regimen that was adequate immediately after processing may not be able to clean dried residue. The maximum storage time after cleaning and before the next use must be determined and validated.

Cleaning may be manual, semiautomated, or fully automated. Manual cleaning may require ongoing verification of operator training and performance. In the case of an operator manually washing tanks, SOPs are required outlining the washing and rinsing procedure for the tank cleaning. The SOPs will require regular review, and operators should be trained on the process at intervals compliant with the company's policies. Thus, it is more labor-intensive but may involve less capital outlay for the manual system. For a fully automated system, SOPs should be in place describing the preparation of the cleaning solutions. This will include the concentrations and temperatures of the solutions. An automated system will need to be programmed for the volume and duration of cleaning and rinse cycles and the pressures and flow rates of these solutions. The software controlling the automated system will require validation. This is an expense not incurred with manual cleaning. Although automated cleaning procedures may be more consistent, in certain applications manual cleaning may be more thorough. If washing machines are used to clean small pieces of equipment, the machines must be validated. Despite which method of cleaning is utilized, the end result of the cleaning will be validated through sampling and assaying for residue of product, contaminants, or cleaning agents.

When cleaning systems and devices, it is critical that the cleaning agents and rinse solutions fill all the interior surfaces of the device and system. This includes module feed and permeate channels and may require (depending on module design and orientation) that lower permeate ports be capped off to ensure filling of the permeate channel with cleaning and rinse solutions. All wetted components of the system must have fluid contact, including but not limited to instruments, piping, pump heads, and any dead legs. Tanks should be given special consideration. Closed tanks may require spray ball cleaning. In the case of fed-batch concentration, the large tank not permanently attached to the system must not be forgotten, nor the piping or pump that connected it to the tank on the system. These components may be cleaned separately or attached to the system for cleaning. If the cleaning reagents are recirculated or reused, the suitability of the fluid for reuse must be assessed. Reuse of cleaning reagents should be based on the worst-case scenario, which is the longest allowable storage time. In this case, the cleaning of the fluid storage containers must also be validated. Cleaning studies should be performed with the process-scale equipment. Any changes in equipment design may affect the cleaning of the system and will probably require revalidation of the cleaning protocol.

7.7.5 Membrane Reuse

Tangential-flow filtration devices have the benefit of reuse. This is a cost savings to the user, but the savings can be offset by the cost of validating a cleaning protocol and a reuse protocol. Many factors are involved in the decision to opt for single use or reuse. The size of the batch and the number of batches per year will usually be the determining factor. For a clarification application, normal flow or tangential flow can be used. A commonly used rule of thumb is to use NFF for batch sizes less than 1000 L or if less than 10 batches are produced per year. TFF becomes more economical with larger batch sizes or frequent processing, in which case the larger initial outlay for the TFF hardware and reuse validation costs are offset by the cost savings of reusing the membranes [39]. Operating costs will include the filter membranes, cleaning reagents, and WFI. Fixed costs include the hardware and validation costs. Because the validation of TFF systems includes cleaning and reuse, there are higher fixed costs associated with TFF. NFF has higher operating costs, since the filters are single use.

Membrane reuse validation studies can be performed at the laboratory scale. When validating membranes for reuse, multiple factors should be considered. System integrity should be monitored before and after each use, and clean-water flux and process flux should be trended over time (see Figure 7.17). Consistent water and process fluxes, coupled with consistent yields, are strong statistics in a membrane reuse validation study. The product retention and contaminant passage must not change over time. Any change in these critical parameters indicates a change in the separation and therefore the process. The validation of membranes for reuse is often performed concurrently to minimize costs and effort. It is important to have an SOP in place allowing rework in the event of a failure. However, reworking requires validation.

When making changes to the system, the amount of revalidation required will be dependent on the impact of the change on the process dynamics. If extra modules are added to a plate-and-frame system, this may not require membrane reuse validation or process revalidation, because no impact would be expected on the lifetime of the membranes if there has been no change in the process or cleaning regimen. The process will not be affected if all the operating parameters are equivalent. However, system cleaning will most likely require revalidation due to the change in system design, which may affect the efficiency of the cleaning step. The additional membrane area may require increased cleaning and flush volumes.

When performing cleaning validation, the worst-case challenge should be used. The worst case will be represented by a lengthy product exposure time prior to cleaning. As mentioned earlier, as residues dry on the system and device components, they fix in place and become more difficult to remove. The type of residue to be removed is crucial — is it soluble, hydrophobic, reactive? The answer to this question will dictate selection of the cleaning agent.

7.7.6 Clean-Water Flux

Clean-water flux, or normalized water permeability (NWP), should not decline drastically throughout the membrane lifetime. A consistent decrease in water flux after processing and cleaning indicates fouling of the membrane and implies that the cleaning step did not remove all of the foulants. A new membrane will show a decrease in water flux after the first use — typically no more than a 10% decrease for cellulosic membranes and a 15–25% decrease for polyethersulfone membranes. This is normal and indicative of the clean membrane becoming conditioned with solutes. After the first cleaning, the water flux value should be consistent, typically within 10% (see Figure 7.20). Any value falling below this range indicates an incomplete cleaning. The cleaning step should be verified to assess whether the step was performed correctly. Were the solutions made as recommended? Was the cleaning time appropriate, and were the correct flow rates, temperature, and pressures used? A continual drastic decline in water flux after multiple uses and cleanings indicates that a new cleaning regimen should be investigated. In some instances,

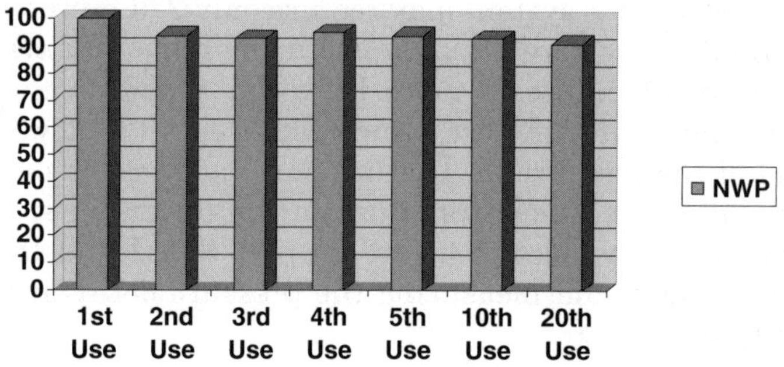

Figure 7.20 Clean water flux values over repeated filter use.

a multi-step cleaning is needed; acids and bases can be used with water flushes in between. Some cleaning agents can be combined for added efficiency. NaOH and NaOCl work well together to clean protein residue from polyethersulfone membranes.

It is important to measure clean-water flux using an appropriate water source, such as microfiltered deionized water, reverse-osmosis permeate, water for injection, or 18-megohm water. Tap water contains organic and inorganic solutes that can foul membranes, resulting in unreproducible measurements [40].

7.7.7 Integrity Testing

TFF devices should be integrity tested *in situ* to show integrity of the filter devices and the system. Acceptable integrity tests include diffusion testing as described in Section 7.3.3 and the pressure hold test. Because TFF devices have an inlet (feed) and an outlet (retentate) port on the upstream side of the filter membrane, either port may be used to introduce gas pressure to the upstream side of the membrane. If the feed port is used to introduce gas pressure, the outlet port (retentate port) must be completely closed to integrity test the device, and vice versa. The membranes must be fully wetted prior to the test. Systems should be stabilized for an appropriate amount of time to ensure even pressure distribution.

A laboratory-scale TFF system may require only 2–3 minutes of stabilization time, whereas a manufacturing-scale TFF system may require 10 minutes or more. Diffusion measurements are taken at the permeate port, which represents the downstream side of the membrane. The pressure hold test is performed by applying a known pressure to the upstream side of the device with the second upstream port closed and the permeate port open, and measuring the pressure decay over a specified time.

7.8 RESIDUE SAMPLING METHODS

ICH Q7A Section 5.25 states, "Acceptance criteria for residues and the choice of cleaning procedures and cleaning agents should be defined and justified." Section 12.74 states, "Residue limits should be practical, achievable, verifiable and based on the most deleterious residue" [2].

A validated protocol must be in place for the sampling and testing of residues and for the determination of the maximum acceptable residue level. Determination of residues after the cleaning and rinse step can be performed multiple ways; however, per Section 12.73, "the sampling methods used should be capable of quantitatively measuring levels of residues remaining on the equipment surfaces after cleaning" [2]. Destructive methods involve dissection of the device followed by visual or FTIR analysis. Obviously this is not an option in a reuse application, so nondestructive methods are employed. Nondestructive methods include direct surface sampling such as swab testing, rinse sampling, coupon sampling, solvent sampling, product sampling, and carryover testing. The advantages and disadvantages of each of these will be discussed, followed by residue limits.

7.8.1 Swab Testing

Swab testing is a direct sample of a specific area; therefore, it yields an accurate assessment of what residue is present in that location. However, many locations in a system are not accessible for swab testing, including within the devices. This limits the usefulness of swab sampling for validation of device cleaning and reuse. Per ICH Q7A Section 12.73, "swab sampling may be impractical when product contact surfaces are not easily accessible due to equipment design" [2]. Swabs may also leave fibers or adhesive residues on the sample site. Rinse samples have the advantage of contacting extensive surface area within the device and system. Samples may be taken of the cleaning solution during the cleaning step or the rinse solution during the rinse step. Rinse samples may also be taken of the last critical flush prior to processing. The disadvantage of rinse sampling is that the origin of the residue obtained in the rinse sample cannot be identified, and there may be residue in the system that cannot be removed by rinse sampling. This is analogous to the dirty pot in the sink: Cooked-on food is on the surface of the pot, but the rinse water remains clear because rinsing is not adequate to remove the residue. The device or the piping may contain surface residue, but the rinse may not be adequate to remove it. The problem here is that the product feed stream may contain agents that extract these residues from the system surfaces, thereby contaminating the product.

7.8.2 Solvent Sampling

Solvent sampling attempts to correct this problem by using a solvent to extract residues. This solvent may be a component of the product feed stream. It is used in the same manner as a rinse sample, so it has the same advantage of contacting extensive surface area throughout the device and system, with the added advantage of solvent extraction of residue. The disadvantage is that the solvent must be removed, and this removal must be validated. Product sampling involves batch analysis for previous batch product residue. The advantage of this is that the product itself is being analyzed for residual, so it is more pertinent to product contamination than analyzing rinse samples. However, how does one determine whether the product is residue from a previous batch or the current batch? One way to overcome this is to run a mock or placebo run, also called carryover testing. The entire process is run except that the feed stream contains the background components and not the product. By simulating the process, any residues on the system that would be removed by the components in the feed stream or the processing times and conditions will be removed in the placebo run. In this method, any residuals found in the placebo product can be identified as carryover residue. Carryover studies must be performed at the process scale.

7.8.3   Coupon Sampling

Coupon sampling uses a sample of the same material of construction that is affixed to an internal surface of the system. The process is duplicated, including cleaning, and the coupon is removed and assessed for residue. A potential problem with coupon sampling is that the coupon itself may interfere with the cleaning process. If an extra piece of filter media is affixed within the system, it may interfere with fluid flow of the cleaning reagents. On the other hand, the coupon may not be subjected to the same cleaning conditions as the filter media within the device. A coupon affixed within the system piping will be contacted by a much higher flow rate since the multiple feed channels within a plate-and-frame device drop the total flow rate by a factor equal to the number of feed channels. Therefore, the coupon may receive a more rigorous cleaning at higher flow rates and show a lower residue level than what is present in the filter device.

7.8.4   Assays

Regardless of what technique is used, the assays for product and contaminant residue testing must be calibrated with known standards. Use specific assays (NIR, HPLC, ELISA) as opposed to nonspecific (TOC, pH, conductivity) in order to identify the residue. If residue is identified by a nonspecific assay such as TOC, the worst-case scenario must be used and all residue identified in the process must be assumed to be that which is most toxic. As well as being a nonspecific assay, TOC testing is restricted to water-soluble species and those containing carbon. As an example, if a rinse sample is taken on a system and analyzed by TOC, no action is required if the residuals are within the specified limit. If the residuals are outside of the specified limit, a specific assay is required to determine whether the residue is product, excipient, or cleaning agent.

If TOC is used, the advantage is that a new procedure does not have to be developed for each new active drug substance manufactured. TOC is sensitive to the ppb range and is less time-consuming and less costly than many other methods. It can be used with direct surface sampling or rinse sampling [41].

7.8.5 Acceptable Residue Limits

PDA Technical Report Number 29 recommends the following formula for determination of maximum allowable carryover [42]:

$$MAC = \frac{TD \times BS \times SF}{LDD}$$

where

    MAC = maximum allowable carryover
      TD = single therapeutic dose
      BS = batch size of next product
      SF = safety factor
    LDD = largest daily dose of next product to be
             manufactured using same equipment

Typical safety factors for injectable products are 1/1,000 to 1/10,000 of a daily dose [42]. The safety factor selected will be dependent on the potency and toxicity of the compound, as well as the analytical limit of detection. Other considerations are the solubility of the product and contaminants in the cleaning reagents, and the cleanability of the system. If the equipment is used to manufacture multiple products, then the effects of cross-contamination must be considered, and limits calculated using the worst-case scenario. The worst-case scenario assumes that any residue present will be the most toxic contaminant present.

An example of a residue limit follows:

- Single therapeutic dose of 100 mg
- Batch size of 10 kg
- Largest daily dose of 800 mg
- Use safety factor of 1/1000

MAC = (100 mg × 10 kg × 0.001)/800 mg = 1250 mg

There are many points to consider in setting residue limits. Limits must be practical with respect to the cleaning situation and verifiable with respect to the assay. An analytical methodology must exist for the specific product, and the rationale behind the chosen limit must be scientifically sound. Bear in mind when calculating residue limits that the total residue should be calculated. Transfer tanks, pumps, and piping must be tested as well as the system. The question of whether all the residues in the process can be identified must be posed. Will partial reactants or by-products be characterized?

7.9 CONCLUSION

The validation effort is ultimately rewarded by a detailed understanding of the process and the product. Through the validation process, control parameters are put in place at each unit operation. These parameters ensure that the process is reproducible and that the process will generate an equivalent product with every batch. As well as establishing limits of normal operation, the outer limits of the process operation are determined, thereby generating a great deal of data describing how the process behaves under varied conditions. A rugged process is much less likely to fail, and in-depth knowledge of the process and how it reacts to minor perturbations allows for monitoring of the process through multiple runs and understanding of why changes are occurring. This allows the opportunity to compensate for and correct for these changes before a batch is lost.

Validation is becoming more of a team approach within drug manufacturing facilities and between drug manufacturers and filter vendors. It is also being incorporated earlier into the drug development phase. The validation department works with R&D, process development, QA and QC, manufacturing, and engineering to ensure that quality is built into the process. Advances in each of these areas are contributing to faster drug development timelines and more quality being built into drug manufacturing processes. For example, the recent integration of process engineering is resulting in improved system designs that minimize system impact on product quality and yield. Advances in assay development are resulting in faster assay turnaround times, which enable faster process times. Vendors are continually providing higher-quality products for use in drug manufacturing processes, such as more robust filter membranes with increased flux to provide faster processing. Disposable products that reduce the burden of cleaning validation, such as disposable capsule filters and bags, are increasing in popularity. Vendors supply validation guides with filter products, which speeds the drug manufacturer's process validation.

The stringency of regulatory requirements is increasing, with emphasis being placed on process characterization and validation. This requires selection of appropriate filtration devices and establishment of acceptable windows of operation for control parameters such as flow rates, pressures, and temperature. These control parameters must meet criteria for yield, quality, purity, and process time. Process development personnel must anticipate the requirements of the full-scale process to ensure that the optimized process is robust, scaleable, and verifiable. Faster process development while investigating a range of control parameters is enabled through factorial design, contributing to speed to market. As technology improves, assays are developed that are more sensitive, allowing for improved product and contaminant characterization and quantification. This advancement in technology may become an obstacle to drug manufacturers, in that as the ability to characterize and quantitate contaminants improves, regulatory agencies may look to drug manufacturers to design processes resulting in higher product purity levels.

More rigorous process characterization, coupled with faster regulatory approval times and improved technology, is resulting in shorter timelines from drug discovery to market. Yet, even with these shorter timelines, more quality is being built into current drug manufacturing processes because of the validation process. This trend will ensure that drug manufacturers will continue to provide safe and effective drug products.

REFERENCES

1. Meltzer, T.H., *Filtration in the Pharmaceutical Industry*, 1st ed., Marcel Dekker, New York, 1987, pp. 532–539.

2. ICH Q7A, Quality of Biotechnological Products: Good Manufacturing Practices Guide for Active Pharmaceutical Ingredients, November 10, 2000.

3. Chao, A.Y., Forbes, F.S.J., Johnson, R.F., and Doehren, P.V., Prospective process validation, in *Pharmaceutical Process Validation*, Nash, R.A., Ed., Marcel Dekker, New York, 2003, pp. 7–30.

4. Morris, G.M., Rozembersky, J., and Schwartz, L., Validation of filtration, in *Biopharmaceutical Process Validation*, Sofer, G. and Zabriskie, D.W., Eds., Marcel Dekker, New York, 2000, pp. 213–233.

5. Carter, J.R. and Levy, R.V., Microbial retention testing in the validation of sterilizing filtration, in *Filtration in the Biopharmaceutical Industry*, Meltzer and Jornitz, Eds., Marcel Dekker, New York, 1998, pp. 577–604.

6. Jornitz, M.W. and Meltzer, T.H., Identifying the sterilizing filter, *Pharm. Technol.*, Sept., 38–44, 2000.

7. Parenteral Drug Association Technical Report No. 26, Supplement Volume 52, Number S1, Sterilizing Filtration of Liquids, 1998.

8. Establishing Product Specific Bubble Point Specifications for Sterilizing-Grade (0.22μm) Durapore® Filters, Millipore Application Note AN1505EN00, rev 2/00.

9. Jornitz, M.W. and Meltzer, T.H., Validation of filtrative sterilizations, in *Filtration in the Biopharmaceutical Industry*, Meltzer and Jornitz, Eds., Marcel Dekker, New York, 1998, pp. 897–924.

10. FDA, Guidelines on validation of the limulus amebocyte lysate test as an end-product endotoxin test for human and animal parenteral drugs, biologicals, and medical devices, Center for Drugs and Biologics and Center for Devices and Radiological Health, Rockville, MD, 1987.

11. Christiansen, G., Monoclonal antibodies, in *Separations Technology*, Olson, W.P., Ed., Interpharm Press, Buffalo Grove, 1995, pp. 353–390.

12. Akers, M.J. and Anderson, N.R., Sterilization validation, in *Pharmaceutical Process Validation*, Nash, R.A., Ed., Marcel Dekker, New York, 2003, pp. 83–157.

13. Stone, T.E., Goel, V., and Leszczak, J., Methodology for analysis of filter extractables: a model stream approach, *Pharm. Technol.*, October 1994.

14. Stone, T.E., Goel, V., Leszczak, J., and Chrai, S., The model stream approach: defining the worst-case conditions, *Pharm. Technol.*, February, 34–51, 1996.

15. USP XXIII, Section 88, Biological Reactivity Tests, *in vivo*, pp. 1699–1703.

16. Reif, O.W., Extractables and compatibilities of filters, in *Filtration in the Biopharmaceutical Industry*, Meltzer and Jornitz, Eds., Marcel Dekker, New York, 1998, pp. 199–244.

17. Kao, Y.-H., Bender, J., Hagewiesche, A., Wong, P., Huang, Y., and Vanderlaan, M., Characterization of filter extractables by proton NMR spectroscopy: studies on intact filters with process buffers, *PDA J.*, 55, 268–277, 2001.

18. Optiseal Cartridges with Hydrophilic Durapore® Membrane, Millipore Validation Guide VG007, rev. 2, Dec. 1999.

19. Badmington, F., Membrane filtration technology, in *Development of Biopharmaceutical Parenteral Dosage Forms*, Bontempo, J.A., Ed., Marcel Dekker, New York, 1997, pp. 171–222.

20. National Institute of Standards and Technology, Standard Reference Material 2806, Medium Test Dust (MTD) in Hydraulic Fluid, 1997.

21. Badmington, F., Prefiltration technology, in *Filtration in the Biopharmaceutical Industry*, Meltzer and Jornitz, Eds., Marcel Dekker, New York, 1998, pp. 783–817.

22. Polysep™ II CGW-Cartridge Filters, Millipore Validation Guide, VG049, rev. A, May 1998.

23. Surface-Type Filters Used in Fluid Clarification, Millipore Technical Brief TB060, Nov. 1991.

24. ICH Q5A, Quality of Biotechnological Products: Viral Safety Evaluation of Biotechnology Products Derived From Cell Lines of Human or Animal Origin, ICH, March 5, 1997 (adopted as a guidance document and published in the Federal Register, September 1998).

25. Brough, H., Antoniou, C., Carter, J., Jakubik, J., Xu, Y., and Lutz, H., Performance of a novel Viresolve NFR virus filter, *Biotechnol. Prog.*, 18, 782–795, 2002.

26. Ensuring Compliance: Regulatory Guidance for Virus Clearance Validation, Millipore Application Note AN1650EN00, rev. 10/02, 2002.

27. Note for Guidance on Virus Validation Studies: The Design, Contribution and Interpretation of Studies Validating the Inactivation and Removal of Viruses, EMEA CPMP BWP, 268/95, 1996.

28. Note for Guidance on Plasma-Derived Medicinal Products, EMEA CPMP BWP, 269/95 rev. 3, 2001.

29. Points to Consider in the Manufacture and Testing of Monoclonal Antibody Products for Human Use, CBER FDA, 1997.

30. Levy, R.V., Phillips, M.W., and Lutz, H., Filtration and the removal of viruses from biopharmaceuticals, in *Filtration in the Biopharmaceutical Industry*, Meltzer and Jornitz, Eds., Marcel Dekker, New York, 1998, pp. 619–646.

31. Industrial Perspective on Validation of Tangential Flow Filtration in Biopharmaceutical Applications, Parenteral Drug Association Technical Report No. 15, 1992, Suppl. Vol. 46, Number S1.

32. Kuwahara, S.S. and Chuan, J.H., Process validation of separation systems, in *Separations Technology*, Olson, W.P., Ed., Interpharm Press, Buffalo Grove, 1995, pp. 427–451.

33. Endotoxin Removal, Millipore Technical Note dTN049, rev. A, March 1997.

34. Sofer, G., Biotechnology product validation. IV. Clearance of impurities from protein and peptide biotherapeutics, *Pharm. Technol. Eur.*, May, 29–32, 1994.

35. Cheryan, M., Membrane properties, in *Ultrafiltration Handbook*, Technomic Publishing Co., Lancaster, 1986, pp. 53–72.

36. Techniques for Demonstrating Cleaning Effectiveness of Ultrafiltration Membranes, Millipore Technical Brief TB1502EN00, Dec. 2000.

37. Hall, W.E., Validation and verification of cleaning processes, in *Pharmaceutical Process Validation*, Nash, R.A., Ed., Marcel Dekker, New York, 2003, pp. 465–506.

38. Michaels, S.L., Michaels, A.S., Antoniou, C., Pearl, S.R., Goel, V., de los Reyes, G., Keating, P., Rudolph, E., Kuriyel, R., and Siwak, M., Tangential flow filtration, in *Separations Technology*, Olson, W.P., Ed., Interpharm Press, Buffalo Grove, 1995, pp. 57–194.

39. Mammalian Cell Culture Clarification, Millipore Application Note AN1511EN00, rev. 3/00.

40. Michaels, S.L., Clean-water permeability as a determinant of cleaning efficiency in tangential-flow filtration systems, *BioPharm*, 7, 38–45, 1994.

41. Clark, K., How to develop and validate a total organic carbon method for cleaning applications, *PDA J.*, 55, 290–293, 2001.

42. Points to Consider for Cleaning Validation, Parenteral Drug Association Technical Report No. 29, Suppl. Vol. 52, No. 6, 1998.

8

Analytical Test Methods for Biological and Biotechnological Products

NADINE RITTER AND JOHN MCENTIRE

CONTENTS

8.1 ANALYTICAL CHARACTERIZATION OF BIOMOLECULAR PRODUCTS

Historically, as technologies were developed that allowed biological or biotechnological materials to be produced in large quantities for pharmaceutical use, the statement was frequently heard in both industry and regulatory circles that "the process is the product." This perspective was based on the understanding that the main production agents — living organisms — produce large quantities of chemically similar material (e.g., proteins) that must undergo a variety of separation steps that can (hopefully) select the greatest yield of the highest purity of a desired molecular entity from the cellular-derived milieu. The separation processes used to sort out the one or more target proteins from other, often copurifying, proteins are optimized, scaled, and validated to reliably achieve the same population of molecular entities from each batch of biologically produced material. The nature of these separation processes is such that even subtle changes in some steps can impart significant variations in the resulting population of proteins. It has been shown repeatedly that successfully defining and controlling the *process* can define and control the *product*, hence the rationale for the phrase [1].

Concurrent with advances in process technologies, analytical technologies have also been emerging that allow biological and biotechnological materials to be scrutinized in ever more sensitive and specific physiochemical and functional detail.

Increasing attention is being given to the tremendous value to be derived from adequate analytical characterization of protein products and, in many cases, critical in-process or intermediate materials. During early product development, in-depth, orthogonal biochemical information gained on the target molecular entity provides a better understanding of the attributes of the product that may contribute to its efficacy. It also allows an assessment of intrinsic product- or process-related impurities that could impact product safety in early clinical trials. As development proceeds and product batches are manufactured, analytical characterization can be used to obtain biomolecular profiles of the product and its impurities in order to evaluate process consistency. Biomolecular characterization techniques are also used to determine the physiochemical comparability of product batches before and after a process change, to assess the success of process scale-up or scale-down, or following technology transfer of the production to a different manufacturing facility.

For these reasons, efforts directed toward the analysis and characterization of the biological/biotechnological *product* have recently achieved a level of significance that was previously considered necessary only for the purification process. In fact, a term now widely used in the biotechnology industry is *well-characterized biological/biotechnological products* or WCBPs (now formally designated by the FDA as *specified products*) [2]. The term reflects the important role of rigorous analytics in ensuring safe and effective products, as has been demonstrated in numerous case studies and discussions at industry-regulatory WCBP meetings (e.g., www.casss.org).

The structural complexity of even simple proteins requires the use of several different analytical technologies to generate a characteristic product "profile." Many of these techniques utilize complex materials and reagents that are relatively labile and subject to manufacturing variability. These features can impact method robustness and the establishment of realistic method performance specifications. There are many factors that should be considered when selecting, optimizing, and validating analytical test methods, and in using test results to establish appropriate specifications. Choices are made during the development cycle regarding the types of standard and state-of-the-art technologies that may be suitable for use with the product. Current regulatory guidance documents and several biotechnology industry publications give considerable information on the typical analytical methods used with different types of WCBPs and other biological products and current expectations for product characterization, release, and stability testing (www.fda.gov; www.ich.org; www.bioprocessintl.com; www.bioprocessing-journal.com; www.biopharm-mag.com). Practical considerations should also be factored into the selection of the methods that will be used for routine quality control testing of product batches. QC analytical methods must be robust enough to function reliably over time under varying operational conditions. *Failure to fully understand the details of the analytical technology and failure to define the intended application of the method are prime reasons for methods that end up in QC laboratories unable to reliably perform to (unsupportable) expectations.*

8.2 PHYSIOCHEMICAL PROFILE OF BIOTECHNOLOGICAL/BIOLOGICAL PRODUCTS

Figure 8.1 highlights elements of the structure of proteins and peptides and the associated physiochemical attributes. To develop a comprehensive profile of a biopharmaceutical product, multiple aspects of the structure require analysis. In addition, tests to determine the product's concentration and potency are conducted to assess functionality. For consistency herein, the terms "method," "technique," and "assay" will be used interchangeably to mean a defined procedure conducted with a designated analytical technology. It is recognized that in certain situations, e.g., compendial monograph specifications, "assay" defines a specific characteristic of a product.

For additional clarity, the differences between *bioanalytical* methods, *biomolecular* methods, and *bioassays* should be noted. Bioanalytical methods are assays used for the quantitative determination of drugs or metabolites in physiological samples derived from animals or humans [3]. Samples analyzed with bioanalytical methods contain the target chemical or biomolecular entity in a complex matrix such as plasma or serum. For chemical drugs, techniques such as solid phase extraction followed by GC, LC, or MS are used to quantify the target entity. For biological drugs, it requires product-specific binding techniques such as immunological methods to quantify the *biological* target in the presence of a *biological* matrix.

Level of Structural Characterization	Analytical Information Obtained

Primary Structure	Protein sequence
	Nucleic acid sequence
	Amino acid composition
	Apparent molecular weight
	Observed molecular mass
	Post-translational modifications:
	  Phosphorylation
	  Glycosylation (monosaccharide composition)

Secondary Structure	Polypeptide chains Peptide fragments Disulfide bond linkages Glycosylation (oligosaccharide structure) Isoforms (e.g., glycoforms)
Tertiary Structure	Receptor-ligand interaction Epitope recognition Cell modulator release Cell differentiation effect Replication competence
Product + Ligand Conjugate	Molar ratios of ligand/product Ligand binding sites

Figure 8.1 Examples of physiochemical characteristics of a biomolecular compound.

The FDA defines bioassays as functional tests used to determine the activity, potency, or biological integrity of a drug product [4]. The WHO/NIBSC developed the following definition of bioassays: "A bioassay is defined as an analytical procedure measuring a biological activity of a test substance based on a specific, functional, biological response of a test system" [5]. Bioassays include *in vitro* methods such as cell culture assays, antiviral assays, infectivity assays, and *in vivo* assays involving animal models.

An additional term, *biomolecular methods*, encompasses the analytical technologies used to perform physiochemical characterization of biological and biotechnological products [6]. Biomolecular methods include various chromatographic, electrophoretic, spectrophotometric, colorimetric, gravimetric, chemical, and compositional technologies. It requires a combination of many of these techniques to adequately establish the physiochemical profile of a biopharmaceutical product.

8.3 ANALYTICAL METHODS USED IN PRODUCTION OPERATIONS

Each unit operation of a validated manufacturing process is supported by specifications to provide assurance that the process is in control. The International Conference on Harmonization (ICH) defines specifications as "the list of tests, references to analytical procedures, and appropriate acceptance criteria which are numerical limits, ranges, or other criteria for tests described. It establishes the set of criteria to which a drug substance, drug product, or materials at other stages of manufacture should conform to be considered acceptable for its intended use. Conformance to specification means that the raw material, product component, drug substance or drug product, when tested according to the listed analytical procedures, will meet the acceptance criteria" [7].

Specifications are considered *contracts* with the regulatory agency whereby the manufacturer agrees to make and test the licensed product as defined in the product submission. The sponsor further agrees to use only those batches of product that pass their given quality control assays. The total quality of a biotechnology product is recognized to be intrinsically linked to a comprehensive strategy that includes specifications, thorough product characterization, compliance with cGMP operational requirements, validated processes, and validated test methods for assessing product release and stability [7]. It is clear that sound analytical methodology is a central tenet of this quality system.

8.3.1 Raw Material Methods

The biopharmaceutical manufacturing process typically encompasses the raw materials used in production (which may include naturally derived "harvest," e.g., plasma, where *in vitro* expression systems are not used to produce the target product), cell culture/fermentation conditions (for expression systems), the purification process, the bulk active product, the formulation of the active product, and the final drug product. Each of these steps requires samples to be taken and data generated to determine whether the materials are suitable for use or whether they should be processed to the next unit operation [8]. In addition, the stability of bulk substance and final drug product must be assessed.

Many methods for the analysis of common raw materials are often compendial, i.e., found in the U.S. Pharmacopoeia [9]. These methods have been validated in large-scale collaborative studies. To implement a compendial method in a user laboratory, the method must be verified under conditions of actual use [10]. The verification study should consist of testing the method with the samples in the buffer or placebo matrix to assess potential matrix interference, with limited repeatability to ensure reliable performance in the user laboratory. Compendial methods for complex or proprietary raw materials (e.g., cell culture media) are not usually available. These materials often require methods that assess critical product attributes such as composition, concentration, and suitable function such as growth promotion or enzymatic activity to assure that each batch is of acceptable quality to be used in the manufacturing process.

While the vendor of the material will have some methods in place for product release, they may not address the same parameters as needed by the specific user for their manufacturing applications. In these cases, it will be necessary for the user to develop and validate the necessary raw materials tests to be performed on each batch of material upon receipt. If vendor testing is suitable to meet the user requirements, the vendor's certificate of analysis may be accepted as the certification of each batch of material quality. However, the vendor should be audited by a qualified entity to assure the user that suitable quality practices are in place to support the integrity of the production and testing of the raw material. The only test required upon receipt of each batch would then be an identity assay to confirm that the correct material was received [11].

8.3.2   In-Process Methods

During cell culture and fermentation steps, critical parameters are measured to ensure adequate control of the processes. Parameters such as pH, O_2 and CO_2 levels, glucose, or other sentinel compounds are monitored to confirm they are within required limits. The assays used to perform these measurements may be simple (e.g., pH or dissolved gas) or more complex (e.g., cell density or target protein concentration). If they are compendial, they may be used with verification, as previously described. If they are noncompendial, they will require validation for routine use under cGMP, as described subsequently.

Product purification is supported with in-process analytical methods to determine the success of a unit operation and the ability to process the material to the next step. In practice, analyte-specific in-process methods are typically developed using purified forms of the target product to measure purity, concentration, or potency. Then, method performance must be verified with actual in-process samples, since much greater amounts of process- and product-related impurities are present in the in-process samples than in the purified product. Also, buffer components and concentrations may be significantly different with in-process samples. For these reasons, it is usually necessary to assess method specificity using test buffer blanks in parallel with test samples from process development experiments to determine the effect on assay performance. The recovery of target protein is usually calculated as a percent of starting material when used to evaluate the optimization and consistency of purification processes.

In 2003, the FDA launched a new initiative termed "Process Analytical Technology" or PAT, which is defined as "a system for designing, analyzing, and controlling manufacturing through timely measurements (i.e., during processing) of critical quality and performance attributes of raw and in-process materials and processes with the goal of ensuring final product quality. The term 'analytical' in PAT is viewed broadly to include chemical, physical, microbiological, mathematical, and risk analysis conducted in an integrated manner" [12]. The concept marries analytical technology, process development tools (such as statistically designed experiments), mathematical modeling, and risk assessment tools (such as failure modes effects analysis) to define the most effective testing and control scheme to best ensure the consistent quality of the manufactured product.

The types of PAT might be categorized according to whether the application is designed to (1) collect test data on a process step where that information is used to make adjustments in real-time to the batch being manufactured; (2) collect test data on a process step from an R&D process model or a scaled production run, where that information is evaluated to better characterize the method of manufacturing, but is not used to immediately alter the batch being sampled; (3) collate historical data from numerous production runs and perform meta-analysis to examine critical process parameters; or (4) evaluate the nature of the process with statistical or other mathematical tools to generate a risk-based assessment of process capability. It is currently a subject of discussion how PAT elements might best be used to develop and improve biopharmaceutical processes. However, any cGMP PAT applications will require appropriate qualification and validation of the test methods used in on-line/at-line operations.

8.3.3 Drug Substance and Drug Product Methods

To determine their acceptable quality, the bulk and final product must be analyzed for identity, purity, impurities, concentration, and potency [7]. Unless the product is listed in a compendial monograph in which regulatory methods for these product attributes are given, the development of noncompendial methods will be necessary. Many historical biological products such as plasma fractionation products (i.e., human serum albumin) and vaccine products do have monograph listings in the USP/NF that must be followed for product release.

However, most biotechnology products are new molecular entities and therefore do not have monograph listings. In the absence of compendial methods, manufacturers of these products must develop and validate their own (noncompendial) analytical methods and product specifications [13]. Manufacturers are also responsible for verifying that analytical methods used for product stability testing are suitably capable of detecting, and as necessary quantifying, degradation products. It should be noted that compendial methods are not necessarily verified to be stability-indicating for the products listed in monographs [9]; the burden is on the user to confirm the appropriate methods for use in stability protocols.

8.4 METHODS USED FOR PRODUCT CHARACTERIZATION, RELEASE, AND STABILITY TESTING

A singular feature of the analysis of biotechnology products — in contrast to small chemical entities — is the diversity of analytical technologies necessary to obtain the physiochemical profile. Characterization of a biopharmaceutical product is considered to be the complete description of its physical, chemical, and biological characteristics [14]. A subset of methods used for product characterization is validated for routine product QC batch release testing. Some of the methods used for product release (e.g., pH, UV, HPLC, SDS-PAGE) are also used as in-process control tests to monitor the characteristics of product intermediates during the manufacturing steps. Some QC release methods are validated to be suitable for use in product stability protocols. Examples of the types of analytical technologies used in the characterization, release, and stability testing of biotechnology products are shown in Figure 8.2. The specific analytical methods required for the characterization, comparability, release, or stability testing of any given biopharmaceutical product are determined by product development studies and discussions with product regulatory reviewers.

METHOD	ATTRIBUTE	TYPICAL USES[a]
pH (if liquid)	General quality	I, C, R, S
Karl Fisher (if lyophilized)	Moisture, stability	C, R, S
Appearance	General quality	I, C, R, S
UV Absorbance	Concentration	I, C, R, S
SDS-PAGE	Identity, purity, stability	I, C, R, S
SEC-HPLC	Identity, purity, stability	I, C, R, S
RP-HPLC, IEX-HPLC, HIC-HPLC	Identity, purity, stability	I, C, R, S
Peptide Mapping	Identity, stability	C, R, S
Mass Spectrometry	Identity, stability	C, R, S
Isoelectric Focusing	Identity, stability	C, R, S
Capillary Electrophoresis	Identity, stability	C, R, S
Immunoassay/ELISA	Identity, stability	C, R, S
Ligand Binding Assay	Identity, potency, stability	C, R, S
In Vitro Bioassay	Identity, potency, stability	C, R, S
N-terminal Sequencing	Identity	C, R
Amino Acid Analysis	Identity, concentration	C, R
Process Residuals (e.g., HCP)	Purity	C, R
Monosaccharides*	Identity	C
Oligosaccharide*	Identity	C
Sialic Acid*	Identity	C
Circular Dichroism	Conformation	C
FTIR	Conformation	C

[a] *I = in-process; C = characterization/comparability; R = QC release; S = stability*

Figure 8.2 Methods frequently used with well-characterized biological/biotechnological products. The intended use of a method depends upon the nature of the product; e.g., *carbohydrate analysis might be validated for release testing of certain glycoproteins.

Comprehensive characterization analysis is typically conducted at key points during the development cycle and after FDA approval. The objective of a characterization study is to provide detailed information from a wide array of techniques in order to provide a thorough understanding of the expected nature of the material. Characterization establishes the physiochemical attributes and biological function of the product and will, and should, have to support its safety and efficacy. When extensive characterization is performed, some "curious discoveries" have been made on the physiochemical nature of biotechnology products [15]. Errors in translation, incorporation of unusual amino acids, novel cross-links, and amino acid substitutions have all been discovered when state-of-the-art analytical methods such as peptide-mapping procedures, mass spectrometry, high-performance liquid chromatography (HPLC), and electrophoretic methods are used to analyze products.

Of particular interest in product characterization is the "fingerprint" of product heterogeneity and product- and process-related impurities of the product. In addition to the major quantitative analyses, qualitative assessment of SDS-PAGE and IEF banding patterns or peptide map and mass spectrophotometric fragment patterns can yield significant information on the capability of the production process to yield material with consistent characteristics, including impurities.

Characterization of the biological function of a product typically requires *in vitro* or *in vivo* bioassays that measure one or more attributes of the product. While it is desirable to utilize a bioassay based on the clinical mechanism of action of the product, in many instances its exact mechanism in humans is not completely defined. In such cases, bioassays serve as surrogate biochemical methods with which to measure the quality and consistency of product functionality.

As discussed in Section 8.9, methods used *only* for drug substance *characterization* generally are not required to be validated in accordance with *all* ICH and FDA guidelines. However, it is expected that these methods should at a minimum be qualified to ensure that they are capable of generating reliable data on the specific material being tested [16].

8.4.1 QC Release Tests — Thumbs Up or Thumbs Down?

Traditional chemical drugs are typically QC release tested for physical description, physical properties (e.g., pH of solution forms, moisture of solid forms, particle size), identity, assay (drug content and purity), process-related impurities (e.g., solvents), microbial limits, and, in some cases, proportion of chiral or polymorphic species [17]. Most of these methods employ spectrophotometric, gravimetric, or chromatographic techniques. Biologically derived pharmaceuticals often require additional immunological, enzymatic, electrophoretic, colorimetric, and cell-based methods for assessing molecular characteristics and complex host- and process-derived impurities. It is expected that no single analytical method can profile all biotechnology product characteristics. Each critical attribute — identity, purity, quality, potency, strength, product- and process-related impurities — is assessed by multiple analytical procedures; each test could yield different results based on differences in method capabilities such as sensitivity and specificity. Figure 8.3 is from USP General Chapter <1045> "Test Procedures for Biotechnology Products" [9]. It illustrates how a variety of biomolecular methods can be utilized to evaluate specific biotechnology product- and process-related impurities.

For biotechnology product QC release testing, it is expected that orthogonal analytical methods will be used for key product attributes [15]. *Orthogonal* refers to methods that exploit different chemical or physical mechanisms for analysis. For example, since SEC-HPLC and RP-HPLC are based on two different separation mechanisms (mass and polarity), they can provide orthogonal chromatographic data on product purity and impurities. Similarly, amino acid sequence (the order of amino acids) and amino acid composition (the total amount of each amino acid) provide orthogonal information on protein identity. Typically, for well-characterized biotechnology products, critical product parameters such as purity and identity are supported with a minimum of two orthogonal QC release methods.

Aggregation: SDS-PAGE, SEC-HPLC, light scattering
Deamidation, Oxidation: Peptide map, HPLC, IEF, MS
Proteolytic Cleavage: Peptide map, SDS-PAGE, HPLC, IEF, MS
Amino Acid Substitutions: AAA, peptide map, MS, protein sequence, CE
Translation Mutations: Peptide map, HPLC, IEF, MS, CE
Host Cell Proteins: SDS-PAGE, Western blot, ELISA
Media Components: SDS-PAGE, Western blot, HPLC, ELISA
Nucleic Acids: DNA hybridization, UV, protein binding
Affinity Antibodies: SDS-PAGE, Western blot, ELISA
Proteases/Nucleases: HPLC, Western blot, ELISA
Leachates/Extractables: HPLC, MS, GC, gravimetric analysis
Process Residuals: Karl Fisher moisture, GC, ion chromatography

Figure 8.3 Analytical methods for biotechnology product impurities. (Adapted from USP <1045> Biotechnology-Derived Articles. Reprinted with permission. © 2005 United States Pharmacopeia. All rights reserved.) Note that the first three sets are often used in assessing protein degradation states.

In product QC testing, it should be noted that no one analytical method is more or less important than another. It is sometimes tempting to think that simple methods (e.g., pH, appearance, UV) are less important to product quality than complex ones (e.g., chromatography or bioassays). In terms of the specifications established for the product — the characteristics, the methodology used to access them, and the criteria for acceptable quality of each characterisic — *every analytical method is uniquely valuable and should be carefully optimized, qualified, and validated to suit its intended use.*

8.4.2   Stability Tests — Looking for Ghosts with Metal Detectors?

For biotechnology/biological products, it is recognized that "the evaluation of stability may necessitate complex analytical methodologies. Appropriate physiochemical, biochemical and immunochemical methods for the analysis of the molecular entity and the quantitative detection of degradation products should also be a part of the stability program whenever purity and molecular characteristics of the product permit use of these methodologies" [18]. Methods used in the stability protocol should detect significant changes in the quality of the product (e.g., purity, potency) with a focus on the ability of the methods to determine product degradation [15]. If the methods have not been experimentally confirmed to demonstrate their ability to detect, and possibly quantify, all potential product degradants, there is a possibility that some forms of product degradation may go undetected. This situation would be analogous to utilizing metal detectors without realizing that the objects of concern are actually ghosts. (Acknowledgments to J.B. Hill for this analogy.)

The best way to demonstrate whether or not a test method is truly capable of detecting or quantifying product degradation is to conduct a *forced degradation study*. Forced degradation studies provide critical information on the inherent stability of the product and its degradation pathways and confirm the capabilities and suitability of the analytical methods to be used in stability testing. This one-time study on a single batch is not considered a part of the normal stability protocol [18]. As shown in Figure 8.4, it should stress the drug

Chemical and Physical Treatments to Promote:

• Aggregation	• Fragmentation
• Precipitation	• Dephosphorylation*
• Deamidation	• Deglycosylation*
• Hydrolysis	• Disulfide bond exchange*
• Oxidation	• Ligand release*

Figure 8.4 Purposeful (forced) degradation conditions typically examined for biotechnology products (* when the product contains these moieties).

substance in several physical and chemical experiments, including various pH solutions, in the presence of oxygen and light, and at elevated temperature and (for lyophilized products) humidity increments. For biotechnology products in solution, it should include agitation stress. For products stored frozen, multiple freeze–thaw cycles should be examined. It is recognized that stress conditions may create product degradants not formed under normal storage, shipping, and handling conditions, but the force-degraded product preparations are considered to be important as reagents used to challenge the potential stability-indicating analytical methods [18].

Whenever significant qualitative or quantitative changes indicative of product degradation are detected during long-term, accelerated, or stress studies, consideration should be given to the potential hazards and to the need for characterization and quantitation of degradants [18]. The goal is to ensure product safety by clearly understanding the physiochemical nature and potential adverse impact of a product's inherent degradation pathway. This is especially true for biotechnology/biological products, where degradants could create new epitopes that could trigger a neoantigenic immune response in patients, such as heat-treating product preparations to achieve viral inactivation [19].

Ideally, initial stress studies should be done early in product development to allow selection of the stability-indicating methods for real-time stability studies [18]. Experiments are designed to cover all potential degradation pathways of a given product, allowing the degradation conditions to proceed and removing sentinel samples at designated points and subjecting them to analysis using orthogonal analytical methods [20]. Accelerated and stress stability experiments can provide valuable information on the degradation pathways and kinetics of degradation [21]. *But unlike chemical pharmaceutical products, shelf-life specifications for biological/biotechnological products cannot be determined from extrapolation of short-term results, but can only be established through real-time stability studies* [18].

8.4.3 Product Potency Assays — Why the Ends Do Not Justify the Means

When discussing release and stability tests for biotechnology products, one frequently heard comment is, "Why can't a potency assay suffice as evidence of product quality and stability? Isn't it the ultimate proof of acceptable product performance?" It is true that biotechnology products may be intrinsically heterogeneous, and the specifications may include designated impurities [7], but it is necessary to ensure continued product safety and efficacy by monitoring and maintaining the degree of heterogeneity and impurities to the levels demonstrated in preclinical and clinical trials.

When choosing a quality control testing scheme, the better question to ask is, "What are the parameters that best demonstrate manufacturing consistency?" These will likely encompass more than just the parameters that are known to impact clinical efficacy, because the first objective of quality control testing is to ensure continued product safety. For biotechnology products, "since the degree of heterogeneity defines their quality, the degree and profile of this heterogeneity should be characterized to ensure lot to lot consistency" [7].

Potency assays generally have greater variability than other physiochemical methods such as chromatography, so changes in product heterogeneity or impurities and degradants might be hidden within, or misinterpreted as, inherent assay variation. Also, because potency assays (and even immunoassays) are based on the measurement of a defined target activity, they can be insensitive to varying levels of impurities unless they interfere with the specific reaction being detected.

8.5 METHODS USED FOR COMPARABILITY ASSESSMENT

There are several points at which it is advantageous to assess the comparability of product batches. At its simplest, a comparability study can be thought of as side-by-side characterization of test materials. That is, test samples from batch A and batch B are assayed in parallel with the types of test methods listed in Figure 8.2 for characterization. While it is possible, it is less desirable to compare test results from samples assayed independently (i.e., on different days, months, or even years), because the effect of intrinsic assay variability can confound the ability to accurately assess the similarities or differences. This is especially true when qualitative "fingerprint" methods are used, because slight variations in method performance can significantly change subtle — but critical — product profile elements. Therefore, the best case for comparability is made when product samples are run together using validated methods. Then, even if the test methods are not fully validated for robustness over time, all of the experimental bias should at least be skewed in the same direction for all samples, allowing more confidence in the interpretation of results.

One key point for comparability assessment is to link safety and efficacy data from all phases of product development to the physiochemical characteristics of the preclinical and clinical lots. Phase I/II drug substance and drug product batches should be compared with the batches used for Phase III to show consistency of manufacturing quality, purity, and potency among them [14]. An effective means by which to make these pre-approval comparisons is to prospectively plan to retain samples of each preclinical and clinical batch of drug substance and drug product at each phase of development, starting with the lots used for toxicology studies. Since these retained samples will be collected and stored before real-time stability studies have been completed, their long-term stability will not be known. However, the effects of degradation on the comparability of lots can be experimentally confirmed with forced degradation analysis. But if batch samples are not retained, the determination of comparability will have to be based on test data collected at different points in time. Any variability in the performance of the method over time, including small method changes made for optimization or validation at each phase, will make the evaluation sample comparability considerably more difficult.

If the characteristics of the lots, particularly in terms of impurities, change dramatically as the process is optimized, it could call into question the applicability of early toxicology and safety test results. That is, if product- or process-related impurities are significantly different from, or greater than, those seen in the product batches used in safety studies conducted in early development, the sponsor may have to repeat some of these earlier studies to ensure that the new or elevated impurities have been experimentally tested for patient safety [22]. Similarly, in drug substance and drug product stability testing, when degradation products result in heterogeneity patterns that differ from those observed in preclinical and clinical development, the significance of these alterations should be evaluated to ensure the continued safety and efficacy of the product [7].

After licensure, continuous improvements in the process, or technology transfer to other manufacturing facilities, can be assessed with FDA-approved Comparability Protocols [30]. A Comparability Protocol is a well-defined, detailed, written plan for assessing the effect of a specific CMC change on the identity, strength, quality, purity, or potency of a specific drug product as these factors relate to the safety and effectiveness of the product [23].

A Comparability Protocol describes the changes that are covered under the protocol and specifies the tests and studies that will be performed, including analytical procedures that will be used, and the acceptance criteria that will be achieved to demonstrate that the specified CMC changes do not adversely affect the product (drug substance, drug product, intermediate, or in-process material) [23].

8.6 DEVELOPMENT, QUALIFICATION, AND VALIDATION OF AN ANALYTICAL METHOD

The objective of method development is to deliver a procedure that is capable of performing reliably to measure a defined attribute of a test sample. Individual firms may use different terminology for some activities (e.g., method optimization, qualification, or validation) or divide parts of the strategy among different operational groups (e.g., analytical development and quality control). The method development strategy can be outlined in terms of questions to be asked. The answers to these questions (and the data to support them) should be captured in writing in method development reports. *Method development reports serve as the historical scientific record of the rationale and justification for how the method was selected and why it is considered suitable for use.* Well-written, comprehensive development reports provide valuable background information to future users of the method. They support the technical content of the chemistry, manufacturing, and controls (CMC) sections of product regulatory filings [24]. In the new 21st century initiatives for cGMP, the FDA acknowledges the key role of product development information in ensuring that quality was "built into" the product design; also, the new initiatives describe a Pharmaceutical Inspectorate composed of technical experts to review specific areas of product quality [25]. Method development reports will likely be of increased interest to regulatory reviewers when they are evaluating the analytical information in product license applications and annual reports.

8.7 TYPICAL ASSAY DEVELOPMENT STRATEGY

1. What is the purpose of the test? Identify the attribute of test samples that requires measurement (e.g., identity, purity, potency, concentration, or other attributes such as moisture).

To do this effectively, consider what statement, or claim, about the test material will be made based on the test results:

"The $A_{280\ nm}$ protein concentration of the product batch is 5.6 mg/ml."

"The purity of product batch 123XYZ is 98.6% by SEC-HPLC."

"The product bands comigrated with the reference standard on SDS-PAGE."

"The product amino acid sequence corresponds to that of curecancerin."

"No single impurity exceeded the limits of quantitation by SEC-HPLC"

"Potency of the batch was 1450 mIU/mg with the chromogenic assay."

"No degradants were detectable by RP-HPLC after 9 months at 5°C."

Understanding the method's intended use is arguably the most critical component of assay development and validation activities [26]. Perhaps because of the wide array of analytical techniques required for the complete analysis of biotechnology and biological products, it is often difficult to dissect the individual intended use for each type of method. *But without clearly defining the method's intended use from the very beginning, the entire process of method development and validation could yield the metaphorical situation of "building the right ladder up the wrong wall."*

For quantitative methods, there is a correlation between the target specifications of the assay's intended use and the capability required of the method to support those specifications [27]. For example, for a specification of 90–110% of a target concentration, the corresponding level of validated assay precision should be less than 5% RSD to reliably achieve accurate results using a minimum of assay replicates (i.e., $n = 3$). Conversely, if the test method can only achieve a validated precision of 10% RSD, the specifications may only be supported for 80–120% unless the number of test replicates is greatly increased. The requirements for method precision are inversely related to accuracy/recovery, i.e., a lower recovery requires a more precise method to support the same claims than a higher recovery method would require. There are published standard probability curves (operating characteristic curves, or OC) that link assay precision capabilities and the number of samples needed to support the desired level of confidence in accuracy [28].

Certain biomolecular techniques can provide information on more than one attribute of the product, such as identity and purity, or identity and potency. If there are multiple intended uses for a single method, these must be investigated individually to ensure the method can support each one adequately. For example, if SDS-PAGE is intended to support claims for purity and identity, the assay procedure should be designed to allow results to be evaluated individually for each attribute. Samples and reference standards might need to be in adjacent lanes on the gels to support the identity claim if comigration of bands is the acceptance criteria. Sample concentration might not be critical as long as the test sample and reference standard were loaded in equivalent amounts and all bands are visible on the gel. In order to obtain purity data, lane order may be flexible but sample loading concentration critical to ensure densitometric scanning values will fall in the linear range of the assay. If an ELISA assay is intended to support claims for identity and potency, the primary antibodies must be demonstrated to be specific for the product to claim immunoidentity, whereas if potency alone were the assay claim, intrinsic background cross-reactivity might be acceptable in the presence of the proper internal controls.

2. How does the test work? Assess the nature of the method technology (immunoreactivity, biochemical activity, quantitation of mass, resolution of polypeptides/impurities, etc.).

If necessary, refer to scientific literature, method books, manufacturer's technical literature, instrument vendor's booklets, etc. to understand exactly how the method — and importantly, the instruments used — technically function. *Each technology has limitations that can significantly impact the ability of the test to meet its intended use.* Edman protein sequencing and mass spectrometry can be very specific for product identity via molecular mass or sequence data, but neither is routinely used in a quantitative manner because the nature of the technologies renders absolute quantitation hard to achieve. SDS-PAGE with Coomassie stain and quantitative image analysis can be developed and validated for purity and impurity determination for many biotechnology products. By comparison, SDS-PAGE using silver staining methods is highly sensitive to low levels of protein and is very useful in product comparability studies, but it is very difficult to reproducibly analyze silver-stained gels using scanning densitometry to establish meaningful quantitative specifications.

If the nature of the technique is well understood and the method's intended use is clearly defined, designing the appropriate development and validation strategy should become a logical exercise to examine those aspects of the technology that are likely to affect the performance of the method for the parameter of interest. A useful exercise is to map out the elements of the procedure, the instruments, the samples, and the reagents with a cause-and-effect diagram to identify the relationship among key elements and to uncover potential sources of variability [29]. Then, experiments can be designed to assess the impact of these variables on the performance of the assay. For quantitative methods, statistically designed experimental (DOE) tools can be highly valuable in assessing the effect of multiple variables simultaneously [30].

> 3. Does the test require special reagents or materials? Identify any reagents or materials that could be critical to the reliable, robust performance of the method (e.g., antibodies, enzymes, substrates, cofactors, commercial kit materials, internal calibration standards, types of cuvettes, specific microtiter plates).

Many biomolecular methods require the use of critical reagents, such as antibodies in immunoassays or cell lines in cell-based assays, which are biologically derived components. Even common materials such as plastics and glass can interact with protein products or the method's biological reagents, and the lot-to-lot or vendor-to-vendor differences in composition can affect successful assay performance. Figure 8.5 lists different types of methods and components that can contribute to variability in method performance. Any of these items can impart a significant degree of variation in test methods unless strategies are in place to prospectively address them [31]. Investigate the impact on assay performance of different lots, or the range handling conditions. Develop an experimental study plan to bridge old lots of critical reagents to new ones before using the new lots in the assay. Include this study plan in the method SOP to ensure that future users will

Biomolecular Assay Type	Potential Batch to Batch Variability
Colorimetric	Unique buffer components Chromogenic reagent Commercial kit active components
Enzymatic	Unique buffer components Substrates Enzymes Cofactors Detection reagents Commercial kit active components
Chromatographic	Unique buffer components Labile mobile phase solvents Chromatography column resin Derivatization or conjugation reagents
Electrophoretic	Unique electrode buffers Gel matrix reagents Sample treatment reagents Staining reagents Commercial kit components
Immunological	Primary antibodies Secondary antibodies Conjugated antibodies Blocking reagents Detection reagents Commercial kit active components Plastic cuvettes or microtiter plates
Ligand Binding	Unique buffer components Target receptor Target ligand Detection reagents Commercial kit active components Plastic cuvettes or microtiter plates
Cell-Based Bioassay	Cell seed stock (homogeneity and viability) Cell culture (passage number and density) Media components Growth factors Antimicrobial agents Harvest reagents (e.g., trypsin) Cell reactants (e.g., induction compounds) Plastic flasks or plates

Figure 8.5   Potentially critical analytical test method components [31].

recognize when and how to perform reagent bridging with the assay.

> 4. What will be used as a reference standard? Determine the appropriate product-specific reference materials for the intended uses of the method.

Check for international standards if the test is to be used with a previously licensed biomolecular entity. Organizations such as the U.S. Pharmacopoeia (USP, www.usp.org) and the National Institute for Biological Standards and Controls (NIBSC, www.nibsc.ac.uk) maintain certified reference standards for many currently licensed biological products and some biotechnology products. For some biologics, the FDA Center for Biologics Evaluation and Research (CBER, www.fda.gov/cber/) has designated reference standards. Reference standards from a certification agency should be used only as primary standards against which in-house working standards are regularly qualified.

Note, however, that international standards for biological products are usually only certified for the calibration of potency or activity, and possibly molecular identity. They may be unsuitable for use in product assays for purity or impurities. In most cases, each biopharmaceutical firm, based on the nature of its purification process and its formulations, must generate its own purity and impurity reference standards. When the product is a new biomolecular entity for which there are no preexisting reference standards, the innovators are responsible for establishing their own reference standards for critical product attributes, including (in some cases) key product degradants [32].

> 5. Can a good test run be distinguished from a bad test run independently of the test sample results? Establish appropriate system suitability controls based on the technology of the method and its intended use.

These are to be included with each run to show that the run was valid. Each analytical test method should incorporate relevant system suitability measures to allow the analyst to verify that the test system is performing to expectations at the time of use [33]. Some system suitability measures are simple (e.g., calibration of a pH meter with standard solutions, or the level of precision among replicates), and others are more complex (e.g., the use of designated reference materials in structural or functional tests).

The inherent value of system suitability is that it provides a mechanism to assess the performance characteristics of the test method at the time and in the location of each use. It has been noted that defining and utilizing appropriate system suitability measures, particularly for nonchromatographic analytical test methods, is one of the most misunderstood aspects of method development and validation [34]. System suitability consists of two parts: (1) the material used in the assessment, and (2) the specifications associated with that material's performance ("validity" criteria). Typical system suitability measures for nonchromatographic methods are in the form of calibrators or controls. For quantitative methods, accuracy and precision are usually confirmed through the use of calibration standards or by the preparation of standard curves. For qualitative methods, positive and negative controls often serve as system suitability measures. In most test methods, a product-specific reference standard is included in the procedure; additional validity criteria can be designed for its use.

Each system suitability measure should have established criteria by which to determine whether the METHOD (not the PRODUCT) meets the specifications that define its suitable performance. These are known as validity criteria; they are the specifications used to determine whether a method is acceptable each time it is performed. For product-specific reference standards, validity criteria can include elution time and peak profile in chromatographic tests, migration distance and banding pattern in gel-based assays, immunoidentity in ELISAs and Western blots, concentration value in protein determination assays, activity values in potency assays, peptide fragment pattern in peptide mapping assays, and composition or fingerprint pattern in assays for posttranslational modifications.

For biomolecular methods, it can be highly valuable to utilize non-product-related test materials as additional system suitability measures. *Test method performance standards, sometimes referred to as "surrogate" or "generic" test method standards, can be selected and validated as a part of development of each method.* To choose the right type of surrogate test method standard, consider the physiochemical nature of the material relative to that of the product and the assay application. For example, if the biotechnology product is an IgG molecule and the assay is SEC-HPLC, a purified commercial IgG might serve as a system suitability control for column performance. If the biotechnology product is a glycoprotein and the assay is for monosaccharide composition, purified bovine fetuin may be included as a system suitability control for accuracy and precision.

Many analytical laboratories have used surrogate test method standards for a variety of biomolecular assays. Bovine serum albumin (BSA) standard reference material from the National Institute of Standards and Technologies (NIST SRM 927c; www.nist.gov) is often used as a system suitability control for the accuracy and precision of amino acid analysis composition and concentration [35]. In a joint project between the NIST and the Association of Biomolecular Resource Facilities (ABRF, www.abrf.org), new biomolecular surrogate test method standards are currently under development [36]. Three synthetic peptides have recently been prepared for potential use as system suitability measures in methods such as mass spectrometry, capillary electrophoresis, amino acid sequencing, amino acid analysis, and HPLC. The USP is in the process of preparing and certifying glycoprotein surrogate test method standards for use in a wide variety of biomolecular methods [37]. Also, a test method reference material was recently established by the Adenovirus Reference Material Working Group (ARWMG) for system suitability use in the analysis of adenoviral gene therapy vectors and is now available from the American Type Culture Collection (ATCC VR-1516, www.atcc.org) [38]. *To best ensure the quality and integrity of surrogate test method standard materials, whenever possible use material that is certified for specified physiochemical properties, such as reference materials from NIST, USP, ATCC, or the NIBSC.* If test method system suitability surrogate standards are obtained from a noncertified source, document the Certificates of Analysis from the vendor for each batch of material.

Demonstrating that each system suitability measure passes its validity criteria confirms that the test method run is valid and that the resulting test sample data can be confidently evaluated.

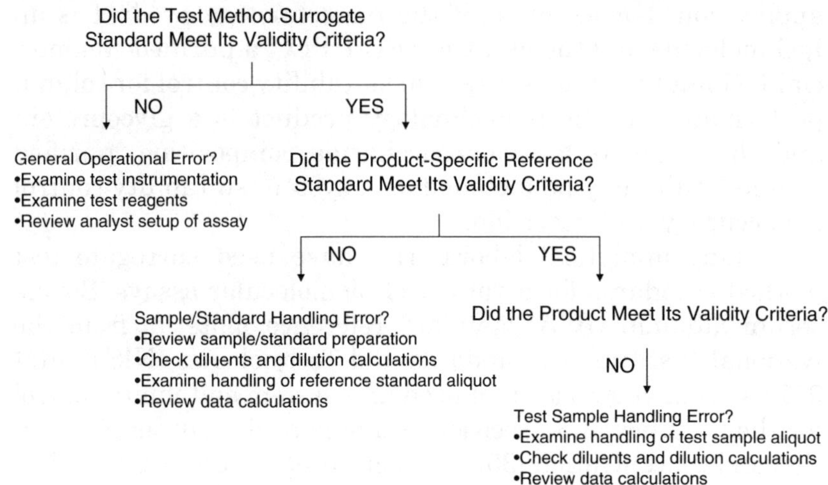

Figure 8.6 Using test method system suitability to isolate assignable cause for an out-of-specification test result.

Figure 8.6 illustrates a decision tree that can be used when investigating an out-of-specification event or an unexpected result by systematically evaluating the test method's system suitability measures. When any part of system suitability fails its validity criteria, the method test run should be critically reviewed to determine and correct the assignable cause. It is considered unacceptable to use the results from invalid test runs in decisions made during cGMP product manufacturing; however, invalidating test data requires a clear justification that is supported by technical evidence [39]. *Building sound system suitability measures into the test method procedure often provides the empirical evidence necessary to quickly and conclusively isolate the source of the assignable cause.*

6. How will the procedure be conducted? Write a draft SOP describing the steps required to perform the method. Include all appropriate system suitability measures (as described above).

Include details on sample preparation, preparation of standards and controls, and system suitability measures. If instruments are used, refer to the appropriate instrument SOPs in the method SOP, or give specific instructions on instrument operation in the method SOP. Specify the number of replicates for each sample/standard, show exactly how to calculate the results, and define how results are to be reported (e.g., significant digits).

When developing and validating analytical methods, it is important to understand the implication of using significant digits in defining reportable values and setting specifications. An all-too-common mistake is to allow extra digits to be reported in the test results or, worse, to incorporate unnecessary digits into the product specification values (S. Kuwahara, personal communication). The number of significant digits that can be accurately reported is related to the level of sensitivity. The method must be sensitive enough to measure differences that are one decimal place beyond the specification.

In addition, the effect of rounding on the outcome of reportable results should be recognized when using additional significant digits. For example, in order to pass a specification of 7.0 to 8.0, assay results of 6.95 to 8.45 are acceptable. However, to pass specifications of 7.00 to 8.00, assay results of 6.995 to 8.004 are necessary. To use these results, the analytical method must be capable of generating accurate and precise values to the thousandth decimal place. The American Society of Test Methods (ASTM, www.astm.org) has published a monograph on the appropriate use of significant digits in test data [40]. The acceptable procedures for rounding values to achieve the desired number of significant digits in reportable assay values have been defined by the USP and the FDA [41]. It may be useful to review practical examples of utilizing suitable significant digits in relation to the capabilities of analytical methods, with applications of consistent rounding rules [42].

Even the wording of the method SOP can impact the ability of different analysts to comparably reproduce the procedure. Figure 8.7 illustrates how a single set of instructions can be easily misconstrued if not clarified. On the left are the SOP instructions. On the right are the various ways in which

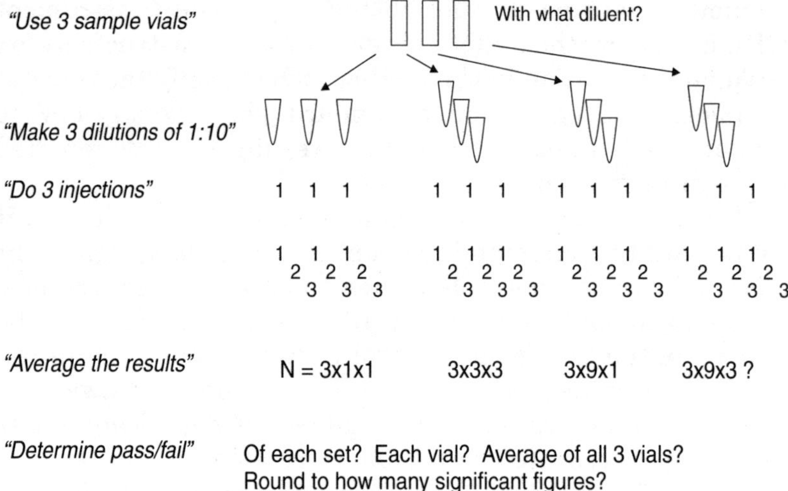

Figure 8.7 Potentially ambiguous test method SOP instructions.

these simple instructions can be interpreted, and where potentially critical information is missing (e.g., sample diluent, averaging methods). Initiators who are very familiar with the method sometimes leave out subtle details that can impact assay performance. The SOP instruction "Vortex the sample" can range operationally from gentle rotation to vigorous agitation, yielding dramatically different outcomes. Also, experienced scientists may inadvertently omit an instruction if it is assumed to be common to the technique. For example, after heating samples for SDS-PAGE, it is common practice to subject the sample to brief microcentrifugation to pool the solution droplets created in the sample vial. Failure to note this "common practice" in the SOP (and failure to specify the time and speed of centrifugation) can propagate sample-handling inconsistencies that may lead to assay problems. The SOP should be as complete and detailed as necessary to allow the method steps to be performed the same way by any analyst, including the data reduction steps. It is a good idea to allow a less-experienced analyst to run through the draft SOPs independently to see if they can complete the procedure solely based on the instructions written in the document. If not, the SOP should be revised until it provides adequate, unambiguous instructions. The best approach is always to (A) *exactly write the procedure to be validated* and (B) *validate the procedure exactly as written.*

> 7. Is the method appropriate for all types of samples to be used? Consider all potential variations in test samples (concentrations, buffers, formulation constituents) that will be included in the intended use of the method.

Run the method per SOP using representative product test materials. Include analysis of buffer or formulation solutions to assess matrix effects. If necessary, optimize assay parameters to achieve suitable preliminary performance. Edit the draft SOP to reflect any changes resulting from optimization experiments.

Most analytical methods for biotechnology products are developed and optimized using samples of the drug substance, since it is often the most suitable material for these studies. But if the method is ultimately intended for use with test samples taken from in-process, conjugation, or formulation steps, it will have to be assessed for performance with those specific types of samples. As shown in Figure 8.8, there are several compounds that can be used in the formulation of biotechnology products [43–46].

Many conjugate reagents or formulation excipients interfere with the analytical methods developed for bulk product. For example, the presence of amino acids can affect compositional analysis, protein concentration assays, and sequencing results. Solubilizers such as Tween can interfere with colorimetric methods at higher concentrations. Sugars can precipitate during HPLC runs if the mobile phase becomes too polar. For both formulated and in-process samples, the concentration of drug substance may be very low (µg/ml), falling below the range of assay linearity where poor accuracy and precision may yield unreliable data. Also, unpredictable interactions between drug substance and excipients may occur. In certain cases, excipient degradation may require its own evaluation

- Osmotic Agents (salts)

- Chelators (EDTA, citrate)

- Cations

- Sugars (mannose, maltose, dextrose)

- Amino Acids (arginine, glycine, glutamic acid)

- Redox Agents (ascorbate, reducing sugars)

- Solubilizers (Tween, Deoxycholate)

- Stabilizers (albumin, lipids)

- Solvents (aqueous, nonaqueous)

Figure 8.8 Typical formulation candidates for proteins and peptides.

and stability testing. For these reasons, analytical methods that were validated for bulk substance may require revalidation for intermediates, conjugates, or formulated product.

> 8. What are the initial performance capabilities of the assay? Conduct an assay qualification or characterization study to systematically investigate the performance ranges of the method for the designated types of samples.

Prior to validating a test method, studies should be conducted to investigate the working ranges of the assay for the parameters that could affect the intended use. *These studies are sometimes called method "qualification" or "characterization" studies* [16]. In most cases, experiments are conducted to assess most of the parameters typically included in a validation study for the type of method such as linearity, accuracy, precision, specificity, etc. Figure 8.9 lists the major test method validation parameters with their ICH definitions.

Experiments performed to assess 1 to 7(a) give an initial indication of the intrinsic performance capabilities of the test

> 1) Accuracy: The closeness of agreement between the value that is accepted either as the conventional true value, or an accepted reference value, and the value measured.
> 2) Specificity: The ability to unequivocally measure the analyte in the presence of components that may be expected to be present.
> 3) Limit of Detection (LOD): The lowest amount of analyte that can be detected, but not necessarily quantified as an exact value.
> 4) Limit of Quantitation (LOQ): The lowest amount of analyte that can be quantified with suitable accuracy and precision.
> 5) Range: The interval between the upper and lower amounts of analyte for which the method has suitable accuracy, precision, and linearity.
> 6) Linearity: The ability within a given range to obtain test results that are directly proportional to the amount of analyte present in a sample.
> 7) Precision: The closeness of agreement between a series of measurements obtained from multiple sampling of the homogeneous sample under prescribed conditions. Three levels of precision may be assessed: (a) repeatability (intra-assay precision); (b) intermediate precision (interassay/ intralaboratory precision); (c) reproducibility (inter-laboratory precision).
> 8) Robustness: A measure of the capacity of the method to remain unaffected by small but deliberate variations in method operational parameters expected during normal usage.

Figure 8.9   Test method validation parameters [50, 51].

method. These results should be compared to the intended application of the assay. If it is seen that method performance is not meeting the requirements of use, optimization experiments are usually conducted until (or unless) the method becomes acceptable. If the method cannot be optimized to meet the initial intended use, either the method will have to be replaced or the acceptance specifications for method performance will have to be reassessed.

The nature and impact of test method variability, particularly with quantitative methods such as those used for purity and potency determinations, should be clearly understood for each method prior to finalizing product acceptance (i.e., pass/fail) specifications for that method. In some cases, an analytical method can demonstrate such inherent variability that it will have to be eliminated from consideration for use with the product and replaced with a technique that can perform appropriately. If not, there will be a statistically predictable percent probability that a given test result will not fall within the product specification range simply due to test method variability [48].

In most cases, the nature and source of test method variability can be identified via a rigorous assay development approach, with attention to even deceptively simple parameters such as test sample preparation and reference standard stability. However, some sources of variation may not be detected until the assay has been used over a long period of time. *Tracking and trending the performance of a new method is a valuable tool to monitor the ongoing reliability of the method for its intended use.* There is a mechanism that can enhance the ability to monitor the performance of the test methods separately from the performance of the samples being tested. Tracking and trending system suitability results independently of the sample results can provide a simple (but powerful) mechanism to distinguish product variability from test method variability. Figure 8.10 illustrates this concept, where parallel tracking charts are generated from assay results.

In Figure 8.10, (A) represents the data obtained from different test samples over time, and (B) represents the results obtained from one or more system suitability measures included in each of those same test runs. It is clear that the shift in performance trend (indicated by the arrows) comparably affects both the test samples and the method system suitability measures. When comparing the product (A) and method (B) data point for point, the general trends are comparably random for the first 11 runs. Then the trends shift from runs 12 to 17. By run 17, the results from both the test

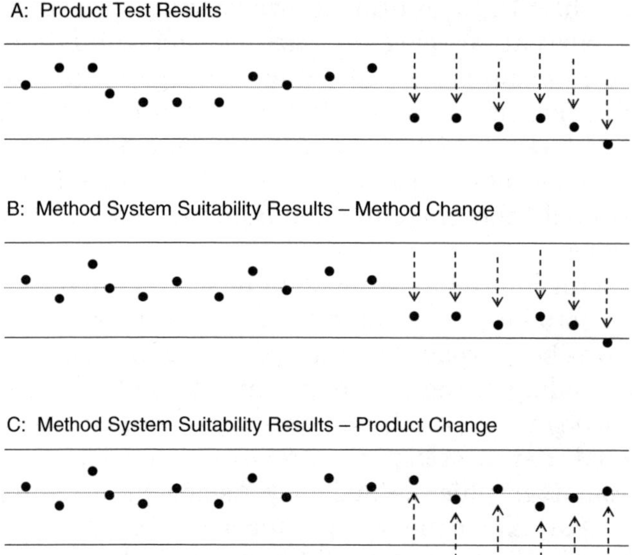

Figure 8.10 Tracking/trending product test sample results vs. method system suitability results.

sample and the method system suitability have fallen out of their specifications. However, if the same 17 test runs produced the data in (A) and (C), where the method system suitability does not show a trend shift, it would imply that something has changed in the product rather than the test.

This kind of method-specific information can be used to rapidly focus troubleshooting investigations to isolate and correct the root cause of change in the data trend.

> 9. Can the method be validated to meet its intended use? Design the validation protocol using sound scientific judgment in alignment with current regulatory expectations.

There are several guidance documents on the current regulatory expectations for test method validation. For QC test methods to be used in cGMP applications, validation studies should follow the guidance given in current ICH and

FDA guidelines [49–51]. In addition, there are many excellent historical and current articles on test method validation, many with specific examples of validation strategies and protocols, with extensive citations for additional reading [52–63]. For bioanalytical test methods to be used in human pharmacology and GLP toxicology and safety studies, assay validation design should follow the current FDA guidance specific for these applications [64].

For those with limited experience in designing qualification or validation studies, it is strongly recommended that each of these references be thoroughly reviewed to obtain a comprehensive understanding of the core requirements and different possible approaches when validating a test method. However, it should be noted that most historical references are based on traditional chromatographic methodology. As shown in Figure 8.2 and Figure 8.3, biotechnology products require a broad range of methods utilizing widely different technologies. For these methods, the principle of a validation study remains the same (i.e., to demonstrate suitability for its intended use), but the experimental design to meet each parameter can differ considerably, based on the nature of the technology.

Currently, there are only a few specific publications on the validation of techniques used specifically for the quality control testing of biotechnology products [65–70]. The USP is in the process of revising chapter <111>, "Design and Analysis of Biological Assays," and has a new chapter in preparation on the validation of bioassays [71]. Figure 8.11 lists the required method validation parameters for different types of test methods as defined by the ICH. Figure 8.12 contrasts these with the required method validation parameters given by the USP. Regardless of which table is used, the parameters must be appropriate to the assay's intended use.

The specific experiments to be conducted to achieve validation of each parameter will be based on the nature of the assay. Most of the aforementioned references have detailed experimental designs for chromatographic assays; these experiments should be adapted for use with other nonchromatographic biomolecular assays for biotechnology products as needed to ensure the assay will meet its intended use.

Analytical Procedure	Identification	Testing for Impurities		Assay
Characteristics		Quantitative	Limit	Content Potency
Accuracy	–	+	–	+
Precision:				
Repeatability	–	+	–	+
Intermediate Precision	–	+ (1)	–	+ (1)
Specificity (2)	+	+	+	+
Detection Limit	–	- (3)	+	–
Quantitation Limit	–	+	–	+
Linearity	–	+	–	+
Range	–	+	–	+

– signifies that this characteristic is not normally evaluated.

+ signifies that this characteristic is normally evaluated.

1) in cases where reproducibility has been performed, intermediate precision is not needed.

2) lack of specificity of one analytical procedure could be compensated by other supporting analytical procedure(s).

3) may be needed in some cases.

Figure 8.11 Validation requirements from ICH validation of analytical procedures.

It should be noted that there are two special applications of assay validation that are distinct from the test method validation strategies previously described. The USP includes a chapter describing the validation studies necessary to have an analytical method accepted into the Pharmacopoeia as a regulatory compendial method [72]. Since compendial methods are intended for application in any analytical laboratory, extensive collaborative studies are needed to verify the repeatability and robustness of the method in order to establish global performance specifications.

Also, validation of an analytical test method for quality-control applications should not be confused with the validation

| | | Assay Category II | | | |
Performance Characteristic	Assay Category I	Quantitative	Limit Tests	Assay Category III	Assay Category IV
Accuracy	Yes	Yes	*	*	No
Precision	Yes	Yes	No	Yes	No
Specificity	Yes	Yes	Yes	*	Yes
Detection Limit	No	No	Yes	*	No
Quantitation Limit	No	Yes	No	*	No
Linearity	Yes	Yes	No	*	No
Range	Yes	Yes	*	*	No

*May be required, depending on the nature ofthe specifictest.

Category I:Methods for quantitation of major components of bulk drug substances or active ingredients (including preservatives) in finished pharmaceutical products.

Category II: Methodsfor determination of impurities in bulk drug substances or degradation compounds in finished pharmaceutical products. These methods include quantitative assays and limit tests.

Category III: Methods for determinationsof performance characteristics (e.g., dissolution, drug release).

Category IV: Identification tests

Figure 8.12 USP data elements required for assay validation. (From Table 2, <1225>. Reprinted with permission. © 2005 United States Pharmacopeia. All rights reserved.)

of assays applied to the detection or quantitation of biological markers in clinical samples. Beyond the parameters such as linearity, accuracy, precision, specificity, and robustness, these biomarker assays also require patient studies that correlate the activity measured *in vitro* with the *in vivo* intended application (such as the designated clinical disease or condition) [73].

If the method is intended to monitor product stability, it should be verified for this capability (as previously described).

10. What if the method validation runs fail to meet performance expectations? Thoroughly investigate the root cause of the failures and determine what corrective actions would prevent the same problem from occurring again.

If the assignable cause for the failure of the method to meet performance requirements is identified, implement the appropriate corrective action and repeat the affected validation runs. If the assignable cause is related to analyst error, it would be wise to immediately address how to prevent propagating the same error in future runs of the validated assay. Sometimes SOP simply requires enhanced clarity, such as more specific instructions or a more logical organization of steps. These document adjustments can usually be justified during validation if they do not change the method itself.

Note that regulatory bodies indicate that laboratory error should be relatively rare [74], so management should be alert to chronic method performance problems that are related solely to laboratory operations. Laboratory variability can usually be minimized with attention to issues such as clearly written SOPs, well-maintained instruments, a meaningful training program, and (arguably) adequate staffing to prevent chronically harried — thereby inadvertently careless — analyst performance. *Regardless of how thoroughly a test method has been validated, if it is not implemented in an adequately controlled laboratory environment, it will not be able to perform reliably. On the other hand, even sound laboratory operations may not be able to compensate for poorly written method SOPs or nonrobust analytical methods.*

It the assignable cause for failure is not identifiable, the assay should not be considered validated. In this case, the assay should be remanded back to the method development process for further assessment of its actual suitability for the intended use. Experience shows that unresolved analytical test method problems that arise during method validation usually continue throughout the life cycle of assay use [75,76].

> 11. When should a validated test method be revalidated? When something changes that could impact its continued suitability for the intended use.

Some firms have a policy of reviewing and revalidating test methods with established frequency (e.g., every 2 years). Routinely reviewing test method SOPs against laboratory practices and test records does have the advantage of maintaining a strong connection between "creeping" performance habits and the actual written steps and can catch disconnects relatively quickly. However, periodic revalidation studies when nothing has changed might not be technically meaningful, and might be more rigorous than most facilities can operationally support. A more effective approach is to look at method revalidation strategies from a risk-based perspective. In other words, when changes do occur, what is the level of risk that the change will impact the state of validation of the assay?

Figure 8.13 lists five categories of change that should trigger a review of the test method and possibly require a measure of revalidation: (1) changes to the product that could affect method performance (e.g., formulation excipients, product concentration), (2) changes in critical assay reagents that cannot meet prior performance requirements (e.g., gel reagents, enzymes, antibodies), (3) changes in instrumentation that cannot meet prior performance settings (e.g., automated amino acid hydrolysis systems), (4) changes in the procedure to

---

Changes to the **product** that could affect method performance (e.g., formulation excipients, product concentration)

Changes in critical assay **reagents** that cannot meet prior specifications   (e.g., gel or blot materials, enzymes)

Changes in **instrumentation** that cannot perform equivalent procedures (e.g., AAA hydrolysis systems)

Changes in the **procedure** to improve robustness of the method (e.g., new qualification procedures for critical reagents, re-optimized sample preparation steps)

Changes in the **product specifications** that go beyond the capabilities of the test method (e.g., specification on quantifying impurities drops from 0.5% to 0.1%; assay limit of quantitation is 0.25%)

Figure 8.13   Potential triggers for method revalidation.

improve robustness of the method (e.g., adding new sample preparation steps), or (5) changes in the product specifications that are beyond the test method capabilities. In most cases, the revalidation may be limited to a set of studies that "bridge" the old part of the procedure to the new part of the procedure. In cases where method performance capabilities are significantly affected and, as a result, will require changes to method specifications, a complete revalidation may be necessary. Regardless of the extent of revalidation needed, it is imperative to confirm that all analysts are sufficiently trained on the new procedure to ensure successful results. It is a useful management tool to monitor trends in method performance (as described previously) following revalidation to spot problems and make the appropriate corrections quickly.

8.8 CONCLUSION

Biological products are macromolecular entities that are considerably larger than most chemical products. With the exception of synthetic oligonucleotides or peptides, living cells — complex metabolic factories — produce them. The target molecules must be isolated from a biochemical milieu consisting of chemical entities relatively similar to the desired product. As such, it may be difficult to completely eliminate impurities derived from the host system. The purified target may comprise several structurally heterogeneous forms, some or all of which might be active. Compared to traditional chemical drugs, biological materials are highly labile, unable to tolerate high temperatures or undue chemical or physical stress. Higher-order biological products (e.g., cells and tissues) may have a very short window of viability. It requires numerous complex analytical methods to provide an effective physio-chemical profile of biotechnology products.

This chapter has presented several factors to consider when selecting the analytical methods to assess the identity, purity, impurities, concentration, potency, stability, and (in some cases) comparability of biotechnology products (Figure 8.14). Since no single method can provide data on all key product parameters, orthogonal analytical methods should be

1. Clearly define the assay's intended use relative to the desired product attribute (e.g., identity, purity, impurities, potency, concentration, stability) and acceptance specification requirements.

2. Understand how the method technology functions to generate data on the parameter of interest.

3. Recognize and control potential sources of method and operational variability that can impact the reproducibility of assay procedure.

4. Assure that assay is robust enough under the conditions of expected use to statistically support the specification requirements for the product.

Figure 8.14 Elements for successful analytical method development and implementation.

used to increase confidence in the quality of the product. Methods used under GLP or cGMP quality practices must be validated for their intended use. The strategies for qualifying and validating biomolecular methods should be based on the type of method, the nature of the product, and the parameter to be evaluated with the data. Laboratories that adopt validated methods (e.g., compendial methods) must experimentally verify the suitable performance of these methods in the user environment. In order to provide a complete product development record, all of these activities must be adequately documented to demonstrate how, when, and by whom they were conducted.

As has been noted, "Some data are worthless; some data are priceless. The conditions and procedures used to find data ultimately determine their value" [77]. All decisions regarding the control of the process and the quality of the product are based on data generated by analytical tests. If there are design flaws in the assays or unrecognized sources of method variation, or if a method is chosen that cannot support the specification requirements, the data will inevitably be inadequate, inaccurate, or unreliable. Therefore, while it is certainly critical to understand the process by which a biological or biotechnological product is produced, it is equally vital to understand the methods of analysis that are applied to the product. Otherwise, it will be very difficult to distinguish between those data that are priceless and those that are worthless.

REFERENCES

1. Comparability Studies for Human Plasma-Derived Therapeutics, FDA Center for Biologics Evaluation and Research and Plasma Protein Therapeutic Association Meeting, Rockville, MD, May 30, 2002.

2. Elimination of Establishment License Application for Specified Biotechnology and Specified Synthetic Biological Products, Federal Register, Vol. 61, No. 94, 24227-24233, May 14, 1996.

3. FDA Guidance for Industry, Bioanalytical Method Validation, May 2001.

4. FDA Guidance Concerning the Comparability of Human Biological Products, Including Therapeutic Biologically-Derived Products, April 1996; FDA Draft Guidance for Industry: Comparability Protocols — Protein Drug Products and Biological Products — Chemistry, Manufacturing and Controls Information, Sept. 2003.

5. WHO/NIBSC, *J. Immunol. Meth.*, 216, 103–116, 1998.

6. McMillen, D., Bibbs, L., Denslow, N., Ivantich, K., Naeve, C., Neice, R., and Tyndall, S., Biotechnology core laboratories: an overview, *J. Biomol. Tech.*, 11, 1–11, 2000.

7. ICH Q6B, Test Methods and Acceptance Specifications for Biological/Biotechnological Products, Aug. 1999.

8. McEntire, J., Biotechnology product validation. V. Selection and validation of analytical techniques, *BioPharm*, June, 68–80, 1994.

9. USP 28/NF 23, 2005.

10. 21 CFR 211.194(a)(2).

11. 21 CFR 211.84 (d)(2).

12. FDA Guidance for Industry: PAT — A Framework for Innovative Pharmaceutical Development, Manufacturing, and Quality Assurance, Sept. 2004.

13. FDA Draft Guidance on Analytical Procedures and Test Method Validation, Aug. 2000.

14. FDA Draft Guidance for Industry: INDs for Phase 2 and 3 Studies of Drugs, Including Specified Therapeutic Biotechnology-Derived Products, CMC Content and Format, Feb. 1999.

15. Canova-Davis, E., Curious Discoveries During the Characterization of Therapeutic Proteins, ARBF News, Sept. 1994.

16. Ritter, N., Advant, S., Hennessey, J., Simmerman, H., McEntire, J., Mire-Sluis, A., and Joneckis, C., What is Test Method Qualification? Proceedings of the WCBP CMC Strategy Forum, July 24, 2003, Bioprocess International, Sept. 2004.

17. ICH Q6A Specifications, Test Procedures and Acceptance Criteria for New Drug Substances and New Drug Products: Chemical Substances, Oct. 1999; ICH Q6B: Test Procedues and Acceptance Criteria for Biotechnological/Biological Products, Aug. 1999.

18. ICH Q5C, Stability Testing of Biotechnology/Biological Products, July 1996.

19. Smales, C., Pepper, D., and James, D., Protein modification during anti-viral heat treatment bioprocessing of factor VIII concentrates, factor IX concentrates, and model proteins in the presence of sucrose, *Biotechnol. Bioeng.*, 77, 38–48, 2001.

20. Yu, J., Intentionally degrading protein pharmaceuticals to validate stability-indicating analytical methods, *BioPharm*, 13, 46–52, 2000.

21. Magari, R., Assessing shelf life using real time and accelerated conditions — although accelerated tests are needed, real time tests are the ultimate proof, *BioPharm Int.*, Nov., 28–32, 2003.

22. Cavagnero, J., Equivalence of Biological and Biotechnological Ingredients and Products, USP Conference on Biological and Biotechnological Drug Substances and Products, Crystal City, VA, Nov. 18–21, 2003.

23. FDA Draft Guidance for Industry, Comparability Protocols: Chemistry, Manufacturing and Controls Information, Nov. 2003 (draft); FDA Guidance Concerning Demonstration of Comparability of Human Biological Products, Including Therapeutic Biotechnology-Derived Products, April 1996.

24. 21 CFR 312.23 (a)(7), IND Content and Format, Chemistry, Manufacturing and Control Information.

25. Pharmaceutical GMPs for the 21st Century: A Risk-Based Approach; Second Progress Report and Implementation Plan, Sept. 3, 2003.

26. McEntire, J., Biotechnology product validation. V. Selection and validation of analytical techniques, *BioPharm*, June, 68–80, 1994.

27. Larry Paul, W., USP perspectives on analytical methods validation, *Pharm. Tech.*, March, 130–141, 1991.

28. Vanderwielen, A.J. and Hardwidge, E.A., Guidelines for assay validation, *Pharm. Tech.*, March, 66–76, 1982.

29. Ishikawa, K., *Guide to Quality Control*, American Society for Quality Press, 1986.

30. Torbeck, L. and Branning, R., Designed experiments: a vital role in validation, *Pharm. Tech.*, June, 108–113, 1998.

31. Ritter, N. and Wiebe, M., Validating critical reagents used in cGMP analytical testing: ensuring method integrity and reliable assay performance, *BioPharm*, May, 12–21, 2001.

32. ICH Q6B, Test Procedures and Acceptance Criteria for Biotechnological/Biological Products, Aug. 1999.

33. Ritter, N.M., Hayes, T., and Dougherty, J., Analytical laboratory quality. II. Analytical method validation, *J. Biomol. Tech.*, 12, 11–15, 2001.

34. Williams, D., Overview of test method validation, *BioPharm*, Oct., 34–51, 1987.

35. Anders, J.C., Parten, B.F., Petrie, G.E., Marlowe, R.L., and McEntire, J.E., Using amino acid analysis to determine molar absorptivity constants: a validation case study using bovine serum albumin, *BioPharm Int.*, Feb. 2003.

36. Remmer, H.A., Ambulos, N.P., Bonewald, L.F., Dougherty, J.J., Eisenstein, E., Fowler, E., Johnson, J., Khatri, A., Lively, M.O., Ritter, N.M., and Weintraub, S.T., Synthetic peptides as certified analytical standards, in *Peptide Revolution: Genomics, Proteomics & Therapeutics*, Chorev, M. and Sawyer, T.K., Eds., American Peptide Society, 2003.

37. USP Conference on Biological and Biotechnological Drug Substances and Products, Arlington, VA, Nov. 18–21, 2003.

38. Sajjadi, N. and Callahan, J., Defining a detailed approach to using the adenovirus reference material (ARM), *Bioprocess. J.*, Sept./Oct., 83–87, 2003.

39. FDA Guidance for Industry Investigating Out of Specification (OOS) Test Results for Pharmaceutical Production, Sept. 1998.

40. ASTM/ANSI EP29-02: Standard Practice for Using Significant Digits in Test Data to Determine Conformance with Specifications, 2003.

41. FDA ORA Laboratory Manual Vol. III: Other Lab Operations, Section 4: Basic Statistics and Data Presentation, Oct. 2003; General Notices: Significant Digits and Tolerances; USP 28/NF 23, 2005.

42. Miller, J.M. and Crowther, J.B., Eds., *Analytical Chemistry in a GMP Environment: A Practical Guide*, John Wiley & Sons, New York, 2000, pp. 79–82.

43. Bontempo, J., Development of biopharmaceutical dosage forms, in *Drugs and the Pharmaceutical Sciences Series*, Vol. 85, Marcel Dekker, New York, 1997.

44. Frokajaer, S. and Hovgaard, L., Eds., *Pharmaceutical Formulation: Development of Proteins and Peptides*, Taylor & Francis, London, 2002.

45. McNally, E., Ed., Protein formulation and delivery, in *Drugs and the Pharmaceutical Sciences Series*, Vol. 99, Marcel Dekker, New York, 1999.

46. Perlman, R. and Wang, Y., *Formulation, Characterization and Stability of Protein Drugs, Case Histories*, Vol. 9, Kluwer Academic Publishers, Dordrecht, 1996.

47. Pess, W.H. et al., Levenberg-Marquardt method as described in Numerical recipes, in *The Art of Scientific Computing*, Cambridge University Press, New York, 1988.

48. Weed, D.H., A statistically-integrated approach to analytical method validation, *Pharm. Tech.*, Oct., 116–129, 1999.

49. FDA Guidance for Industry, Analytical Procedures and Method Validation, Chemistry, Manufacturing and Controls Documentation, Aug. 2000 (draft).

50. ICH Q2A Text on the Validation of Analytical Procedures, May 1995.

51. ICH Q2B Validation of Analytical Procedures: Methodology, Nov. 1996.

52. McEntire, J., Selection and validation of analytical techniques, *BioPharm*, June, 68–80, 1994.

53. Torbeck, L. and Branning, R., Designed experiments: a vital role in validation, *Pharm. Tech.*, June, 1088–1114, 1996.

54. Weed, D., A statistically-integrated approach to analytical method validation, *Pharm. Tech.*, Oct., 116–129, 1999.

55. Green, J., A practical guide to analytical method validation, *Anal. Chem.*, 68, 305A–309A, 1996.

56. Krause, S., Good analytical method validation practice: setting up for compliance and efficiency. I, *J. Validation Technol.*, 9, 23–32, 2002.

57. Krause, S., Good analytical method validation practice: deriving acceptance criteria for the AMV protocol. II, *J. Validation Technol.*, 9, 162–178, 2003.

58. Snyder, L., Kirkland, J., and Glajch, J., Eds., Completing the method: validation and transfer, in *Practical HPLC Method Development*, 2nd ed., John Wiley & Sons, New York, 1997, pp. 685–712.

59. Swartz, M. and Krull, I., Eds., Method development, optimization and validation approaches, in *Analytical Method Development and Validation*, Marcel Dekker, New York, 1997, pp. 25–39.

60. Vanderwielen, A. and Hardwidge, E., Guidelines for assay validation, *Pharm. Tech.*, March, 66–76, 1982.

61. Williams, D., An overview of test method validation, *BioPharm*, Nov., 34–51, 1987.

62. Paul, W., USP perspectives on analytical methods validation, *Pharm. Tech.*, March, 130–141, 1991.

63. Layloff, T., Nasr, M., Baldwin, R., Caphart, M., Drew, H., Hanig, J., Holberg, C., Koepke, S., Lunn, G., MacGregor, J., Mille, Y., Murphy, R., Ng, L., Rajagopalan, R., Sheinen, E., Smela, M., Weischenbach, M., Winkie, H., and Williams, R., The FDA regulatory methods validation program for new and abbreviated new drug applications, *BioPharm*, Jan., 30–38, 2000.

64. FDA Guidance for Industry Bioanalytical Method Validation, May 2001.

65. Anders, J., Parten, B., Petrie, G., Marlowe, R., and McEntire, J., Using amino acid analysis to determine absorptivity constants: a validation case study using bovine serum albumin, *BioPharm Int.*, Feb., 30–37, 2003.

66. Allen, D., Baffi, R., Bausch, J., Bongers, J., Costello, M., Dougherty, J., Jr., Federici, M., Garnick, R., Peterson, S., Riggins, R., Sewerin, K., and Tuis, J., Validation of peptide mapping for protein identity and genetic stability, *Biologicals*, 24, 255–275, 1999.

67. McEntire, J., Selection and validation of analytical techniques, *BioPharm*, June, 68–80, 1994.

68. Ritter, N., Hayes, T., and Dougherty, J., Analytical laboratory quality. II. Analytical method validation, *J. Biomol. Techn.*, 12, 11–15, 2001.

69. Patel, U., Meeting the challenges of enzyme assay validation, *BioPharm*, July, 48–52, 2000.

70. Findlay, J.W.A., Smith, W.C., Lee, J.W., Nordblom, G.D., Das, I., DeSilva, B.S., Khan, M.N., and Bowsher, R.R., Validation of immunoassays for bioanalysis: a pharmaceutical industry perspective, *J. Pharm. Biomed. Anal.*, 21, 1249–1273, 2000.

71. USP Conference on Biological and Biotechnological Drug Substances and Products, Crystal City, VA, Nov. 18–21, 2003.

72. USP 28/NF 23 (2005) <1225> Assay Validation.

73. Bowsher, R. and Smith, W., Practical approach for clinical drug development: analytical validation of assays for novel biomarkers, *AAPS Newsmagazine*, June, 18–25, 2002.

74. FDA Guidance for Industry Investigating Out of Specification (OOS) Test Results for Pharmaceutical Production, September 1998.

75. Hokanson, G.A., Life-cycle approach to the validation of analytical methods during pharmaceutical development, *Pharm. Tech.*, Aug., 118–130, 1994.

76. Miller, J. and Crowther, J., Eds., *Analytical Chemistry in a GMP Environment: A Practical Guide*, John Wiley & Sons, New York, 2000.

77. Torbeck, L.D. and Branning, R.C., Designed experiments — a vital role in validation, *Pharm. Tech.*, June, 108–114, 1996.

9

Facility Design Issues —
A Regulatory Perspective

NANCY ROSCIOLI AND SUSAN VARGO

CONTENTS

9.1 INTRODUCTION

Properly designed manufacturing facilities are critical to the successful approval of biotechnology-derived (biotech) products. The Food and Drug Administration (FDA) has established regulations that govern establishments used to manufacture biological products. These include the Code of Federal Regulations (CFR), Title 21, Part 600, Subpart B Establishment Standards [1] and Parts 210 and 211 of current Good Manufacturing Practice (cGMP) regulations [2]. These regulations were established prior to the advent of biotech products. The intent of the regulations, however, is applicable to facilities designed to produce biotech products.

The FDA's guidance on aseptic processing [3] and the National Institutes of Health (NIH) guidelines on research involving recombinant DNA (rDNA) molecules [4] are useful in designing manufacturing facilities. The latter document provides information on the physical containment requirements for large-scale processes. The International Conference on Harmonization (ICH) issued cGMP guidance [5] applicable to manufacturers of active pharmaceutical ingredients (API), which contains information on buildings and facilities. Other organizations that have published standards relevant to facility design criteria include the International Society for Pharmaceutical Engineers (ISPE) [6] and the International Organization for Standardization (ISO) [7,8].

For the most part, these regulations and guidance documents provide general information with regard to facility design criteria, the reason being there is no one floor plan that is suitable for the manufacture of all biotech products. It is important to understand the principles described in these references and apply them appropriately to your manufacturing process and facility design. In general, manufacturers should design a facility that can be validated and can be maintained at a level of compliance consistent with the requirements of cGMP. The facility design should ensure that the manufacturer's product could be produced in a consistent and controlled manner. The final goal is a product that meets its established quality attributes of safety, purity, potency, identity, and efficacy.

In this chapter, we will discuss the current regulatory criteria as applied to facilities designed to produce biotechnology-derived products.

9.2 REGULATORY REQUIREMENTS

The CFR, Title 21 Part 600, Subpart B [1] contains the establishment standards for biological products. Section 600.10 describes the requirements for personnel working in a manufacturing facility. Included in this section are the requirements for adequately trained personnel; rules prohibiting personnel from entering a manufacturing area who may adversely affect the safety and purity of a product; gowning requirements for personnel working in aseptic manufacturing and in manufacturing involving live vaccine production; and the exclusion of personnel who work with pathogenic viruses, spore-bearing microorganisms, or other infectious agents or animals from working in other manufacturing areas on the same day. Section 600.11 describes the requirements for the physical establishment. Included in this section are the requirements for facility cleanliness and appearance; precautions for exclusion of extraneous infectious agents; adequately designed air systems to prevent the dissemination of microorganisms from one manufacturing area to another and to supply air quality sufficient to ensure product quality; and maintenance of localized temperature-controlled areas (e.g., incubators, freezers). Specific equipment requirements noted in this section include the use of sterilizing equipment, which is capable (i.e., validated) of destruction of contaminating organisms; specific temperature requirements for both saturated steam and dry heat sterilization; and the recommendation that equipment design and construction should permit thorough cleaning (and the ability to inspect for cleanliness). Several subsections within Section 600.11 describe the requirements for use of animals in production (including animal care, quarantine procedures, immunization, and bleeding areas). Finally, requirements still exist for the segregation and containment of production areas utilizing live virus or spore-bearing organisms. The general intent of these regulations is the protection of the product through adequate facility design and adequate training of personnel. For these reasons, the Establishment Standards remain applicable to all biological biotech products.

In conjunction with the Establishment Standards, the CFR, Title 21 Part 211 [2] Subparts B, C, and D provide requirements for organization and personnel, buildings and facilities, and equipment as part of the cGMP regulations. These regulations apply to all biological products. Again, the intention is to ensure product quality through adequate facility design and adequate training of personnel. For biological products, the more restrictive regulation will apply. For this reason, it is most important that manufacturers of biological products become familiar with both sets of regulations and apply them accordingly.

While not a regulation, the ICH published guidance for industry on cGMP for API production [5]. In many ways, this document parallels Part 211 with regard to sections on personnel, buildings, and facilities and process equipment. The document also contains information on validation (specifically, process validation and cleaning validation). Finally, there is a section on APIs manufactured by cell culture/fermentation (i.e., biotech products). The ICH does not intend for this to be an independent section, but rather a section to discuss (in general terms) the differences in levels of control between classical fermentation and fermentation as part of a biotech process. The ICH clearly states that cGMP principles apply to APIs derived from biotechnology processes. Again, the emphasis is on adequate facility design to prevent contamination and cross-contamination, thereby ensuring a product that will meet its predetermined quality requirements.

9.3 FACILITY INFORMATION REQUIRED FOR BIOLOGICS LICENSE APPLICATIONS AND NEW DRUG APPLICATIONS

Biotech products are submitted to the FDA for licensure using a Biologics License Application (BLA) or for approval using a New Drug Application (NDA) depending on the type of product. Limited facility information is required as part of the Chemistry Manufacturing and Controls (CMC) information submitted with either type of application.

9.3.1 Chemistry Manufacturing and Controls

There are a number of CMC guidance documents available from the FDA to assist applicants in filing BLAs for various types of products. These documents are available on the FDA's Web site and include guidance documents for therapeutic recombinant DNA-derived products and monoclonal antibody products for *in vivo* use [9]; autologous somatic cell therapy products [10]; human plasma-derived biological products or animal plasma- or serum-derived products [11]; synthetic peptide substances [12]; human blood and blood components intended for transfusion or for further manufacture [13]; allergenic products [14]; biological *in vitro* diagnostics [15]; and vaccines [16].

Most of the CMC guidance documents for BLA submissions are divided into two sections on drug substance and drug product. The facility information requested in both the drug substance and drug product sections includes information regarding all manufacturers involved in the manufacture, testing, and packaging of the drug substance and product; floor diagrams of each manufacturing facility; and a description of the manufacture of other products in the same facility including their developmental status and their relationship to the product that is the subject of the application. In addition, both drug substance and drug product sections require a description of the contamination precautions in place with regard to facility design, equipment features, and manufacturing practices designed to prevent contamination and cross-contamination. It is important to note that the drug substance facility information required for biotech products submitted in BLAs is not required for the applications for those products submitted in NDAs.

The drug product section of the CMC documents for BLA submission reference an FDA guidance document that requests additional facility information regarding equipment placement; heating, ventilation, and air conditioning (HVAC) and water systems; environmental and water monitoring programs; and sterilization methods and validation. Extensive information regarding the media fill validation of aseptic processes, investigations of media fill failures, stability, and the container closure system is also requested. The FDA guidance document is entitled "Guidance for Industry for the Submission of Documentation for Sterilization Process Validation in Applications for Human and Veterinary Drug Products" [17] and is available on the FDA's Web site. This information on sterilization process validation is also required for drugs filed as NDAs.

There is a second FDA guidance document that specifically addresses aseptic processing including environmental requirements, media fills, and allowable contamination rates.

This document is entitled "Guideline for Sterile Drug Products Produced by Aseptic Processing" [3]. Recently, the FDA published a revised guidance document on asceptic processing. The Aseptic Processing Guideline [18] is currently available on the FDA's Web site.

9.3.2 Establishment Description

A description of manufacturing facilities as well as plant systems and other related facility features is required for all biological products except for specified biotechnology-derived therapeutic products including rDNA products, monoclonal antibodies, and synthetic peptides, as well as rDNA vaccines. Any biotech products that do not fall into these categories, such as vaccines made by recombinant technology, must also file an Establishment Description in addition to the CMC section.

An Establishment Description [10,11,13–16] guidance document is provided as a companion to all CMC guidance documents for products that require establishment descriptions. The Establishment Description requires the applicant to submit general facility information as well as limited information on major plant utilities and systems. General facility information includes simple floor diagrams depicting general facility layout as well as product, personnel, equipment, waste, and airflow. An illustration or diagram that depicts the areas served by each air-handling unit and air pressure differentials is also required.

A section on water systems requests a general description of the water system, water quality, and use and a certification that installation and operational qualification have been performed. A summary of the validation protocol and data as well as an overview of the routine monitoring program are also requested.

Similar information is required for the HVAC system. A general description of the HVAC system, as well as containment and segregation features, must be provided as well as a summary of the HVAC system validation and routine environmental monitoring program. Guidance regarding air and water specifications, limits and monitoring parameters, and frequencies is provided in the section of this chapter on environmental monitoring (see Section 9.7).

Any computer systems that control critical processes must be described, as well as a summary of the qualification and validation for each system.

The Establishment Description also contains a section on contamination and cross-contamination issues. This section requests information on cleaning procedures, cleaning validation, and containment features that are designed to prevent contamination and cross-contamination. Some of the information requested here is identical to that requested in the CMC section, and it is permissible to cross-reference the CMC section rather than to repeat the same information.

9.3.3 CBER/CDER Reorganization

FDA has completed the third phase of its implementation of the transfer of certain product reviews from CBER to CDER. The products transferred include the following classes of therapeutic products: monoclonal antibodies; cytokines, growth factors, and interferons; proteins extracted from animals or microorganisms intended for therapeutic use; and therapeutic immunotherapies [19].

The FDA has emphasized that under the new structure, the biological products transferred to CDER will continue to be regulated as licensed biologics. Thus, the CMC guidance documents referenced previously and the guidance provided in the remainder of this chapter should remain applicable after the products are transferred from CBER to CDER.

9.4 FACILITY DESIGN

9.4.1 General Considerations

Facilities designed to manufacture biotech products, to the drug substance stage, have the following manufacturing areas:

- Cell inoculum suites

- Fermentation/harvest area
- Purification areas
- Bulk filtration area
- Support areas (component preparation, media preparation, buffer preparation)

These areas are standard within the industry [5,20,21]. Design considerations have not varied tremendously except for more extensive use of closed systems (refer to Section 9.4.2). Validated closed systems have allowed manufacturers to reduce room environmental classifications (e.g., the use of gray space) and to minimize the level of gowning for their operators.

9.4.1.1 Cell Inoculum Suites

With all biological products that are biotechnology-derived, the first step in production is the expansion of an ampoule of cells taken from a fully released Working Cell Bank (WCB). The implementation of GMP begins at this stage for biologicals of this nature. Cell inoculum suites are highly controlled areas from an environmental standpoint because these operations are considered "open." The manufacturer must take a prospective approach to prevent contamination and cross-contamination (see Section 9.8) in the cell inoculum suites. Mammalian cell culture inoculum suites tend to meet Class 10,000 (ISO 7), while microbial seed inoculum suites tend to meet Class 100,000 (ISO 8). In both cases, all open manipulations of the mammalian cells or microbial seeds are performed in a certified laminar airflow hood (LAF) or biological safety cabinet (BSC) supplied with HEPA-filtered, Class 100 (ISO 5) air. The areas have terminal high-efficiency particulate air (HEPA) filtration with low-level returns. The pressure cascades are determined by the level of containment required; however, the majority of these suites operate with positive pressure cascades. Room surfaces are smooth and nonporous and are on a rigorous cleaning schedule. Operators have a high level of gowning, which includes a bunny suit, shoe covers, head cover, safety glasses, gloves, and mask. When performing manipulations in the LAF or BSC, operators will add sterile sleeves and a second pair of gloves before beginning work.

9.4.1.2 Fermentation/Harvest Areas

Fermentation/harvest areas contain the majority of closed-system operations within a manufacturing facility. Manufacturers have been able to validate their fermentation trains as closed, thereby assuring the FDA that the environment should have no impact on the required quality of the product at this stage of production. As a result, most manufacturers design these areas to meet Class 100,000 (ISO 8) standards but do not operate within the specifications of Class 100,000. These areas tend to have more exposed piping and floor drains. Most manufacturers continue to use HEPA-filtration (either in-line or terminal) with low-level returns (high-level returns are generally not found in newly designed facilities). The pressure cascade will be dependent on the required level of containment. Room surfaces are smooth and nonporous and are cleaned per a predefined schedule. Operators have a moderate level of gowning, which includes a plant uniform with shoe covers, safety glasses, and head cover. Some manufacturers will add a laboratory coat to the initial gowning. Also, gloves are used for operations such as removing sample bottles from the fermenter.

Areas used for the harvesting process are either part of the fermenter hall or are in a separate area adjacent to the fermenter hall. In general, these areas meet the same design criteria as those specified for the fermenter halls. One area of concern is the harvesting of live organisms and the potential for generating aerosols through centrifugation or homogenization. The manufacturer is encouraged to include closed systems in the design criteria for these types of operations. The use of negative pressure cascades and additional gowning (e.g., bunny suit) for the operators may be required for these types of processes.

9.4.1.3 Purification Areas

All biotech products require some level of purification. Typically, these processes include column chromatography and ultrafiltration. While not sterile, these processes are considered clean and should be designed to minimize the addition of bioburden and endotoxin. The use of presterilized bags or tanks that can be sterilized and the development of processes designed to collect product pools and not fractions have allowed manufacturers to operate these areas as Class 100,000 (ISO 8). To support the use of a Class 100,000 environment, the manufacturer should have bioburden and endotoxin data (from process streams) indicating that the environment has no impact on the product. If the process data do not support the use of a Class 100,000 environment or if the process design is open (e.g., fraction collection), the environmental classification will be more restrictive (i.e., Class 10,000 or ISO 7) with the open manipulations performed in an LAF or BSC supplied with HEPA-filtered, Class 100 (ISO 5) air. Purification areas will have terminal HEPA filtration with low-level returns and positive pressure cascades. Room surfaces are smooth and nonporous and are cleaned on a rigorous schedule. Operators (even in a Class 100,000 environment) have a high level of gowning, which includes a bunny suit, shoe covers, safety glasses, and a head cover. Some manufacturers include masks and gloves as part of the gowning requirements for purification.

Viral inactivation (for mammalian cell culture processes) steps are part of the purification process. Manufacturers must design the purification areas to prevent the potential of viral contamination from the previral processing areas to the postviral processing areas [5,22]. Complete physical separation (including once-through air or a separate recirculating air handler) is the easiest way to prevent viral contamination.

9.4.1.4 Bulk Filtration Areas

Bulk filtration areas are designed for the purpose of 0.22-μm filtration of the drug substance prior to storage and shipment to a contract filler or prior to storage and formulation in an on-site formulation/fill suite. This is not considered a sterile filtration, but a bioburden-minimizing filtration. Manufacturers design these areas to the highest environmental standard within a bulk manufacturing facility. Room classification meets either Class 10,000 (ISO 7) or Class 1,000 (ISO 6) with all open manipulations performed in an LAF or BSC supplied with HEPA-filtered, Class 100 (ISO 5) air. These areas have terminal HEPA filtration with low-level returns and positive pressure cascades. Room surfaces are smooth and nonporous and are cleaned on a rigorous schedule. Operator gowning is at a high level, which includes a bunny suit, knee boots, hood, safety glasses, mask, gloves, and sterile sleeves. In general, typical bioburden specifications for the drug substance post-filtration are 0 CFU/ml or < 1 CFU/ml.

Recently, several manufactures have designed and validated closed systems for the filtration of the drug substance. These manufacturers have been approved to perform this step in a Class 100,000 (ISO 8) environment with reduced operator gowning.

9.4.1.5 Support Areas

Support areas include equipment preparation, media preparation, and buffer preparation. Equipment preparation areas typically consist of three contiguous suites: dirty equipment staging and washing, clean equipment storage and preparation for sterilization, and storage of sterilized equipment. Ideally, these suites should be designed with pass-through washers and autoclaves, and operators should not be allowed to move from the equipment wash area to the clean areas without changing gowns. A one-way flow is strongly encouraged to prevent mix-ups of dirty, clean, and sterile equipment. Depending on the quantity of equipment that is reused and the number of products in the facility, a manufacturer may have one or two equipment preparation areas. Many manufacturing facilities have an equipment preparation area for upstream operations and one for downstream operations. This type of design will allow more flexibility and efficiency of operation while providing a higher level of separation between upstream and downstream equipment. Manufacturers who use a majority of disposables and fixed equipment tend to design facilities with one equipment preparation area. In this case, scheduling is used to separate upstream and downstream equipment. Generally, these areas are designed to meet Class 100,000 (ISO 8) standards. The clean equipment storage/preparation area and the sterile equipment storage area are required to meet this standard during operations. The clean areas will have HEPA filtration (either in-line or terminal) with low-level returns and positive pressure cascades. Room surfaces are smooth and nonporous and are cleaned on a predefined schedule. The equipment wash area tends to operate under less-restrictive environmental controls. Some manufacturers design this area with a negative pressure cascade.

Both media and buffer preparation areas should be designed to meet Class 100,000 (ISO 8) standards. Media preparation will require dust control measures and an area for the sterile filtration and bottling of small-volume media and other nutrients required for mammalian cell culture operations or microbial seed operations. Media preparation areas have a higher level of environmental control and a greater use of closed systems than in the past. Several viral and mycoplasma contamination events were attributed to practices in the media preparation area. Cleaning of this area is more rigorous, open additions and mixing activities are eliminated or minimized, and operator gowning includes gloves and a mask. Many of these areas have terminal HEPA filtration with low-level returns and positive pressure cascades. Buffer preparation areas will meet the same design criteria.

Most facilities will have an area for media preparation and an area for buffer preparation. Some manufacturers have decided to use one area for both activities. Before deciding on this type of design, the manufacturer should consider the overall impact on the efficiency of operation and the extent of cleaning validation that will be required to use tanks for both media and buffer (refer to Section 9.8).

9.4.2 Specific Considerations

Three areas that have affected facility design considerations include the use of closed systems, the use of gray space, and the addition of Good Large-Scale Practice (GLSP) [4] to the list of biocontainment levels.

9.4.2.1 Closed Systems

As stated previously, the use of closed systems has allowed manufacturers to operate under less-restrictive environmental conditions. Closed systems are designed to protect the product from the immediate environment. Process additives, such as nutrient feeds, antifoam, and processes gases, may be introduced during production. However, these additions are done in a tightly controlled manner such that the product is not adversely affected and the closed system is not open to the environment. The same is true for the removal of in-process samples for process monitoring purposes.

In general, closed systems are cleaned in place (CIP) and sterilized in place (SIP) with extensive use of hard piping and transfer panels. There should be minimal human intervention (specifically with regard to making and breaking connections). Validating these systems can be a challenge for a manufacturer. The validation of a closed system should include SIP assessment and media hold studies. The manufacturer should be able to demonstrate the integrity of the system through pressure hold tests and filter integrity tests. Other means of assessment include the overall contamination rate attributed to a closed system operation and the level of the calibration and preventive maintenance programs to ensure that the system will not fail.

Some manufacturers have made extensive use of flexible tubing and tubing welders to establish a closed system. This type of system is more difficult to validate as "closed" and to ensure consistency of operation. Operators must be rigorously trained to ensure that the welds are acceptable. Bad welds can open the system to the environment and increase the rate of contamination. In addition, if the tubing welder reuses the blades, the operator must document the number of uses. Blades should be discarded before they fail.

9.4.2.2 Gray Space

Closed systems have offered the advantage for some manufacturing activities to occur in gray space. Gray space has minimal requirements for environmental control. Surfaces do not need to meet the requirements as stated in the cGMP regulations [2] nor is high-quality air required for this type of environment. Generally, gray space has been approved for use in areas where there is no potential for adding or removing materials. An example is the buffer hold operation. The operation itself is completely closed with buffers delivered to the tanks and from the tanks using hard pipe delivery systems. There will be occasions when these tanks are opened. Typically, these are during maintenance activities. Manufacturers must be able to return the tanks to the level of cleanliness required to protect the quality of the buffer. These tanks should have both CIP and SIP capabilities.

Another scenario for the use of gray space involves the fermentation operation. A few manufacturers have been approved to locate the fermenter in gray space; however, the location of the addition and removal ports had to be in classified space.

9.4.2.3 Good Large-Scale Practice

The July 1991 update [23] to the NIH guidelines for research involving the use of recombinant DNA organisms included a new category called Good Large-Scale Practice. Essentially, organisms that meet the criteria for GLSP could be released into the environment without undergoing inactivation. This meant that manufacturers using GLSP organisms did not have to install, validate, and maintain an inactivation system (local state or city laws could override this provision). GLSP organisms are described as those viable, recombinant strains derived from host organisms which are nonpathogenic and nontoxigenic and have a long history of safe use at large scale [23]. As an example, the majority of recombinant *E. coli* strains meet these criteria.

Biosafety levels 1–3 (biosafety level 4 is atypical for a biotech product) apply to increasing hazard levels of host organisms with regard to potential harmful impact to personnel and to the environment. These biosafety levels and their requirements are defined in the April 2002 update to the NIH guideline for research involving recombinant DNA organisms [4]. The overall goal is to ensure that the viable host organisms are maintained within a defined closed system and that environmental contaminants are prevented from entering the system. Design features may include the following:

- Negative pressure cascades
- Use of airlocks
- Once-through air with HEPA filtration on the air supply and (depending on the biosafety level) the air exhaust
- Equipment/system for the inactivation/decontamination of process materials (specifically, process fluids containing viable cells and materials that may have come in contact with viable cells)
- Established spill procedures
- Appropriate levels of gowning for operators

9.5 UTILITIES: DESIGN AND OPERATION

The design and installation of high-quality, reliable plant utilities are crucial to the operation of a GMP facility for the manufacture of biotech products. Plant utilities include water and clean-steam systems, HVAC systems, sterilization systems, and decontamination and waste treatment systems. This section will focus on water systems and HVAC systems, but many of the principles of qualification, maintenance, and operation of these systems can be applied to all plant systems.

9.5.1 Water Systems

Water is an essential component of parenteral products and probably accounts for the largest component volume utilized in manufacturing operations. The quality and consistency of high-purity water appropriate for manufacturing operations depends on several factors including (1) the quality and source of the incoming potable water, (2) choice of treatment and water purification steps, (3) design and construction features of the water system including storage and distribution components, and (4) the effectiveness of routine monitoring, preventive maintenance, and calibration programs [24].

9.5.1.1 Incoming Potable Water

The incoming potable water is required to meet the Environmental Protection Agency's National Drinking Water Regulations as set forth in Title 40 of the CFR, Part 141 [25]. These regulations specify maximum contaminant levels for organic and inorganic chemicals, turbidity, and microorganisms. It is also required by these regulations that the water be supplied under continuous positive pressure in a plumbing system free of defects that could contribute to contamination of a drug product.

Because the incoming water quality can vary considerably, influenced by factors such as rainfall and seasonal variations, most water systems begin with a series of pretreatment steps that are chosen based on the characteristics of the incoming water. Pretreatment systems usually consist of one or more different types of filters designed to reduce chlorine, chemicals, and bioburden levels [26]. Prior to primary water purification, softening may be necessary as the final pretreatment step to substitute sodium ions for minerals containing magnesium or calcium, in order to prevent the buildup of insoluble precipitates.

9.5.1.2 Water Purification Systems

Water purification systems may follow the initial pretreatment steps in various sequences depending on the characteristics of the water and the design of the system. Reverse-osmosis (RO) and deionization (DI) are common water purification steps. RO is often the first system in this series. RO systems remove a large percentage of the total dissolved solids, as well as bacteria and endotoxin, from the feed water. A well-designed, single-pass RO system will typically reject up to 95% of dissolved solids and 99% of microorganisms and endotoxin by pumping water through a semipermeable membrane from a high-solids solution to a low-solids solution, allowing water to pass and retaining the dissolved solids, organic matter, and bacteria [27].

Since RO membranes retain highly charged salt ions to a greater extent than weakly ionized monovalent ions, it is often desirable to follow the RO system with an ion-exchange unit. DI water is produced by passing water through either a mixed-bed or a two-bed cation-anion exchanger to remove residual ionic components. The type of deionizer and resin capacities should be chosen based on the quality of water that is desired, the quality of the feed water, and the anticipated water volume throughput. The preinstallation analysis should also take into account the surface area of the ion-exchange resin beds, the temperature range of the system water, the operational range of the flow rates, the frequency of use of the system, the type of regenerant chemicals, and the proposed method of steam sterilization or sanitization. Such analysis will help determine how often beds will need to be regenerated and will assist in the development of maintenance schedules for the system [27].

Other systems that may be a part of the water purification system include ultraviolet (UV) sterilizing units and ultrafiltration (UF) systems. The purpose of UV irradiation is to damage bacterial DNA to control bacterial growth, and these units are often located downstream of the DI unit since deionization does not remove microbial contamination. A UF unit may be placed in a water system to remove nonviable particles and bacteria as well as organic and colloidal material. UF employs the use of a variety of membranes whose pores range in size from approximately 0.003 to 0.006 μm in diameter [24,27]. Ultrafilters are often intended to remove pyrogens whose sizes generally range from 1.5 to 3000 kDa molecular weight.

Water that has been purified by RO or DI systems is often intended to meet the U.S. Pharmacopoeia (USP) Purified Water (PW) specifications and may be used for a number of applications. These applications may include initial cleaning of equipment, preparation of bacteriological media for fermentation, and feed water for the system intended to produce water for injection (WFI) [24].

9.5.1.3 Distillation

Distillation is the most common method for production of WFI from feed water that generally meets USP PW specifications. There are three system areas to be considered in the construction and design of the WFI system: the WFI purification unit, the distribution system, and the storage system for the water. Water purification by distillation is accomplished by heating to convert water into vapor, which then passes over a condenser and is cooled to liquid [26]. Dissolved mineral matter is not volatile at the boiling point of water and remains behind. There are various types of distillation stills including single-effect, multiple-effect, and vapor recompression stills.

9.5.1.4 Storage and Distribution Systems

The distribution system design is critical to the overall performance of the WFI system. Probably the most common system design is composed of a distribution loop that recirculates water at 80°C with point-of-use heat exchangers to cool the water to the appropriate temperature for the desired operations and a storage tank of adequate size to meet the greatest water demands that may be anticipated [24]. Cold or ambient distribution loops are sometimes employed when large volumes of water are needed for production steps such as media and buffer preparation. A dual hot loop/cold loop may be designed to maintain a comparatively large inventory of 80°C WFI in a recirculating loop, while a smaller inventory of cool water is circulated in a separate loop. There should be provisions for ambient or cold loops to be maintained at 80°C during periods of nonuse to inhibit microbial growth [24]. The period of time the water must be elevated to 80°C should be based on validation data. Finally, the distribution system should be capable of sanitization, preferably by steam sterilization.

9.5.1.5 Materials of Construction

Materials of construction for the piping and distribution systems must be resistant to corrosion and should minimize contamination [28]. Ideally, stainless steel piping should be used throughout the system to meet these requirements; however, plastic piping is less expensive and is often used in the systems that produce feed water for the distillation unit. The recommended composition of the distillation unit as well as its storage and distribution systems is stainless steel AISI grade 316L or better, *L* referring to low carbon grade [28]. Tubing and the fittings of the distribution should have interior surfaces that are smooth, uniform, and free of pits and crevices where organic matter could lodge and contaminate the system. The smooth interior surface is achieved through mechanical polishing and generally followed by electropolishing, which removes the surface layer and its impurities. The components of the distribution and storage systems should be permanently joined in a sanitary manner. A welding method that produces welds that are smooth and free of defects such as automatic orbital welding should be employed. The locations of all welds should be documented on system blueprints and all welds should be inspected for defects as part of the water system validation.

Fittings in the system should be of sanitary design and should meet the 3-A sanitary design and component standards [28]. Joints in the WFI system should be minimized to prevent leaks and bacterial growth. Stainless steel diaphragm valves are recommended.

Proper design of the piping distribution system should facilitate water circulation. Dead legs of more than six pipe diameters are not permitted in order to prevent areas of stagnant water where bacterial contamination may occur.

Piping must be sloped to ensure proper drainage of water, and sufficient pressure must be supplied to maintain turbulent flow [28].

9.5.1.6 Passivation

Once installed, the system should be cleaned and passivated. Passivation is a method by which chemical agents react with metal surfaces to render the surfaces nonreactive. Following cleaning and passivation, the water system should be qualified and validated to ensure that it consistently produces water of the appropriate quality [24].

9.5.1.7 Water System Qualification

Operational checks of all components of the water system should be performed using calibrated monitoring instruments including conductivity meters, temperature-sensing devices, pressure-sensing devices, and flow meters [26]. Temperatures in loops and storage tanks, as well as during sanitization or steam sterilization procedures, should be monitored. Performance qualification should include intense monitoring of all use points on the system as well as other key sites including the incoming potable water source, feed water to the still, the still outlet, and storage tanks. The water quality following each pretreatment and purification step should also be monitored. After the initial performance qualification, a routine monitoring schedule should be established for all of these components [24]. Routine monitoring of the water system is discussed in more detail in Section 9.7.

9.5.2 Heating Ventilation and Air-Conditioning (HVAC) Systems

Both the cGMP regulations for finished pharmaceuticals [2] and the biologics standards sections [1] of the CFR specify the requirement for a system to provide ventilation, air filtration, air heating, and cooling to manufacturing areas to allow for adequate ventilation; equipment for control over pressure, microbes, dust, humidity, and temperature; air filtration systems consisting of prefilters and particle filters; and adequate control over recirculated air and adequate exhaust. Separate air-handling units should be supplied for areas where different products are handled, and adequate containment should be provided as required.

Facility design and operation must be considered in the design and operation of an appropriate HVAC system including the room classification requirements, whether the facility will contain a single product or multiple products, whether simultaneous or campaigned manufacturing of more than one product will be performed, and whether the product has any containment requirements. Other considerations include segregation requirements for personnel, product, materials, waste materials, and clean and dirty equipment, as well as temperature, humidity, and pressure differential requirements between rooms and suites.

The air classification required for a manufacturing process is largely determined by the type of product and the degree of product exposure to the environment (see Section 9.4). Since biotech products generally support microbial growth, most manufacturing operations must take place under controlled environmental conditions, or Class 100,000 (ISO 8) conditions, at a minimum. Exceptions include certain "closed" systems that have been validated to be closed to the surrounding environment. Downstream purification steps that are not closed or where open manipulations in laminar flow hoods take place may be performed in Class 10,000 (ISO 7) environments, and "critical areas" where the sterilized dosage form, containers, and closures are exposed to the environment must meet Class 100 (ISO 5) requirements (see Section 9.7). Air supplied to adjacent areas of different classifications must also be segregated by maintaining pressure differentials of 0.05 inch of water, with the "cleaner" areas being positive, to less clean areas [3]. Exceptions include containment areas where live agents are handled in areas that are negative to surrounding areas.

The HVAC system must be capable of reliably meeting these requirements, maintaining adequate air quality, segregation, and containment. The fundamental goal of an HVAC system is to bring fresh air into a facility, mix it with recirculated air whenever possible, and then condition the air through filtration, heating, cooling, and humidification or dehumidification. The system also supplies air to work areas and then recovers it for partial or total exhaustion into the atmosphere.

9.5.2.1 HVAC Components

Basic HVAC components include a prefilter bank composed of 30% ASHRAE and 85% ASHRAE filters, preheat coils, cooling coils, fans, components for humidification and dehumidification, and a final filter bank including terminal HEPA filters [29]. Other HVAC components include sealed or welded ductwork and monitoring devices for temperature, pressure, and humidity. The HVAC system and its components can be designed to maintain cleanliness and minimize contamination. For example, placement of air inlets in the ceiling and low wall returns creates an airflow pattern with a sweeping action to minimize particulate contamination [3]. Restrictions on the volume of air supplied from outside, high filtration standards, and well-established airflow direction also can help decrease contamination. The series of filters in each air-handling unit (AHU) of the HVAC system filter contaminants from the air, with final filtration through a terminal HEPA filter.

9.5.2.2 Recirculated versus Once-Through Systems

In a recirculating system, exhausted air is directed into a ducted return system where it is combined with exhausted air from other rooms, drawn through dust collectors and filtering systems, mixed with a percentage of makeup air, and then recirculated to various rooms [29]. Recirculating systems provide for economical use of filters as well as the systems that provide heating, cooling, and humidification.

Once-through systems utilize 100% outside air. The once-through system is most frequently used in those manufacturing applications having the greatest risk of cross-contamination. In this system, air is taken in from the outside environment, conditioned, distributed through the facility, and then exhausted. These systems typically require the use of reheating coils in individual zones in order to maintain temperatures under all load conditions; thus, energy costs are very high [29].

Recirculating and once-through systems can be combined to meet the needs of the manufacturing facility. For example, containment areas may be supplied with once-through air to minimize the chance of cross-contamination. Other areas in the same facility may be supplied with recirculated air.

9.5.2.3 HVAC Requirements for Aseptic Processing

There are special HVAC requirements for aseptic processing facilities. Not only must critical areas be supplied with HEPA-filtered air that meets Class 100 (ISO 5) requirements, but laminar flow as well as minimum airflow velocities must be maintained to ensure that contaminants are efficiently swept away from the product [3,18]. Smoke testing must be performed as part of the initial HVAC qualification and periodically thereafter to confirm appropriate control over direction of airflow. It is generally recommended that the AHU that supplies aseptic processing areas be dedicated to those areas to prevent any contaminants present in earlier processing steps from being introduced into the aseptic environment.

9.5.2.4 HVAC System Qualification and Monitoring

Installation and operation of all components of the HVAC system must be verified once the system is installed. HEPA filters must be tested for integrity and efficiency. Integrity testing ensures that there are no leaks, and efficiency testing ensures that HEPA filters are capable of retaining particles ≥ 0.3 μm with an efficiency of 99.97% [3,18]. Filter testing must be repeated at least semiannually. The performance of the HVAC system is initially evaluated as part of the environmental qualification of the facility, and the continued performance of the system is monitored through a comprehensive environmental monitoring program (see Section 9.7).

9.6 FACILITY CLEANING

The GMP regulations for finished pharmaceuticals [2] and the biologics establishment standards [1] both stress the importance of maintaining clean facilities and incorporating design features (e.g., coved corners; smooth, hard, nonporous surfaces) that allow for easy cleaning. It is important to establish facility cleaning procedures that specify daily, weekly, and monthly cleaning activities. Related procedures that should be developed include cleaning procedures that are performed following a plant shutdown or as part of recommissioning activities following facility construction or modifications. Facility disinfecting agents must be validated for effectiveness and should include effectiveness testing against any live organisms manufactured in the facility. Finally, facility cleaning procedures should be qualified with postcleaning environmental monitoring to ensure they are effective.

9.6.1 Cleaning Procedures

There are generally two types of daily cleaning that occur in manufacturing facilities. At the conclusion of a shift or at the conclusion of operations in a particular area, production operators perform a number of cleaning and room clearance tasks in accordance with written procedures. These tasks often include removal of waste, components, materials, and equipment from the area that is to be discarded, cleaned, decontaminated, sterilized, or returned to stock. The area is inspected for any residual materials or product from the day's operations, and the surfaces (lab benches, equipment surfaces) are cleaned and disinfected. The operators may also disinfect other items such as doorknobs and cabinets. A logbook or other documentation is generally completed, signed, and dated to document that the daily cleaning has been performed.

In addition to operator cleaning at the conclusion of production or other operations, a cleaning crew or contracted cleaning service may also perform additional activities after hours each day such as floor and wall cleaning and removal of trash from the facility. Cleaning personnel, whether they are company employees or from a contracted cleaning company, must follow written procedures and should be trained on their responsibilities as well as on other facility or company procedures applicable to their work such as gowning procedures that are required and basic GMPs that apply to their specific activities. All cleaning activities performed by cleaning personnel or a contract cleaning service must also be documented, signed, and dated.

Additional, more rigorous cleaning activities are often performed on a less frequent basis such as weekly or monthly. These activities may include cleaning of ceilings, exposed piping, and lighting panels. Some of these activities may be scheduled during plant shutdowns.

9.6.2 Cleaning Agents and Equipment

The mops, cloths, and buckets used for facility cleaning should be stored and cared for so that they do not contaminate the area during cleaning. For example, all mop heads and cloths used for cleaning surfaces should be made of low-particulate-shedding material. Mops, buckets, and other cleaning supplies should be dedicated to particular manufacturing areas to prevent cross-contamination between areas. In aseptic areas, mop heads and other cleaning equipment may be autoclaved before use.

Disinfectants used in manufacturing facilities are chosen based on their ability to kill a broad spectrum of contaminants including bacteria, molds, and spores. It is common to rotate the use of two or more disinfectants to prevent the growth of resistant organisms. Another common approach is to use one broad-spectrum disinfectant routinely with the use of a second disinfectant periodically to prevent mold or spore growth.

Whatever the disinfectant or combination of disinfectants chosen, disinfectant effectiveness studies must be performed to validate their effectiveness. FDA investigators generally expect disinfectant effectiveness studies to include the application of challenge organisms to coupons of the surfaces to be disinfected. Disinfectants are applied for a defined period of time and their effectiveness is determined. Challenge organisms generally include standard organisms used for sterility and growth promotion testing as well as common environmental isolates and any host organisms used in the manufacturing process. The results of disinfectant effectiveness studies may be used to determine the best combination of disinfectants, the most effective rotation of disinfectants, minimum contact times, and other aspects of disinfectant use. It is important to note that investigators conducting FDA inspections commonly request disinfectant effectiveness studies.

9.6.3 Monitoring Cleaning Effectiveness

It is prudent to incorporate some measure of cleaning effectiveness into the facility's environmental monitoring program to ensure continued effectiveness of the cleaning program and personnel adherence to cleaning procedures [30]. In order to accomplish this, postcleaning environmental monitoring should be performed periodically (e.g., monthly or quarterly). Postuse environmental monitoring should focus on surface sampling from floors, walls, doors, equipment, lab benches, and other surfaces. If unacceptable levels of contaminants are found in postcleaning samples, corrective actions may include retraining of personnel or modifications of cleaning agents or procedures [30].

9.6.4 Recommissioning Activities

Following plant shutdowns or major facility or utility modifications or maintenance, a number of activities must be performed to bring the facility back on-line. There should be written procedures for these activities as well as documentation of all activities performed followed by review and approval by the unit responsible for quality assurance to effectively release the areas for GMP manufacturing. Recommissioning procedures should include specific cleaning procedures as well as environmental monitoring procedures to ensure that the facility environment is under an appropriate level of control for GMP manufacturing.

9.7 ENVIRONMENTAL MONITORING

Maintaining control over manufacturing processes is a key element in the consistent production of a product that is safe, pure, and effective. Environmental control is specifically mandated by the cGMP regulations [2] for aseptic processing operations. However, environmental control for bulk manufacturing operations for biological products including products produced by biotechnology is also required due to the nature of these products. These products are composed of proteins and other biological components that may support microbial growth. Furthermore, such products cannot withstand terminal heat sterilization.

A comprehensive environmental monitoring program for biological and biotechnology bulk and final product manufacturing is necessary to ensure that the environment is sufficiently controlled during manufacturing operations. Environmental monitoring should include scheduled monitoring of airborne viable and nonviable particulate levels, pressure differentials, direction of airflow, temperature, humidity, and microbial contaminants on personnel, equipment, work surfaces, floors, and walls. Monitoring of the water and clean steam that supply the manufacturing facilities is also required [30].

Several guidance documents, including FDA-issued documents, specify environmental requirements for aseptic processing areas [3,7,8,18]. Many of the concepts described in these documents can also be applied to bulk manufacturing facilities for biotech products.

9.7.1 Nonviable Particulate Monitoring

Airborne nonviable particulates should be controlled and monitored in all critical and controlled manufacturing environments. Air in aseptic processing areas where final drug products are filled is generally monitored continuously for nonviable particulates. Nonviable particulate monitoring frequencies in other areas vary based on the nature of the operations (open or closed to the environment), susceptibility of the product to contamination, and whether there are subsequent steps designed to remove contaminants from the product [30]. Airborne nonviable particulate monitoring should generally be performed during manufacturing to ensure that the environment is under a sufficient level of control while operations are ongoing. In addition to detecting nonviable contaminant levels, nonviable particulate monitoring also provides a good indication of the microbial quality of the environment since microbial contaminants are generally associated with dust particles or water droplets. Static particulate monitoring (performed when an area is at rest) is important for establishing a baseline with which to compare nonviable particulate levels during operations [30].

Nonviable particulate levels are expressed in numbers of particles per cubic foot or meter. Nonviable particulate levels are expressed as airborne particulate cleanliness classes that represent the maximum number of particles at ≥ 0.5 µm per cubic foot or cubic meter (see Table 9.1) [30]. Most controlled bulk manufacturing operations are performed in Class 100,000 (ISO 8) environments with those requiring cleaner conditions (such as open manipulations within an LAF) occurring in Class 10,000 (ISO 7) environments. Final product manufacturing steps, where sterilized product is exposed to the environment (e.g., filling and lyophilization operations), must be performed in Class 100 (ISO 5) laminar airflow environments [3,18]. The area surrounding Class 100 (ISO 5) aseptic processing areas may be Class 1000 (ISO 6) or Class 10,000 (ISO 7).

9.7.2 Airborne Viable Microbial Monitoring

Microbial monitoring methods include quantitative, volumetric air sampling, quantitative surface monitoring, and personnel monitoring. Quantitative sampling of manufacturing environments for viable airborne contaminants requires the

TABLE 9.1 Airborne Nonviable Particulate Classes and Viable Contaminant Limits

Classification			Nonviable (particles ≥0.5 μm)		Viable (colony-forming units [CFUs])	
			ft³	m³	CFU/ft³	CFU/m³
U.S.	EU	ISO[a]				
Class 100	Class A	5	100	3,530	0.1	1
Class 10,000	Class B	7	10,000	353,000	0.5	7
Class 100,000	Class C	8	100,000	3,530,000	2.5	100
—	Class D[b]	—	100,000	3,530,000	2.5	100

[a] ISO 14644-1 designations [7] provide uniform particle concentration values for cleanrooms. ISO 5 particle concentration is equivalent to Class 100 and EU Grade A.

[b] European Class D particulate limits must only be achieved during "at rest" conditions. All other air classifications listed in the above table represent limits that must be maintained during operations.

use of a volumetric sampling device that draws in a specific volume of air and captures microorganisms, usually impinging them onto an agar surface [30]. Like nonviable particulate monitoring, viable airborne contaminants should be monitored during manufacturing operations to ensure that products are not exposed to unacceptable levels of microbial contamination during manufacturing. For bulk manufacturing operations, airborne microbial sampling is often scheduled during specific manipulations such as inoculations, transfers, and sampling steps. Aseptic processing of the final product requires a representative number of samples covering the entire process.

Acceptable limits for airborne microbial monitoring are provided for each nonviable air cleanliness classification in Table 9.1 [30].

9.7.3 Contact Plates and Swabs

Contact plates (agar plates designed such that the agar surface can directly contact the surface to be sampled) and swabs are useful indicators of contaminant levels on equipment, work surfaces, floors, walls, and personnel [30]. Surface sampling should be performed following operations but before cleaning to determine contaminant levels that existed during operations. Likewise, personnel monitoring should be performed immediately following operations and prior to disinfecting gloves and gowns. Special care should be taken to thoroughly clean all surfaces following sampling to ensure that any residual microbiological media from contact plates and swabs is removed.

Monitoring locations on walls, floors, and other surfaces should include "high-traffic" areas such as doorknobs, pass-throughs, and floor samples proximal to doorways, cold rooms, etc. There are no clear recommendations for either monitoring limits or frequencies for surface monitoring in bulk manufacturing areas. It is recommended that such limits be set after compiling and reviewing microbiological monitoring data gathered during controlled GMP manufacturing operations. Surface monitoring frequencies usually follow the same schedules as those for nonviable and viable airborne contaminants.

Routine personnel monitoring is usually limited to aseptic processing or final product manufacturing steps. Other critical steps such as bulk filtration, when open manipulations with product may occur, should also include personnel monitoring. Monitoring sites for aseptic processing personnel should include, at a minimum, gloves, chest, forearms, and face mask. Personnel must be monitored following each aseptic operation, including aseptic media fills.

9.7.4 Temperature and Humidity Monitoring

Temperature control and monitoring is required by the cGMP regulations for finished pharmaceuticals [2]. Temperature should be monitored and regulated in all areas of the facility, including the warehouse, to protect products, raw materials, and components from extremes in temperature that may affect their quality. It is equally important to ensure personnel comfort, especially in areas where workers are required to wear gowns, in order to reduce perspiration and shedding in controlled manufacturing areas.

The cGMP regulations for finished pharmaceuticals [2] also require humidity to be monitored in aseptic processing areas. The regulations do not prescribe an acceptable humidity range, but it should be set sufficiently low to discourage the growth of molds. In addition to aseptic processing areas, humidity should be monitored in all warehouses where raw materials and other components are stored. While humidity control in such areas is not required, humidity limits should be set so that raw materials and components sensitive to extremes in humidity can be moved out of the area or destroyed as necessary when unacceptable humidity levels are reached.

9.7.5 Gowning Qualification

In addition to routine personnel monitoring, personnel monitoring is an important component of the gowning qualification program. It is recommended that all personnel who gown to enter controlled manufacturing environments undergo gowning training and qualification, including environmental monitoring, to ensure that personnel gown properly and do not inadvertently introduce contaminants into the manufacturing environment [30].

9.7.6 Water Monitoring

Water and clean steam used in manufacturing facilities must also be routinely monitored. All components of water pretreatment and purification should also be monitored as part of a comprehensive water-monitoring program. Unlike other types of environmental monitoring, specifications have been established in the USP [31] for water that is used for pharmaceutical purposes. In addition, the potable feed water provided by municipalities to manufacturing facilities must meet 40 CFR Part 141, which sets forth the National Drinking Water Regulations [25] including maximum contaminant levels for organic and inorganic chemicals, turbidity, microorganisms, and coliform bacteria.

The USP [31] describes minimum requirements for PW, WFI, and Sterile Water for Injection. The two types of water

TABLE 9.2 Specifications for USP Purified Water and Water for Injection

Test	Suggested Minimum Testing Frequency	Specification
	Purified Water	
Total organic carbon	Weekly	500 ppb
Conductivity	Weekly	See USP 28 (specification is temperature dependent)
Bioburden	Weekly	100 CFU/ml
	Water for Injection	
Total organic carbon	Weekly	500 ppb
Conductivity	Weekly	See USP 28 (specification is temperature dependent)
Bioburden	System daily/each port weekly	10 CFU/100ml
Endotoxin	System daily/each port weekly	0.25 EU/ml

most commonly used in biotech and other pharmaceutical facilities are PW and WFI. Both PW and WFI have specifications for total organic carbon (TOC), conductivity, and microbial quality. In addition, WFI also has an endotoxin specification. Specifications for PW and WFI may be found in Table 9.2. For biotech products, PW may be used for initial cleaning of equipment and product contact surfaces, as well as for bacterial fermentation media preparation. WFI must be used for final rinsing of all equipment and other product contact surfaces, as well as for all other product manufacturing steps (for example, buffer preparation, mammalian cell culture media preparation).

While water specifications are clearly established, monitoring frequencies for water are not specified in regulations or guidance documents. However, monitoring frequencies for both PW and WFI systems have been well established by industry practice. Purified water systems are monitored not less than once monthly for TOC and conductivity and not less than weekly for microbial quality. Worst-case points on the system (usually those points furthest from the water purification systems) are usually chosen for sampling. Microbial monitoring samples are sometimes taken from various points on the water distribution system to ensure that there are no pockets of microbial contamination or biofilm formation in the system.

Monitoring of WFI systems is more rigorous. TOC and conductivity monitoring occurs not less than weekly, usually from worst-case locations. Microbial and endotoxin monitoring should be performed daily, rotating sampling points so that each point on the system is monitored at least weekly.

9.7.7 Data Management and Trending

Alert and action limits for contaminants should be established for each manufacturing area based on the nature of the operations that occur in the area, whether the steps are open or closed to the surrounding environment, and the ability of subsequent validated steps to remove microbial contaminants and endotoxin. It is important that alert limits be based on historical data obtained during actual controlled manufacturing conditions. Trend analysis of data should be performed to detect developing problems before they become detrimental to the safety or purity of the product. Action limits should also reflect historical data and, for critical and controlled manufacturing areas, should be set according to acceptable numbers of contaminants recommended for each air classification in accordance with the ISO standards [7,8].

Corrective actions should be established for implementation when action limits are exceeded. Corrective actions may also be warranted following several consecutive alert limit excursions. Environmental monitoring procedures should include instructions for documenting excursions, investigating and determining the root cause of excursions, and assessing the product impact. Identification of the contaminants, to the species level if possible, should be one of the first steps of the investigation. Investigations should also include a review of activities that took place during the time of the excursion, cleaning records, and data trends from the area where the excursion occurred as well as data from other adjacent areas and should take into account the possibility of sampling and testing errors. Based on the results of an investigation, corrective actions may include sanitization, retraining, maintenance, modification of cleaning and other procedures, requalification, or revalidation.

Although the causes of excursions cannot always be anticipated, corrective actions should be predetermined to the extent possible to ensure consistent and efficient resolution. Courses of action and resolution should include appropriate oversight and concurrence by the unit responsible for quality assurance. The quality assurance unit should always make the final determination as to whether an environmental monitoring excursion resulted in product impact. In fact, routine environmental monitoring results and any associated deviations and investigation reports should be easily correlated to batch production records and reviewed as part of the final batch record review and release to assess the impact of the environment on product safety and quality.

The environmental monitoring concepts and recommendations should be considered when developing a comprehensive facility monitoring program. They represent requirements dictated by regulations, FDA guidance recommendations, and industry standard practices. However, some aspects of the environmental monitoring program for a particular facility will also be unique based on facility and equipment design, the manufacturing process, and many other factors [30]. For example, many bulk and final process manufacturing steps can now be performed in systems that are validated to be completely closed to the outside environment. In such cases, a reduced amount of monitoring may be acceptable to the FDA if a company presents compelling data validating the integrity of their closed systems. Finally, probably the most important point to keep in mind while designing environmental monitoring programs and procedures is that environmental monitoring should provide useful product- and process-related data that help ensure the safety and purity of products.

9.8 MULTIPRODUCT CONSIDERATIONS

The emergence of biotech products ushered in the increased use of multiproduct manufacturing facilities [20,21,32]. It is rare to find a manufacturing facility that is dedicated to the production of a single product. Dedicated manufacturing facilities, however, are required for certain product types (e.g., penicillin, cephalosporin) [2] or if there is no reasonable method of cleaning to remove product residuals. While it is more cost-effective for a manufacturer to build a single facility capable of producing multiple products, these facilities bring a higher level of regulatory risk (Table 9.3). The FDA's primary concerns, for multiproduct facilities, are increased risk for product contamination, product cross-contamination, and product mix-ups. It becomes the manufacturer's challenge to design a facility that will prospectively eliminate or minimize these concerns.

9.8.1 Types of Multiproduct Facilities

There are two major categories that define a multiproduct facility (Table 9.4). Campaign manufacturing is the most common mode of operating a multiproduct facility. A single lot of product is manufactured at any one time in the facility. Products manufactured could include both approved and unapproved products. The facility would then be "changed over" for the next product type. For the most part, campaigning has included a single host type (e.g., CHO-derived products). Recently, manufacturers have expanded the concept to include multiple host types (e.g., both CHO-derived and *E. coli*-derived products). This type of scenario includes separate

TABLE 9.3 Regulatory Concerns Associated with Multiproduct Facilities

---

Cross-contamination between products

Contaminants/residuals introduced into the product, which are difficult to detect

Production of unapproved products in a licensed production facility

Workers alternating between two or more processes or products

TABLE 9.4   Categories of Multiproduct Facilities

Campaign Manufacturing

Production of a single product, derived from the same type of host cell,
  at any one time
Production of a single product, derived from different types of host cells,
  at any one time

Simultaneous Manufacturing

Production of two different products at the same time
Production of two lots of the same product (same stage of production) at
  the same time
Production of two lots of the same product (different stage of production)
  at the same time

manufacturing suites, with dedicated product equipment for
each host type. Sharing product contact equipment between
multiple host types has caused concern on the part of the
FDA. The FDA's major reservations for this type of manufacturing include adventitious agent issues (transfer from mammalian cell culture to microbial cell culture), endotoxin
residual issues (transfer from microbial cell culture to mammalian cell culture), viricidal capability of equipment cleaning
agents, and potential toxicity (i.e., virulence factors) associated with certain microbial strains. For the FDA to consider
this type of manufacturing arrangement, the manufacturer
will have to demonstrate full knowledge of adventitious
agents associated with the mammalian cell banks; effectiveness of viral inactivation/clearance steps; viricidal capability
of product contact cleaning agents (to inactivate potential
viruses associated with the specific mammalian cell culture);
effectiveness of the cleaning agents to remove residual endotoxin from product contact equipment; effectiveness of cleaning agents to inactivate toxic/virulence factors that may be
associated with microbial strains; and the presence of validated analytical methods capable of detecting these types of
residuals.

The second category of multiproduct facility operation is
the simultaneous mode. In this scenario, a manufacturer may
be producing two lots of the same product or two different

products at the same time. Generally, this scenario requires the use of closed systems (refer to Section 9.4). Also, any open product manipulations (e.g., sampling, seed inoculum transfer) must be limited to one lot of one product at a time. Simultaneous manufacturing is most often found in fermentation halls (i.e., operating multiple fermenter trains simultaneously) and occasionally in cell culture suites. In the latter scenario, only one product lot would be manipulated in an LAF at any given time. The LAF would be wiped down and all materials used for the manipulation would be cleared from the LAF before the next product lot would be placed in the LAF. Typically, there are multiple incubators to accommodate the different products in the cell culture suites.

9.8.2 Design Considerations

Good facility design is instrumental in achieving the appropriate level of segregation required to operate a multiproduct facility. When designing a facility, the manufacturer should consider the potential for interactions between personnel, product, equipment, and the environment. Good design will allow the following:

- Separation of function
- Separation of different products or different lots of the same product
- Flow patterns that will prevent mix-ups
- Sufficient space for all operations to be performed
- Sufficient space for storage of equipment/components not in use
- Easily cleanable and maintainable walls, floors, and work surfaces
- Separate air-handling systems (where appropriate) to prevent cross-contamination
- Appropriate validation of processes/procedures (e.g., cleaning), systems (e.g., HVAC), and equipment (e.g., fermenters)

While simplistic in nature, the aforementioned elements require careful planning on the part of the manufacturer. The first (and most important) question a manufacturer must answer before these elements can be addressed is, "What type of products will be manufactured in this facility?" In many instances, manufacturers attempt to design a facility without carefully considering the types of products that one could produce in the facility. Also, no single facility can produce all types of products.

Design criteria (particularly for simultaneous production) should ensure sufficient space to allow for separation of functions and products. If physical separation is not achieved through design, then the manufacturer must rely on operational controls. Controls of this nature rely heavily upon operator training, clear labeling, and precise scheduling. The concept of separation can be extended to support areas, too. For example, a facility with a single component/equipment preparation area may operate on a campaign basis to ensure that components/equipment from one product are cleaned in separate loads. This should reduce the chance of mix-ups. Prevention of mix-ups in media and buffer preparation areas is critical, too. In cases where a single area/equipment is used for both media and buffer preparation (particularly if animal-derived components are used in media preparation), the manufacturer will be challenged to ensure that the cleaning procedures are capable of removing residuals.

A second concern with regard to space is storage. When equipment is not in use, it should be stored properly. Corridors and material transfer airlocks are not acceptable places for the storage of equipment. In addition, staging areas should be sized sufficiently to hold equipment that needs to be cleaned or to store media/buffers that will be used in production. Again, the more activity in a facility, the greater the chance for mix-ups.

In addition to space, flow patterns and air-handling systems are used to ensure proper separation. The most direct way to ensure separation via flow is to design a two-corridor system with one-way flow. There should be a clean corridor for entry into the manufacturing areas with a return corridor for movement of personnel and equipment out of the manufacturing areas. This is the "gold standard" for flow patterns within a multiproduct facility. One-way flow, however, may not (in all cases) be the most practical. If a single-corridor system is designed for the facility, then the manufacturer should employ the appropriate operational controls to prevent cross-contamination and mix-ups. Manufacturing suite entry gown rooms may be necessary to ensure adequate separation between employees (particularly for those involved with open product manipulations).

Separation through air systems (refer to Section 9.5) can be achieved through the use of once-through air or the use of multiple air handlers with recirculation of air within the room. Recirculation of filtered air in a multiproduct facility is not recommended. The potential for cross-contamination exists, and proving that cross-contamination will not occur with this type of system is extremely difficult. Also, the efficiency of operation could be affected with this type of a system. For example, if two cell culture suites are being supplied by a recirculating system, it is possible that only one suite at a time may be used for open manipulations of product. Pressure cascades are important in these facilities from a product protection standpoint. The extent of the cascade should be taken into consideration during the design phase. Again, defining prospectively the types of products and processes that will be introduced into the facility will assist in determining the required level of environmental cleanliness.

9.8.3 Product Changeover Procedures

The product changeover (PCO) standard operating procedure is a staple in all multiproduct facilities. The extent of the PCO is dependent on the type and number of shared pieces of equipment within the manufacturing suite. Typically, the following items are found in a PCO:

- Removal of all product (including intermediates), process materials (including media, buffers, raw materials), and disposable equipment from the processing area that will not be used for the next product.
- Equipment that is dedicated to single product (e.g., chromatography resins) is adequately identified,

cleaned, and removed from the area to a proper storage location.

- Equipment that is shared between products is cleaned using validated cleaning procedures. In many cases, all soft parts are removed and replaced prior to introducing the next product. Either rinse water or swab samples are taken and analyzed for residual product and cleaning agent.
- Facility cleaning (see Section 9.6), which may include walls and certain work surfaces such as the interior of incubators, is performed prior to introducing the next product.

The process of PCO is documented (most manufacturers use a checklist approach) by manufacturing. PCO, however, is not complete until Quality Assurance reviews the area, the documentation, and the residual test results and approves the area/equipment ready for production of the next product.

9.8.4 Cleaning Validation

Clean equipment is a requirement of the cGMP regulations [2]. The intent of this regulation is to prevent contamination or adulteration of drug products. The increased use of multi-product facilities heightened the FDA's concern with regard to contamination and cross-contamination of products through the use of shared equipment. The FDA issued a series of inspectional guidance documents with direction to agency inspectors on evaluating cleaning validation [22,33–35]. In addition, the ICH cGMP guidance document for API manufacturers [5] contains a section on cleaning validation. One of the most comprehensive sources on cleaning validation issues associated with biotech products is the Parenteral Drug Association's (PDA) technical document on cleaning and cleaning validation [36].

Clearly, this concept of clean equipment and the ability to validate the cleaning processes is critical in ensuring a safe product. Of all the requirements a manufacturer must meet to gain approval for a multiproduct facility, a successful cleaning validation program is the most important in receiving

TABLE 9.5 Goals of a Cleaning Validation Program

Minimize bioburden and endotoxin levels
Ensure product purity
Prevent cross-contamination of products
Adequate removal of product and cleaning agents
Assays capable of monitoring the effectiveness of the cleaning procedures

FDA approval. In addition to establishing procedures for cleaning equipment, the manufacturer must develop and validate procedures for cleaning the facility. Facility cleaning issues were discussed in Section 9.6.

9.8.4.1 Goals of a Cleaning Validation

The goals of cleaning validation are summarized in Table 9.5. In essence, the manufacturer should ensure that the cleaning process is both consistent and effective. Consistency is determined by evaluating the system used to clean the equipment. Typically, the manufacturer performs an installation qualification (IQ) and an operational qualification (OQ) to verify a repeatable system performance. A list of potential validation parameters is presented in Table 9.6. Measuring the removal of both the cleaning agent and the product assesses cleaning effectiveness. When designing a protocol for evaluating effectiveness, the manufacturer should take into consideration the stage of production, equipment design, method of cleaning,

TABLE 9.6 Potential Cleaning Process
Validation Parameters

Wash and rinse volumes
Water temperature
Water quality
Flow rate and pressure
Time and sequence of steps
Time elapsed prior to cleaning
Agitation rate
Coverage of the system/equipment being cleaned
Concentration of the cleaning agent

the analytical methods that will be used to detect residues, and appropriate acceptance criteria. Residues for both the cleaning agent and the product must meet predetermined acceptance criteria.

9.8.4.1.1 Stage of Production

The major stages of production for a biotech product include cell culture/fermentation, harvesting, and purification. The residuals from each of these stages will be different and, therefore, should be taken into account when developing the cleaning validation protocol [36]. As an example, fermentation residuals can include the recombinant cells and their metabolic by-products, media components, other nutrients such as glucose feeds, antifoam, and cleaning agents (e.g., detergents, acids). The manufacturer should determine which of these residuals will have the greatest impact on the subsequent product lot in terms of cell growth/metabolism and downstream operations. If the downstream operations have been validated to remove process contaminants such as host cell proteins/residual DNA, then these components may be less of a concern. Generally, it is difficult to perform specific product residual testing on samples from a fermenter. It is more typical to assess for overall cleanliness using a general but sensitive assay such as total protein or TOC (Table 9.7) [37,38]. Conductivity and pH are used to assess for removal of the cleaning agents.

For the purification stage, the potential contaminant is the product. With most of today's processes, the first step in purification clears a large percentage of the process contaminants from the fermentation stage. As the process moves forward, the type and concentration of process contaminants decrease while the purity and yield of the product increase. It is standard practice to assess for residuals using product-specific assays (Table 9.7). Conductivity and pH, as with fermentation samples, are used to assess for removal of cleaning agents.

TABLE 9.7 Examples of Analytical Methods Used to Detect Product and Cleaning Agent Residuals

Method	Advantage	Disadvantage
HPLC	Very specific; moderate to high sensitivity; quantitative	Expensive
TOC	Broad spectrum; low-level detection; on-line capability; rapid turnaround; quantitative	Nonspecific; aqueous-soluble samples only
EIA/SDS-PAGE	Specific for biologicals; very sensitive	Long turnaround time; labor intensive; problems with denatured proteins
pH/Conductivity	Rapid; inexpensive; on-line capability; quantitative	Nonspecific; limited sensitivity
Visual inspection	Immediate results; good for general screening	Not quantitative; subjective

9.8.4.1.2 Equipment Design

The equipment design has a large impact on the type of sample one can take during cleaning validation. Equipment size, configuration, and materials of construction are important in determining where and how a piece of equipment will be sampled during the validation study [36]. Manufacturers should strive to include visual examination, swab samples, and rinse water samples in the cleaning validation study. Spray pattern studies can determine sites that may be difficult to reach with cleaning agents. Tops of tanks, sight glasses, and soft parts are often considered worst-case scenarios for sampling because of their location or their porosity. In one study, cleaning of the sight glass was not achieved via CIP methods [39]. A manual cleaning procedure had to be developed (and validated) for the sight glass.

A more recent consideration for multiproduct facilities is the use of disposable bags. Many manufacturers have implemented the use of bags for storage of media, buffers, and product intermediates. The use of bags has minimized the need for cleaning validation for many manufacturers. The FDA, however, does require compatibility studies and container/closure studies [9–16] for bags used in the manufacturing process.

9.8.4.1.3   Method of Cleaning

CIP systems are most commonly used to clean larger, fixed pieces of equipment. These systems may be easier to validate and to ensure consistency of operation because they are automated and they eliminate the human factor. Table 9.6 identifies numerous parameters that should be taken into consideration when validating a CIP system. The most critical of these parameters are time, temperature, flow rate, concentration of the cleaning agent, and surface contact time of the cleaning solution [36]. Generally, these parameters are evaluated during the system OQ.

Manual cleaning methods are also used in multiproduct facilities. These methods are more difficult to validate because of the human factor. The difficulty lies in the ability to demonstrate consistency in the manual cleaning process from operator to operator. The validation study should include multiple operators cleaning the same equipment by the same procedure. Manual cleaning validation requires a rigorous training program and periodic verification of the operators to ensure that the cleaning procedure continues to be effective and consistent.

9.8.4.1.4   Analytical Methods

As listed in Table 9.7, there are various methods used to detect cleaning agents and product residuals. The FDA does not mandate the use of any one method. The requirements the FDA imposes on manufacturers include the following [5,33]:

- That the method can be validated
- That the method is quantifiable

- That the specificity and sensitivity of the method are relevant to the stage in production from which the sample was taken
- That the analytical method in combination with the sampling method has been challenged to demonstrate that residuals can be recovered from the surface

These four criteria should be taken into consideration when choosing a method for detection of residuals.

9.8.4.1.5   Acceptance Criteria

Without a doubt, establishing predetermined acceptance criteria for a cleaning validation protocol is the most difficult aspect of developing the protocol. Again, the FDA does not impose acceptance criteria but provides guidance [5,33]. The FDA indicates that it is impractical for them to set criteria due to the variety of products and processes. Instead, they ask the manufacturer, based on the manufacturer's specific knowledge of the product and the process, to set acceptance criteria that are "practical, achievable, and verifiable" [33]. The rationale for the acceptance criteria is the responsibility of the manufacturer.

9.8.4.2 Common Inspectional Pitfalls

FDA inspectors are instructed to review cleaning validation protocols and final reports during preapproval and regular biennial inspections [33]. The following is a list of common 483 observations directed to the cleaning validation program:

- Analytical methods used to measure product residuals were not validated.
- Cleaning validation for the worst-case products is inconclusive in that swab recovery studies had not been performed.
- Cleaning procedures were not validated for the removal of both the cleaning agent and the residual product.

- Rinse solutions were not analyzed for the active ingredient during the cleaning validation of formulation tank.
- Cleaning validation was incomplete in that the minimal drug substance residue level was not determined.
- Test method validation for cleaning validation studies did not include determination for the limit of detection.
- Cleaning validation protocol did not specify the responsibility for performing and approving the study.
- Cleaning validation did not account for hold times for equipment prior to cleaning or for hold times of equipment following cleaning.
- Cleaning validation protocol did not address the requirement for revalidation.
- Spray ball pattern studies were not done as part of the cleaning validation for the production fermenter.

9.8.5 Introduction of New Products into a Multiproduct Facility

With the elimination of the requirement for the Establishment License Application [40] came a reduction in preapproval supplement reporting requirements with regard to changes to a manufacturing facility. One change that may still require a preapproval supplement is changing a manufacturing facility from a dedicated product facility to a multiproduct facility [41]. A reduction in reporting requirement can be achieved through establishing a policy for the introduction of new products into a multiproduct facility (assuming a manufacturer has requested and received approval to operate a multiproduct facility) and receiving approval from the FDA on this policy. From the FDA's perspective, the approved product in a multiproduct facility will take priority over clinical and toxicology product lots made in the same facility (specifically using shared equipment). Essentially, this means that all other products will be required to meet the same standard as an approved product. The following items should be considered when developing a policy to evaluate introducing new products into a multiproduct facility:

- Safety is the primary concern. Only fully qualified (mammalian and microbial) cell lines [42,43] should be introduced into the facility. Cell lines with bacterial, fungal, or mycoplasma contamination should not be allowed into the facility. Cell lines that harbor a virus that cannot be removed or inactivated by the production process and by the established equipment cleaning and sterilization methods should not be allowed into the facility. Potential pathogenicity (associated virulence factors) and toxicity should be evaluated for new microbial hosts. Host/toxin inactivation methods should be a part of the safety evaluation.

- The safety profile of the new product should be considered during the evaluation. Information on effective dose, pharmacology, and potential allergic or anaphylactic reactions should be included in the review.

- The ability to clean your shared equipment using your current approved cleaning methods is critical to this evaluation. A major change to your approved cleaning methods could constitute a preapproval supplement. Part of the cleaning evaluation should be assessing the potential for carryover of host/product residuals and determining whether you have the analytical methods to test for the new host/product residuals.

- The capacity to store dedicated product contact equipment should be considered during this evaluation.

- The design of the facility should be considered when introducing a new product. Does the product "fit" into the design/operational plan for the facility? Will it be necessary to change approved flow patterns to accommodate the new product?

- Raw materials used in the manufacture of the new product must meet the established quality requirements of those used in the production of the approved products.

- New products may require new documentation (certainly, a new batch record) and additional training for the staff.

- Any new equipment that may be required for the new product should meet the minimum standards of an IQ/OQ and appropriate calibration and preventive maintenance schedules. Even though the new product may not be approved, the manufacturing is occurring in an approved facility. Consequently, GMP compliance is necessary.

Individuals who are typically involved in this type of an evaluation include quality, manufacturing, development, and regulatory personnel.

9.9 CONTRACT MANUFACTURING

By definition, contract manufacturing denotes a situation in which a potential license applicant contracts with one or more separate manufacturing entities to perform a part of or all of the manufacturing steps, as a paid service, for the potential license holder. Prior to May 14, 1996, contract manufacturing (for biological products) included only those manufacturing activities that did not warrant a license (e.g., sterile filling) [44]. Contract manufacturers performing manufacturing steps such as fermentation/harvest and purification were required to hold a separate license. The FDA considered steps of this nature to be critical and capable of impacting the product structure and specificity. This policy meant that companies who were product innovators but did not have the capability to manufacture their own products could not hold a license. The Federal Register Notice (61 FR 24227) of May 14, 1996 [40], changed the FDA's policy on contract manufacturing and broadened its scope. This notice included a change in the definition of *manufacturer* to include "any legal person or entity who is an applicant for a license where the applicant assumes responsibility for compliance with applicable product and establishment standards" [45]. By broadening the definition of manufacturer, the FDA agreed that a license applicant who did not own the manufacturing facility performing critical manufacturing steps could hold the license. This also eliminated the requirement for each contract manufacturing facility performing critical operations to hold a separate license. Contract manufacturers must, however, continue to register with the FDA per the registration and listing provisions in the CFR, Title 21 Parts 207 and 607 [46].

9.9.1 Regulatory Issues

The change in definition of manufacturer expanded the use of contract manufacturing by companies desiring to produce biological products. In addition, there was a shift in regulatory responsibilities. Responsibility for ensuring compliance and disclosure of confidential information, as part of a license application, were affected by the change in definition of manufacturer.

9.9.1.1 Compliance Issues

Even though the contract manufacturer is responsible for compliance under the Food, Drug, and Cosmetic Act (FD&C Act, 21 USC 301) [47], the license holder (or client) assumes responsibility for compliance with the applicable regulations and standards. The license holder must be able to ensure that his product meets the provisions as stated in his license application and is manufactured in accordance with cGMP regulations [48]. Essentially, this means the license holder must have access to pertinent facility and operational information. Information deemed critical includes (but is not limited to) the following:

- Floor plans (including flow patterns and placement of equipment)
- Equipment validation
- Utilities/systems validation
- Calibration and preventive maintenance programs
- Multiproduct policies (product changeover procedures, cleaning procedures, policies for introducing new cell lines or products into the facility)
- GMP training program
- Quality systems

There are several approaches used to ensure compliance and to ensure access to critical information. These include periodic audits, "person in the plant," and the Quality Agreement. Typically, all three are used in a contract manufacturing arrangement.

9.9.1.1.1 Periodic Audits

Auditing, by the license holder, can be an extremely useful tool in determining the capability of the contract manufacturer to produce the product and the contract manufacturer's level of compliance. The license holder should, at a minimum, review the following areas:

- Facilities and equipment (overall appearance and cleanliness; status of equipment/utilities/systems with regard to validation, calibration, and preventive maintenance; facility design with regard to prevention of contamination and cross-contamination)
- Quality unit and systems (independent reporting structure; critical quality systems established such as change control, deviation management, and failure investigations; established auditing programs, including the ability to manage inspections by the FDA and other regulatory agencies)
- Document control (procedures for establishing, revising, and issuing SOPs and batch records; procedures for batch record review; access-controlled areas for storage of documents)
- Personnel (adequate staff in terms of expertise and numbers; established GMP and on-the-job training programs)
- Regulatory (overall expertise and level of experience with the FDA and other regulatory agencies)

It is in the license holder's best interest to be on site during key stages of the contract manufacturing arrangement. These include, but are not limited to, the following:

- Initial technology transfer to the contract manufacturer
- Manufacture of "shake down" lots

- Process validation
- Manufacture of lots to support the license application
- Preapproval inspection

Typically, the number of site visits will diminish as confidence in both the ability to manufacture the product and the ability to maintain an adequate level of compliance is achieved by the contract manufacturer. At a minimum, the license holder should perform an annual audit of the contract manufacturer to ensure an adequate level of compliance [5,48]. Compliance actions can be initiated against both the license holder and the contract manufacturer for failure of the contract manufacturer to adhere to the requirements of the license or for failure to comply with the cGMP regulations.

9.9.1.1.2 *"Person in the Plant"*

The "person in the plant" is an employee of the license holder who is on site at the contract manufacturing location. This individual may be present during all or some of the manufacturing activities. Having an employee on site can be beneficial for both parties, particularly if the manufacturing process is complex or if there is a large geographical distance between the license holder and the contract manufacturer. To be effective, the "person in the plant" must understand the manufacturing process and should be able to assist in making decisions that could impact the quality of the product. In addition, this individual can participate in review of associated documentation (e.g., deviation reports and batch records).

9.9.1.1.3 *Quality Agreements*

Quality agreements have become the cornerstone of contract manufacturing arrangements. This agreement documents the roles and responsibilities of the license holder and the contract manufacturer [49]. This document can be requested during the FDA's review of the license application or during the FDA's inspection. For these reasons, it is recommended to separate the quality agreement from the contractual details of the business arrangement between the two companies.

The content of the quality agreement may vary between companies. In general, the following roles and responsibilities are defined in the document:

- A general statement of work including manufacturing site location and the responsibilities of each party
- Type of documentation to be issued at the completion of manufacture, including review time for the batch record by the contract manufacturer and documentation audit provisions for the license holder
- Record retention requirements
- Sample retention requirements (including storage locations)
- Training specifications
- Raw material supply (including vendor audits and raw material certification [50])
- Planned and unplanned deviation management (including specified time for notification to the license holder)
- Validation activities specific to the license holder's product (including review and approval of validation protocols and reports)
- Validation activities specific to the manufacturing facility (including assurance from the contract manufacturer to maintain the facility and equipment in a validated state)
- Inspections by regulatory agencies
- Periodic audits by the license holder (compliance assessment)
- Notification of changes that could impact the approved license (including sufficient time for the license holder to notify the FDA of the impending change [51])
- Product release responsibilities
- Product specifications
- Product shipping requirements

Signatures on this document include representatives of both companies from their respective quality, manufacturing, and regulatory organizations. These agreements should be revisited on a periodic basis to ensure that the roles and responsibilities have not changed and that both companies are meeting the current compliance standards.

9.9.1.2 Confidentiality Issues

The second regulatory area affected by the change in definition of manufacturer is the issue of introducing information into a license application without breaching confidentiality. This was not an issue prior to May 14, 1996, because manufacturers who performed critical steps in production were required to file a separate license application. Proprietary information was maintained in these license applications. To assist in this matter, the FDA has recommended the use of Type V Master Files [52] as a vehicle for submission of proprietary information. The FDA suggests that information such as a listing of all products manufactured in the facility and a listing of noncompendial test procedures be filed in a Type V Master File. The license holder, however, must have sufficient information from the contract manufacturer to make informed decisions on the adequacy of the product changeover and cleaning validation programs. Both the license holder and the contract manufacturer are responsible for the quality of the product (per the requirements of the license).

9.10 FACILITY INSPECTIONS

9.10.1 History and Statutory Requirements for Facility Inspections

Section 704 of the FD&C Act [53] sets forth the FDA's statutory authority to conduct inspections of any factory, warehouse, or establishment where food, drugs, devices, or cosmetics are manufactured, processed, packed, or held. In addition, Section 351 of the Public Health Service (PHS) Act [54] requires the FDA to conduct inspections of establishments for the propagation or manufacture and preparation of biological products prior to the issuance of a license.

Over the past 10 years, FDA inspections for biological products, including those for biological products produced by biotechnology, have undergone dramatic changes prompted by both reorganizations within the FDA as well as by a number of regulatory initiatives [55]. Prior to this, virtually all biologics inspections were performed by CBER personnel and were primarily focused on the scientific principles supporting the manufacturing process and the resulting product. Regulatory initiatives, perhaps beginning with a CBER reorganization that took place in January 1993, have resulted in inspections that remain scientifically based with a renewed emphasis on the application of GMPs in the evaluation of all manufacturing and testing operations.

Regulatory initiatives, beginning with the Elimination of the ELA Rule in 1996 [40], followed by the rollout of the BLA for all biological products [9–16], completed in 1999, further aligned the mechanisms for ensuring GMP compliance for drugs and biologics. In 1997, a major FDA compliance initiative [56] was launched. A cadre of FDA investigators, known as Team Biologics, was trained and assembled to begin leading routine biologics inspections under the direction of the FDA's Office of Regulatory Affairs (ORA) to further align biologics inspections with other FDA inspections, which are managed by ORA.

Finally, in 2002, the FDA decided to consolidate the reviews of certain therapeutic products. On September 6, 2002, the FDA announced that responsibility for reviewing new biological drugs, other than those for vaccines, blood, tissues, gene therapy, and related products, would be transferred from CBER to CDER [19]. The product categories transferred from CBER to CDER include monoclonal antibodies; cytokines, growth factors, enzymes, and interferons (including recombinant versions); proteins intended for therapeutic use that are extracted from animals or microorganisms; and therapeutic immunotherapies. The intent of this initiative is to improve consistency between the regulation of these categories of products and other, similar products already regulated by CDER. CBER remains primarily responsible for CBER's public health responsibilities, namely, the regulation of vaccines and ensuring the safety of the nation's blood supply. The impact of these recent changes on the inspection program cannot yet be assessed, but the focus of these inspections is likely to remain on compliance with the cGMP regulations [2] to ensure the consistent production of products that meet all of their quality attributes of safety, purity, potency, and efficacy.

Finally, another FDA initiative that may help shape the future of inspections is the introduction of systems-based inspections for pharmaceutical GMP inspections [57]. A similar quality-systems-based inspection program was implemented by the Center for Devices and Radiological Health several years ago. While the current initiative does not formally include biologics inspections, inspectors of biological products are already including systems-based reviews in their product inspections [55].

The systems-based approach focuses on the adequacy of the systems in place to prevent and resolve problems. Investigators first evaluate a firm's quality system and at least one of five other major GMP systems including facilities and equipment, materials, production, packaging and labeling, and laboratory control [57].

The benefits of the new inspection approach are anticipated to include increased efficiency, enhanced communications, and clarified enforcement processes. Enhanced communications are expected to result from the clearer organization of the inspection findings and their broader applicability to the overall GMP status of the firm, so that the enforcement process becomes more transparent [57].

9.10.2 Current Focus of Inspections

The issues on which FDA investigators tend to focus a great deal of attention may be predicted by their recent compliance history. The preamble of the proposed revision to the cGMP regulations, published in 1996 (61 FR 20103), summarizes the FDA's current thinking. This summary articulates the FDA's current expectations with regard to GMP compliance. The proposed revisions, which were prompted by the FDA's regulatory and enforcement activities, indicated a lack of understanding among some manufacturers with respect to certain cGMP regulations [58]. The proposed revisions primarily address deficiencies in the areas of process validation, analytical methods validation, contamination/cross-contamination, and testing. The FDA also emphasizes the importance of the quality assurance functions of the quality control unit in ensuring GMP compliance. For example, the FDA suggests that the quality control unit be responsible for ensuring that validation procedures are current and for reviewing changes and determining when revalidation is necessary.

Current areas of concern that have the greatest impact on facilities and facility design include process validation, contamination and cross-contamination issues, and quality assurance oversight. Common FDA citations that relate to facilities are described in the following sections.

9.10.2.1 Process Validation

The FDA's recent compliance history includes numerous citations related to process validation. The following commonly noted observations provide some insight into the FDA's expectations: failure to validate all manufacturing operations including qualification of all processing equipment; failure to validate changes in manufacturing operations including all related equipment and utility changes; failure to justify deviations that occurred during validation or qualification activities; failure to establish all appropriate specifications and acceptance criteria in validation and qualification protocols prior to initiating validation; and failure to incorporate worst-case and challenge conditions in validation and qualification protocols for products, equipment, and utilities [55].

Process validation is considered to be the cornerstone of ensuring consistent product quality, but FDA investigators continue to find firms that have failed to validate or revalidate their processes, equipment, and systems.

9.10.2.2 Contamination and Cross-Contamination

Contamination has always been a concern for biological products. The cGMP regulations [2] address the control and prevention of contamination. Prevention of contamination and cross-contamination remains a focus of FDA regulatory and compliance activities. With the increased number of multiproduct facilities as well as increased use of contract manufacturing, the potential sources of contamination and cross-contamination have increased dramatically [55]. Potential contaminants include product and cleaning residuals (from multiproduct equipment, for example) and unknown adventitious contaminants introduced from other products. In addition to these contamination sources, other sources of product contamination may include contaminants removed in an earlier manufacturing step or adventitious contaminants from starting materials of human or animal origin [55].

Procedures and controls in place to prevent contamination and cross-contamination are closely evaluated by investigators and may include (but are not limited to) the following: process validation of manufacturing steps for the removal or inactivation of adventitious agents; validation of cleaning procedures for removal of product and cleaning agent residuals; validation of column sanitization procedures for removal of column contaminants; qualification and certification of HVAC systems, air pressure differentials between areas, and the environmental monitoring program including some representative data; facility cleaning and changeover procedures between products, as applicable; facility and equipment cleaning and usage documentation procedures (cleaning and usage logs); disinfectant effectiveness studies; gowning procedures and personnel training programs; flow patterns for personnel, product, materials, and waste throughout the facility; and labeling and segregation procedures [55].

9.10.2.3 Quality Assurance Functions

Again, due to the FDA's recent compliance history and the fact that a large number of FDA observations stem from inadequacies in one or more quality control or quality assurance functions, the proposed cGMP regulations [58] emphasize the importance of the quality control unit. The quality control unit is charged with quality assurance responsibilities including change control and oversight of validation procedures.

Some of the quality assurance programs and responsibilities likely to be reviewed by investigators are described as follows. Change control procedures are required to include adequate oversight to ensure that requalification or revalidation is performed as necessary and to ensure that the FDA is notified of changes as necessary in accordance with the regulations [51,59].

Deviation reporting and investigation procedures are required, including evaluation of corrective actions to ensure their effectiveness in preventing deviations and failures from recurring. Investigators often request a history of all investigations that have been initiated within a particular time period, determine whether investigations are completed within a reasonable time frame, and choose specific investigations for review. Investigators will expect a procedure for error and accident reporting to be in place that specifies the criteria used to determine which errors and accidents should be reported to the FDA.

Document review and document control procedures must be in place, including procedures for review of batch records, test records, validation protocols and reports, and all other manufacturing and testing documentation. Document control procedures refer to those procedures used to create and review new documents, make revisions to existing documents, approve new and revised documents, and implement new and revised procedures, including documented training of personnel [55].

The aforementioned five areas certainly represent areas of focus for FDA investigators, but inspections are usually quite comprehensive and cover a myriad of other topics. The scope of regular biennial and preapproval biologics inspections generally includes the following: observation of manufacturing operations; inspection of all warehousing, manufacturing, labeling, packaging, testing, storage, and support facilities; review of all production and process controls and process and methods validation; review of inspection of plant systems and utilities, including supportive qualification, validation, maintenance, and routine monitoring data; aseptic processing validation; and review of the GMP training program and assessment of its effectiveness [55].

In addition to the examples of common observations presented here, other sources of information that may be useful in understanding the FDA's current compliance concerns are the FDA-483s issued to the industry. These documents list the observations made by FDA investigators during inspections. They are available upon request in accordance with the Freedom of Information (FOI) Act [60]. Warning letters, which are issued when FDA-483 observations warrant official FDA action, are also available. These are published on the FDA's Web site and do not require FOI requests.

In summary, many FDA regulatory and compliance initiatives have shaped the current face of the FDA inspection. The scope of an inspection is generally comprehensive and may take several weeks to complete. Although the list of possible areas of review is exhaustive, the FDA is looking for a few basic principles to be present throughout the manufacturing and testing operations: validation; control of the manufacturing process, including contamination control and control of the manufacturing environments; and quality assurance oversight of all manufacturing, testing, and validation activities.

9.11 SUMMARY

While facility design has evolved, the basic regulatory principles governing design criteria remain the same. The FDA continues to require that manufacturers design facilities to prevent adverse impact on the predefined quality of the products manufactured within the facility. Despite certain regulatory and compliance initiatives or changes to the regulations, the bottom line for facility design criteria remains the prevention of contamination and cross-contamination.

REFERENCES

1. Code of Federal Regulations, Title 21, Part 600, Subpart B.

2. Code of Federal Regulations, Title 21, Parts 210 and 211.

3. Guideline on Sterile Drug Products Produced by Aseptic Processing, Center for Drugs and Biologics, June 1987.

4. NIH Guidelines for Research Involving Recombinant DNA Molecules, Appendix K, Physical Containment for Large Scale Uses of Organisms Containing Recombinant DNA Molecules, April 2002.

5. Guidance for Industry Q7a Good Manufacturing Practice Guidance for Active Pharmaceutical Ingredients, Center for Drug Evaluation and Research, Center for Biologics Evaluation and Research, ICH, August 2001.

6. Sterile Manufacturing Facilities Baseline® Guide, Volume 3, ISPE, January 1999.

7. Cleanrooms and associated controlled environments — Part 1: Classification of air cleanliness, ISO 14644-1, ISO, May 1, 1999.

8. Cleanrooms and associated controlled environments — Part 2: Specifications for testing and monitoring to prove continued compliance with ISO 14644-1, ISO 14644-2, ISO, September 15, 2000.

9. Guidance for Industry: Content and Format of Chemistry, Manufacturing and Controls Information for Recombinant DNA-Derived Products or a Monoclonal Antibody Product for *in vivo* Use, Center for Biologics Evaluation and Research, August 1996.

10. Guidance for the Submission of Chemistry, Manufacturing and Controls Information and Establishment Description for Autologous Somatic Cell Therapy, Center for Biologics Evaluation and Research, January 1997.

11. Guidance for Industry: For the Submission of Chemistry, Manufacturing and Controls Information and Establishment Description Information for Human Plasma-Derived Biological Products, Animal Plasma or Serum-Derived Products, Center for Biologics Evaluation and Research, February 1999.

12. Guidance for Industry for the Submission of Chemistry, Manufacturing and Controls Information for Synthetic Peptide Substances, Center for Biologics Evaluation and Research, 1994.

13. Guidance for Industry for the Submission of Chemistry, Manufacturing and Controls and Establishment Description Information for Human Blood and Blood Components Intended for Transfusion for Further Manufacture and for the Completion of Form 356h, Application to Market a New Drug, Biologic or Antibiotic Drug for Human Use, Center for Biologics Evaluation and Research, May 1999.

14. Guidance for Industry: Content and Format of Chemistry, Manufacturing and Controls Information and Establishment Description Information for Allergenic Extract or Allergen Patch Test, Center for Biologics Evaluation and Research, April 1999.

15. Guidance for Industry: Content and Format of Chemistry, Manufacturing and Controls Information and Establishment Description Information for a Biological *in vitro* Diagnostic Product, Center for Biologics Evaluation and Research, March 1999.

16. Guidance for Industry for the Submission of Chemistry, Manufacturing and Controls Information and Establishment Description Information for a Vaccine or Related Product, Center for Biologics Evaluation and Research, January 1999.

17. Guidance for Industry for the Submission Documentation for Sterilization Process Validation in Applications for Human and Veterinary Drug Products, Center for Drug Evaluation and Research, Center for Veterinary Medicine, November 1994.

18. Guidance for Industry: Sterile Drug Products Produced by Aseptic Processing — Current Good Manufacturing Practice, Center for Biologics Evaluation and Research, Center for Drug Evaluation and Research, September 2002.

19. FDA Consolidation of Review of Certain Therapeutic Products, Food and Drug Administration, September 2002.

20. Hill, D. and Beatrice, M., Facility requirements for biotech plants, *Pharm. Eng.*, 9, 35–41, 1989.

21. Devine, R.A., Licensing biotechnology facilities, in *Regulatory Practice for Biopharmaceutical Production*, Lubiniecki, A.S. and Vargo, S.A., Eds., Wiley-Liss, New York, 1994, pp. 357–381.

22. FDA, Therapeutic Products, Inspections of Licensed Therapeutic Drug Products, Program 7341.001, Compliance Program Guidance Manual, chap. 41, October 1, 1998.

23. Recombinant DNA Research; Actions Under Guidelines; Notices, *Federal Register*, 56 (138), July 18, 1991.

24. Roscioli, N.A., Scott, A.M., and Beatrice, M.G., Water systems for biotechnology facilities, in *Regulatory Practice for Biopharmaceutical Production*, Lubiniecki, A.S. and Vargo, S.A., Eds., Wiley-Liss, New York, 1994, pp. 383–405.

25. Code of Federal Regulations, Title 40, Part 141, National Drinking Water Regulations.

26. Parenteral Drug Association Design Concepts for the Validation of a Water for Injection System Technical Report Number 4.

27. Meyrick, C.E., Practical design of a high purity water system, *Pharm. Eng.*, 9, 20–27, 1989.

28. Materials, Surfaces, Finishes and Components for Sanitary Applications, Pharmaceutical Manufacturers Association Water Seminar, Atlanta, GA, 1982.

29. del Valle, M.A., HVAC systems for biopharmaceutical manufacturing plants, *BioPharm*, 2, 28–42, 1989.

30. Roscioli, N.A., Renshaw, C.A., Gilbert, A.A., Kerry, C.F., and Probst, P.G., Environmental monitoring considerations for biological manufacturing, *BioPharm*, 9, 32–40, 1996.

31. The United States Pharmacopoeia, 28th rev., 2005.

32. Bader, F.G., Blum, A., Garfinkle, B.D., MacFarland, D., Massa, T., and Copmann, T.L., Multiuse manufacturing facilities for biologicals, *BioPharm*, 5, 34–42, 1992.

33. Guide to Inspections of Validation of Cleaning Processes, Division of Field Investigations, Office of Regional Operations, Office of Regulatory Affairs, FDA, July 1993.

34. FDA, Blood and Blood Products, Inspection of Plasma Derivatives of Human Origin, Program 7342.006, Compliance Program Guidance Manual, chap. 42.

35. FDA, Vaccines and Allergenic Products, Inspections of Licensed Vaccines, Program 7345.002, Compliance Program Guidance Manual, chap. 45, October 1, 1999.

36. Brunkow, R., DeLucia, D., Green, G., Haft, S., Hyde, J., Lindsay, J., Myers, J., Murphy, R., McEntire, J., Nichols, K., Prasad, R., Terranova, B., Voss, J., Weil, C., and White, E., Cleaning and Cleaning Validation: A Biotechnology Perspective, PDA Technical Document, 1995.

37. Baffi, R., Dolch, G., Garnick, R., Mar, B., Matsuhiro, D., Niepelt, B., Parra, C., and Stephan, M., A total organic carbon analysis method for validating cleaning between products in biopharmaceutical manufacturing, *J. Parenteral Sci. Technol.*, 45, 13–19, 1991.

38. Jenkins, K.M., Vanderwielen, A.J., Armstrong, J.A., Leonard, L.M., Murphy, G.P., and Piros, N.A., Application of total organic carbon analysis to cleaning validation, *J. Parenteral Sci. Technol.*, 50, 6–15, 1996.

39. Sherwood, D., Fisher, D., Clifford, J., and Slade, S., Experiences with clean-in-place validation in a multiproduct biopharmaceutical manufacturing facility, *Eur. J. Parenteral Sci.*, 1, 35–41, 1996.

40. Elimination of Establishment License Application for Specified Biotechnology and Specified Synthetic Biological Products; Final Rule, *Federal Register*, 61(94), May 14, 1996.

41. Guidance for Industry Changes to an Approved Application for Specified Biotechnology and Specified Synthetic Biological Products, Center for Biological Evaluation and Research, Center for Drug Evaluation and Research, July 1997.

42. Points to Consider in the Characterization of Cell Lines Used to Produce Biologicals, Center for Biologics Evaluation and Research, July 1993.

43. Guidance on Quality of Biotechnological/Biological Products: Derivation and Characterization of Cell Substrates Used for Production of Biotechnological/Biological Products, Center for Biologics Evaluation and Research, ICH, September 1998.

44. FDA's Policy Statement Concerning Cooperative Manufacturing Arrangements for Licensed Biologics; Notice, *Federal Register*, 57, November 25, 1992.

45. Code of Federal Regulations, Title 21, Part 600, Section 600.3 (t).

46. Code of Federal Regulations, Title 21, Parts 207 and 607.

47. Federal Food, Drug and Cosmetic Act, Prohibited Acts, Section 301.

48. Ryan, C.S. and Wan, M., Risk management and liability for biologicals, *BioPharm*, 13, 40–42, 2000.

49. Carter-Hamm, B. and Vinson, G., Facilitating client audits: The contract laboratory perspective, *BioPharm*, 15, 12–16, 2002.

50. Young, T. and Douglas, R., Managing raw materials in a contract manufacturing facility, *BioProcess. J.*, 2, 47–49, 2003.

51. Guidance for Industry, Changes to an Approved Application for Specified Biotechnology and Specified Synthetic Biological Products and Biological Products; Final Rule and Notices, *Federal Register*, 62(142), July 24, 1997.

52. Guidance for Industry (draft), Submitting Type V Drug Master Files to the Center for Biologics Evaluation and Research, Center for Biologics Evaluation and Research, August 2001.

53. Federal Food, Drug and Cosmetic Act, Factory Inspection, Section 704.

54. Public Health Service Act, Biological Products, Section 351.

55. Roscioli, N.A., The evolution of biologics inspection, *Reg. Affairs Focus*, 5, 25–27, 2000.

56. Team Biologics: A Plan for Reinventing FDA's Ability to Optimize Compliance of Regulated Biologics Industries, Office of Regulatory Affairs, Food and Drug Administration, 1997.

57. FDA, All Human Drugs, Drug Manufacturing Inspections (Pilot Program), Program 7356.002, Compliance Program Guidance Manual, January 1, 2001.

58. Code of Federal Regulations, Title 21, Parts 210 and 211, Current Good Manufacturing Practice: Amendment of Certain Requirements for Finished Pharmaceuticals, Proposed Rule, *Federal Register*, 61(87) 20103-20115, May 3, 1996.

59. Guidance for Industry, Changes to an Approved Application Biological Products, Center for Biologics Evaluation and Research, July 1997.

60. Code of Federal Regulations, Title 5, Part 552, Freedom of Information.

10

Validation of Computerized Systems

MONICA J. CAHILLY

CONTENTS

10.1 INTRODUCTION

Computerized systems validation (CSV) represents one of several foundational quality systems necessary to ensure the overall integrity of the biopharmaceutical manufacturing, testing, packaging, and holding process — and thereby meet the ultimate goal of ensuring biopharmaceuticals provided to patients are safe and effective. CSV strategies must meet the needs of a competitive business environment characterized by complex and rapidly changing technologies. As such, CSV strategies should be streamlined, yet effective, and tailored to the specific risks posed by individual types of computerized systems. An appropriate CSV program truly adds value to the biopharmaceutical manufacturing process and is not — as is frequently misconstrued — a mere documentation exercise.

10.2 HISTORICAL OVERVIEW

Computerized system validation has emerged as a cornerstone of process validation with changing regulatory expectations and technologies. Computerized systems were not widely used at the time the United States Food and Drug Administration (FDA) first published what are now referred to as the "predicate rules" governing pharmaceutical and biopharmaceutical manufacture and testing. These FDA predicate rules include, but are not limited to, Good Manufacturing Practice (GMP) regulations that govern manufacture, processing, packing, and holding of drugs/biologics; Good Laboratory Practice (GLP) regulations that govern the conduct of nonclinical drug/biologic safety studies; Good Clinical Practices

(GCPs) that govern the conduct of clinical trials; and the Quality System Regulation (QSR) that governs the design, manufacture, packaging, labeling, storage, installation, and servicing of medical devices intended for human use. Although these FDA predicate rules do not explicitly describe all requirements for computerized systems validation, FDA inspectional requirements, expressed as early as 1983 in FDA's *Blue Book* entitled *Guide to Inspection of Computerized Systems in Drug Processing* [1], include the expectation that computerized systems used for FDA-related activities will be validated for their intended use.

During the time period from the early 1980s to the late 1990s, pharmaceutical firms* implemented varying degrees of computerization, largely depending on the firm's management style, i.e., whether management was innovative, moderate, or conservative. The vignettes that follow, although an oversimplification of reality, provide some illustration of the challenges faced by the industry during this era.

Innovative firms embraced change and technological advancements and opted to automate production and laboratory functions to the greatest extent possible given available technologies. Some innovative firms even introduced — and validated — the use of robotics in the production areas. In order to accomplish these objectives efficiently, these firms instituted global CSV policies and procedures to create a corporate culture that endorsed and promoted unified strategies for CSV. To achieve these benefits, resource requirements could be relatively high. To implement and sustain innovative strategies, firms required not only state-of-the-art technological and material resources, but also a relatively high degree of internal expertise and the work environment and financial resources necessary to attract and retain these "high performers." There was measurable risk associated with

---

* For simplicity, the term *pharmaceutical* may be used to more broadly refer to both pharmaceuticals and biopharmaceuticals.

implementing technologies that had not yet been "proven" or demonstrated as "tried and true" in the marketplace. Problems often had to be resolved from within the firm since solutions were not readily available elsewhere. During this era, the path of innovation could be demanding — and lonely, since many peer pharmaceutical manufacturers were unwilling to take similar risks.

Many firms chose the more moderate approach of purchasing and validating only a few primary computerized systems, such as large data management systems (e.g., Laboratory Information Management Systems [LIMS] or Clinical Data Management Systems [CDMS]). In these firms, validation was frequently decentralized and viewed as a "one-off" exercise that was largely outsourced to consulting firms. This approach allowed the benefit of some computerization without the high material and technological resources required by more innovative strategies. In addition, moderate approaches also minimized requirements for internal expertise and broadscale internal CSV training initiatives.

However, the more moderate approach was not without its attendant costs. Due to limitations in available technology or budget, firms operated with "hybrid" environments, i.e., utilizing numerous interfacing paper and electronic record-keeping systems, that created inefficiencies and opportunities for error. In addition, with visible inconsistencies in computerization and validation and insufficient training, some firms failed to instill in their employees a true "validation mindset." As a result, employees were not aware of the need to be fully involved in the validation process, to assume sincere ownership of their FDA-related computerized systems, and to consistently use them in an appropriately controlled manner. In addition, unaware employees could use readily available desktop productivity programs to create a plethora of spreadsheets and databases as ancillary electronic systems for supporting FDA-related activities — without understanding the need to validate these programs for their intended use. Internal Quality Assurance (QA) personnel who lacked sufficient validation awareness focused auditing on paper systems and available printouts from electronic systems and failed to directly inspect desktop and network server systems. As a result, QA often overlooked compliance deficiencies associated with computerized systems. These inconsistent approaches resulted in compliance consequences for many firms, as evidenced by FDA Form 483 observations and warning letters related to failure to appropriately validate and control computerized systems [2].

During this time period, other firms followed a more conservative approach and responded to perceived compliance risks associated with FDA regulatory expectations for computerized systems and the costs associated with validation — historically estimated to be as high as 50% of the overall cost of purchase and installation of the computerized system — by avoiding or limiting the use of computerized systems, particularly in the production areas. These firms continued to use paper-based systems or rudimentary and antiquated automated systems.

In some scenarios, firms chose the ill-advised route of purchasing and operating an unvalidated computerized system (e.g., a computerized inventory control system), identified to FDA during an inspection as a "management tool," in parallel with a redundant manual system (e.g., paper inventory control cards), identified to FDA as the "primary data capture system." Although this practice could provide some short-term benefits, the long-term costs could be significant. Software systems implemented without appropriate development controls were error-prone and unreliable and frequently a source of frustration for users who complained that the system did not adequately meet their needs. The availability of dual record-keeping systems and inconsistent user training also led to tedious, and oftentimes futile, attempts to reconcile data discrepancies between the electronic and paper records. Moreover, these scenarios inculcated an employee mindset that paper record-keeping systems were paramount and that a computerized system was an "add-on" to the business process rather than an integral, foundational component of the business process. These firms failed to gain internal technological and validation expertise, leaving them wholly unprepared to benefit from the current advent of broadscale technologies for efficient automated production of high-quality pharmaceuticals.

Perhaps due at least in part to avoidance strategies and the consequent lack of market demand by pharmaceutical manufacturers, diverse technological solutions to fully automate pharmaceutical production and testing processes were not readily available until more recently. Changing regulatory expectations have helped fuel a dramatic shift in the availability and use of innovative software solutions and, in turn, more consistent and comprehensive approaches to CSV.

In 1997, the FDA issued *Title 21 Part 11 of the Code of Federal Regulations (CFR) the Electronic Records; Electronic Signatures Rule* [3], a regulation that applies to all FDA-related computerized systems that create, modify, maintain, archive, retrieve, or distribute electronic records in fulfillment of any of the requirements of any FDA regulation, (i.e., FDA "predicate rules") or that are intended for direct inclusion in a submission to the FDA under the requirements of the United States Federal Food, Drug and Cosmetic Act and the Public Health Service Act, even if such electronic records are not specifically identified in FDA regulations. 21 CFR Part 11 (commonly referred to simply as "Part 11") sets forth the minimum standards that must be met in order for the FDA to consider electronic records and electronic signatures to be trustworthy, reliable, and generally equivalent to paper records and handwritten signatures executed on paper.

Part 11 reiterates several requirements for computerized systems that have been defined for decades in FDA predicate rules. These include historical requirements for validation of computerized systems, security of computerized systems, training of personnel that use and maintain computerized systems, maintenance of backup copies of electronic records, and the need for written policies and procedures. However, Part 11 also requires that software used for FDA-related purposes provide technical features that had not previously been required by regulation, including such features as computer-generated audit trails, device checks, operational system checks, sequencing checks, and others. In addition, Part 11 dictates technical features required for electronic signatures should a firm choose to employ these in lieu of handwritten signatures.

Although the industry initiated meetings with FDA in 1991 to create a rule that would permit use of electronic signatures in electronic submissions, when Part 11 was finally issued in March 1997, there was a strong negative reaction within industry, as expressed by the Pharmaceutical Research and Manufacturers of America (PhRMA) in a white paper submitted to FDA in 1999 [4]. Industry's primary complaints included the following: the cost of compliance with Part 11 (estimated by several firms to be in excess of $150 million); the impracticality of bringing all computerized systems, including legacy systems (i.e., systems implemented prior to August 20, 1997, and still in operation for FDA-related purposes after that date), into compliance with Part 11 by the effective date of August 20, 1997; the relative scarcity of vendor-supplied software solutions that included all of the technical features required by Part 11 and the complexity and expense of retrofitting existing software systems to include these features; and the general confusion and lack of clear guidance on interpreting and applying the rule both within industry and by FDA investigators in the field.

Part 11 brought computerized systems compliance to the fore at all firms. Most firms started their Part 11 compliance program by inventorying all FDA-related software systems at the firm and determining the baseline level of compliance of each. Many firms faced the disconcerting realization that numerous FDA-related software systems were in use without predicate rule controls, such as validation, security, and backup of electronic records, much less the Part 11 technical controls such as audit trails and electronic signature capabilities. Several firms discovered hundreds of uncontrolled spreadsheets and databases that had been used or were in use for FDA-related purposes. Many firms realized they lacked comprehensive internal expertise in CSV and that written CSV procedures were woefully out-of-date or nonexistent. Employees lacked sufficient training in CSV and in proper ways to use and control the specific software systems they were using for FDA-related purposes. The spotlight revealed that many had not yet even achieved a defensible baseline level of compliance with predicate rule requirements for computerized systems. In short, the computer compliance problem was much bigger than Part 11.

The magnitude of this problem brought great opportunity for each firm to dramatically reinvent its approach to record keeping and technology. Part 11 required the minimum controls necessary to rely on electronic records and electronic signatures in lieu of paper records and handwritten signatures. Part 11 thus laid the foundation for a paradigm shift from paper-based manufacturing, testing, and control to paperless operations. Visions of sitting at a computer screen and querying databases to quickly assess a product's history and quality throughout development, clinical trial, manufacturing, testing, distribution, and shelf life seemed realistic and attainable. Computers could be envisioned assessing product quality in continuous real time during manufacture — thereby yielding a higher-quality product with more efficiency and predictably lower costs. Laboratories could be run with handheld wireless devices that prompt analysts to follow step-by-step analytical instructions from downloaded procedures and that automatically capture and evaluate results from a fully integrated suite of instruments. Even more futuristic visions saw the processing power of computers being applied to evaluate contextual information associated with complex data sets stored in multiple interrelated databases to rapidly diagnose potential quality issues or predict trends. These visions could not be realized with antiquated and isolated computerized systems that could not effectively "talk" to each other or with disparate piles of paper records. The vision demanded seamlessly integrated computerized systems and the necessary fuzzy logic to quickly cull data and discern patterns.

The question then was how to achieve these possibilities given the current state of affairs. The entire pharmaceutical industry demanded that software vendors supply solutions with the necessary features for Part 11 compliance. This sparked an incredible surge in the availability and variety of software solutions. Part 11 had helped fuel a technology revolution. From scarcity to abundance, pharmaceutical manufacturers now primarily faced the dilemma of choice.

The path from unwieldy "hybrid" environments of separate computerized and paper systems to futuristic, fully electronic operations was fraught not only with technological challenges, but with numerous compliance hurdles as well. Many firms fell into the trap of not having an ultimate vision or global computing technology strategy and instead basing decisions primarily on the perceived compliance threat associated with Part 11. In a reactive mode, many firms purchased and validated expensive third-party Part 11 add-ons to existing software systems only to realize soon afterwards that the awkward conglomeration could not be effectively interfaced with other major software systems at the firm or that the cumbersome mix was rendered obsolete by new releases of core software that fully incorporated Part 11 technical controls. A more effective strategy was fundamentally based on risk assessment and balanced short-term needs with long-term goals. Following this more tactical approach to Part 11 compliance, firms would triage compliance issues associated with the existing hybrid environment while at the same time select and validate computerized system upgrades that were consistent with the firm's ultimate vision for fully integrated, paperless operations.

At the turn of the millennium, growing public concern over the cost of pharmaceuticals and the remarkable fact that pharmaceutical manufacturing processes were generally much less automated than comparable manufacturing processes in other nonregulated industries suggested that too many costly decisions might have been made on the basis of fear of compliance ramifications and not on good science, good technology, and clear assessment of risk to product quality. In August 2002, FDA acknowledged this concern in a new initiative, *Pharmaceutical cGMPs for the 21st Century: A Risk-Based Approach* [5]. This initiative promised changes in approaches to pharmaceutical manufacture and regulation that would merge science-based risk management with an integrated quality systems approach. Ultimately, FDA hoped to encourage the "latest scientific advances in pharmaceutical manufacturing and technology...while continuing to ensure pharmaceutical product quality" [5].

One of the first agenda items for FDA's new compliance initiative was to reexamine Part 11 and address concerns that certain interpretations of Part 11 would unnecessarily restrict the use of electronic technology, significantly increase the cost of compliance, and discourage innovation without significant public health benefit. In August 2003, FDA issued guidance on Part 11 that further clarified its intended scope and application [6]. The guidance also stated FDA's intent to exercise enforcement discretion with regard to certain Part 11 requirements during the period of time that FDA reexamined Part 11. As of this writing, the reexamination of Part 11 was still underway.

These actions documented FDA's support of the wisdom that pharmaceutical manufacturers needed a more tactical approach to computerized systems compliance. The FDA initiative essentially encourages firms to triage compliance issues associated with the existing hybrid environment in accordance with risk posed to product quality, patient safety, and data integrity. It simultaneously encourages firms to pursue the latest computerized system technologies — including those that may ultimately provide fully integrated, paperless operations.

Finally, current regulatory trends outside of FDA also encourage pharmaceutical manufacturers to use technological solutions to fully automate operations and, in turn, necessitate more consistent and comprehensive approaches to CSV. Two examples of recent rulings that impact computerized systems used within the pharmaceutical industry include the U.S. Health and Human Services patient privacy regulations, effective April 2003 and promulgated under the Health Insurance Portability and Accountability Act (HIPAA) of 1996 [7], and the U.S. Securities and Exchange Commission rules governing financial reporting under the Sarbanes–Oxley Act of 2002 [8]. HIPAA applies to organizations handling patient records, such as clinical sites and pharmaceutical companies sponsoring the clinical trials, and requires computing standards that protect the confidentiality, integrity, and availability of electronic protected health information. Sarbanes–Oxley is legislation directed at publicly traded companies and contains provisions for financial electronic records intended to protect investors by improving the accuracy and reliability of corporate disclosures required by securities laws and for other purposes. The rulings under both of these acts require Part 11-type controls for applicable computerized systems and associated electronic records.

The trend of outside agencies requiring control over the pharmaceutical industry's computerized systems and electronic records is expected to continue as automation becomes more widespread. Gone are the days when firms could elect to validate only a few select computerized systems within the firm or a few select modules within computerized systems because they were used for FDA purposes. Good business practices in this electronic era dictate that every computerized system within the firm should be brought into a defensible state of control commensurate with its intended use and relative risk. For these reasons, creating a corporate culture that promotes and sustains computerized systems compliance and developing streamlined, risk-based approaches to CSV are a must.

10.3 CREATING A CORPORATE CULTURE FOR COMPUTERIZED SYSTEMS COMPLIANCE

The term *computerized systems validation* may be used to refer to different concepts. Some use the term to simply describe the testing associated with releasing a new software system. With this viewpoint, a firm might narrowly focus on testing and documenting individual computerized systems one-by-one in hope of eventually achieving compliance with FDA predicate rules and Part 11. This linear approach to validation compliance is costly and generally cannot be sustained beyond the initial release of each system since it overlooks meaningful development of comprehensive supporting quality systems. It fails to cultivate the necessary environment for sustained computerized systems compliance.

In this chapter, the term *computerized systems validation* will instead be used to describe a holistic, interrelated set of processes and controls designed for the purpose of specifying, developing, testing, implementing, and maintaining a computerized system in a manner that ensures it is fit — and continues to be fit — for its intended use. As such, CSV must take place in a business environment that nourishes computerized systems compliance. That is, firms must build a holistic framework of interrelated quality processes and controls that support the use of electronic records and electronic signatures in lieu of paper records and handwritten signatures.

To do this, many firms might need to reinvent themselves, their computerized systems compliance program, and their attitudes toward technology and thereby shift each employee's mindset. This transformation starts with an examination of existing computerized processes and all functional areas that support any FDA-related process. Using this awareness, firms then radically reconceptualize the business, imagining future technologies, personnel roles, and quality systems that will provide efficient, paperless operations while continuing to ensure the production of high-quality pharmaceuticals. This vision would then be imparted to each employee through a variety of training initiatives as work begins to revitalize quality systems and introduce new technologies.

Example activities necessary to effect this change are described in the following sections.

10.3.1 Develop a Global Computing Vision with Short-Term and Long-Term Milestones, and Implement Technologies to Fully Automate All Functional Areas in Accordance with the Firm's Global Computing Vision

Information Technology (IT)/Information Systems (IS) personnel drive this planning by defining common data and computing architectures, identifying key global computing systems slated for near-term and long-term purchase and installation, and defining necessary network infrastructure elements for increasing integration and security. The planning process should encourage imagination of technologies that do not yet exist. The plan should be flexible and allow for dynamic adaptation to superior emerging technologies as they become available. In the near term, IT/IS personnel must assume a central role in decision making for all software and hardware purchases at the firm to ensure that purchases contain necessary elements for Part 11 compliance and are consistent with the global computing vision. Then, all future software purchases should be aligned with the dynamic, global computing plan.

10.3.2 Document a Risk-Based Approach to Compliance That Identifies Key Vulnerabilities, Control Points, and the Risk Management Approach and Objectives

The firm's documented risk assessment/risk management approach to control of computerized systems may guide the overall scope and depth of validation, remediation, and change control activities and therefore enhance efficiencies.

10.3.3 Train All Personnel to Shift Their Mental Paradigm from a Paper-Based World to Thinking in Terms of Paperless Operations, and Build Internal Expertise in Computerized Systems Compliance

This training may be conducted as "21 CFR Part 11 Awareness Training" but should not be presented from the perspective of introducing yet another FDA regulation. The training of all employees, agents, and representatives of the firm must communicate the essence of the Part 11 rule — i.e., the paradigm shift from paper as "raw data" to electronic records as "raw data," the need to establish and maintain security and access controls, and the awareness of the legally binding nature of electronic signatures. Training of Senior Management must emphasize the need for a corporate shift from paper-based business strategies and practices to paperless/electronic business practices. Training of supervisory/data review personnel should emphasize the importance of reviewing electronic records and relevant metadata, such as audit trails — instead of incomplete printouts — prior to approving results generated by the FDA-related computerized system. QA personnel must be trained to perform in-depth inspections of computerized systems, their configuration controls, and their associated FDA-related electronic records — instead of limiting the internal audit process to the more superficial review of computerized system printouts and externally visible controls.

To build internal expertise in computerized systems compliance, the firm must establish core computerized systems training curricula for all employees that include, as a minimum, training in CSV, change control, reporting of computer-related incidents, and computerized systems security and password policies. In order to control the proliferation of unqualified spreadsheets, databases, and electronic document systems, all employees must be trained in the requirements of properly managing and controlling these systems when used for FDA-related purposes. Employees must also be made aware that FDA-related electronic records must not be stored on local or stand-alone drives that are not secured or routinely backed up.

Computerized systems compliance expertise might need to be enhanced in both the IT/IS and QA departments. To do so, the firm should hire, or train as necessary, additional staff for the IT/IS department to establish expertise in both technologies and FDA requirements, including predicate rule and 21 CFR Part 11 requirements. Technical training should include, as necessary, skills related to corporate computing standards, the common security architecture, and computerized system administration. Internal Quality personnel should obtain in-depth training in current industry standards for CSV and 21 CFR Part 11, as well as in the necessary technology skills required to effectively inspect computerized systems and associated specifications.

10.3.4   Reorganize Personnel and Responsibilities
to Institute Global Authority with
Distributed Local Control

Global or centralized personnel should set policy, actively influence decisions at the corporate level, maintain a bird's-eye view of global/corporate issues, and immediately report issues of concern to the Senior Management team. Supporting personnel, distributed locally within individual functional areas, should conduct more focused, detailed, and specific functions in support of local operations, monitor local areas for issues, and report issues of concern to the global or centralized authority. For computer compliance initiatives, this model is one of several possibilities that can be applied to expand and stratify Quality and IT functions and expertise throughout the organization. Doing so promises to enhance effectiveness and efficiency of the overall computer compliance program. The potential models are illustrated in the following sections.

10.3.4.1   Centralized/Distributed Quality Model

QA resources for consistent, effective, and efficient oversight of computer compliance-related activities have traditionally been limited. In many organizations, QA personnel, and their compliance expertise, were maintained in a silo outside of functional areas. In these instances, QA would periodically visit functional areas for brief inspections and then submit a report to management based on this limited sample. Often-times, the inspected groups complained that QA lacked the expertise to effectively inspect the science and technology behind the processes and, instead, focused on superficial documentation issues. The perceived or real lack of technical expertise within QA was exacerbated by the organization's formal separation of QA from day-to-day functional operations. QA, in turn, was often frustrated by the lack of compliance expertise and compliance initiatives within the functional areas. These views and realities must change if effective quality oversight of computerized systems is to be established. A robust computer compliance program requires dedicated and skilled quality involvement in several efforts, including CSV, change control, internal inspections of computerized systems, computerized system incident handling, audits of vendors of critical software systems, conducting periodic reviews of validation documentation, and conducting audits of contract manufacturers and contract laboratories to ensure the adequacy of their program for compliance with Part 11.

In the distributed model, quality/compliance resources are *embedded within* local functional areas, such as within the IT/IS area and Engineering, to ensure appropriate skill development and the active and efficient oversight of individual system implementation projects within those functional areas. Distributed quality personnel champion quality and compliance initiatives from within organizational units and are responsible for more day-to-day systems-related issues. For example, local quality/compliance personnel in the IT/IS Compliance Group would participate in computerized system validation projects, change control, audits of software vendors, management of IT/IS documents, conducting of IT/IS compliance training, development of IT/IS compliance procedures, handling of computer-related incidents, and other local computer compliance-related activities.

Likewise, the Engineering Department would create an internal Engineering Compliance Group with roles and responsibilities for control systems compliance analogous to the roles and responsibilities that the IT/IS Compliance Group assumes for software systems compliance. For example, the Engineering Compliance Group would coordinate day-to-day qualification, change control, and incident handling for manufacturing and facilities control systems/equipment. For those manufacturing systems that have both software and control system components, such as Supervisory Control and Data Acquisition (SCADA) systems, the combined software validation/equipment qualification effort would require harmonized participation by the System Owner (e.g., the Production Manager), IT/IS Compliance, Engineering Compliance, and, if warranted due to system criticality, the central or global QA.

Distributed quality personnel would submit regular status reports to the central or global QA who, in turn, would report critical issues or apparent trends of concern to the Senior Management team. Using a risk-based approach to personnel distribution, the central QA authority would be tasked with issuing global policies and procedures and oversight of larger initiatives and systems-related issues deemed to be "critical." For example, the central QA authority would be actively involved in the following: all critical computerized system-related incidents (e.g., a broadscale infection of the firm's network with a damaging virus); all critical computerized system change controls (e.g., major modification of the security administration module for a critical software system); the purchase and implementation of all critical computerized systems (e.g., a global, remote Electronic Data Capture system); qualification of critical contract facilities (e.g., a primary contract manufacturing site); etc.

10.3.4.2 Centralized/Distributed IT/IS Model

Historically, at most firms, the IT/IS role has been limited to deployment and support of network systems and software classified as "business systems" (generally large data management systems such as Enterprise Resource Planning [ERP] systems). The purview of IT/IS control and expertise historically did not extend into production areas or to laboratory areas where many of the firm's most critical software systems with direct impact on product quality, patient safety, and data integrity (such as computerized production equipment and computerized laboratory instruments) were located.

In the centralized/distributed IT/IS model, these critical software systems are brought fully under the purview of the IT/IS organization for important IT/IS functions, such as validation, change control, security administration, disaster recovery, incident handling, storage of application code, and management of electronic records. To effect this change, sufficient IT/IS personnel and material resources need to be allocated for local functions, such as security administration of software systems, that may be currently under the purview of Engineering, Facilities and Maintenance, or Laboratory personnel. IT/IS personnel should also ensure that electronic records from all FDA-related computerized systems throughout the firm — including nonnetworked systems in the production, facilities, and laboratory areas — are appropriately backed up and maintained.

This model endorses the organizational placement of the System Administrator for each production and laboratory system in the IT/IS department for the following reasons: (1) to function organizationally independent of the system user group and thereby avoid conflicts of interest over the abilities to delete electronic records and alter user access rights; (2) to better harmonize IT/IS efforts to network all computerized systems; (3) to centralize efforts to perform daily system backups; and (4) to centralize efforts to activate or revoke user access rights for all computerized systems upon changes in a given user's employment status.

Central IT/IS assumes final approval authority for computing decisions. Operational units must be prohibited from introducing software into the firm without approval by the central IT/IS function to ensure that any new software provides the technical features required for Part 11 compliance and is consistent with and can be appropriately integrated into the firm's long-term computing vision. The central IT/IS unit also maintains a controlled, up-to-date reference list of all software systems within the firm.

10.3.5 Centralize and Automate Quality Systems Support Operations

Paper-based systems or combinations of paper and electronic record-keeping systems are inefficient and often ineffective as a result of the difficulty of querying records to quickly tabulate information and discern trends. Moreover, it is difficult to implement any major initiative without efficient support operations. For example, deploying a Part 11 compliance program necessitates revision or creation of thousands of controlled documents such as policies, procedures, and individual system-related validation documents. Inefficiencies in document management frustrate timely achievement of Part 11 compliance objectives. Even worse, addressing administrative bottlenecks divert valuable personnel resources from more important activities related to ensuring product quality, patient safety, and data integrity.

Examples of support operations that might need to be established or revitalized are described in the following sections.

10.3.5.1 Document Management

The firm should have a centralized department and global computerized system, i.e., an Electronic Document Management System (EDMS), for distributing, electronically approving, and controlling revision of documents, such as policies and procedures. The implementation of an EDMS greatly facilitates efficient deployment and secure revision control of all policies and procedures, including those issued for CSV/Part 11 compliance.

Document support operations should also include creation of global policies and procedures that define computerized systems maintenance and control, addressing topics that include, but are not necessarily limited to, the following:

- Computerized system validation
- Qualification and control of desktop productivity programs (spreadsheets, databases)
- Computerized system change control
- Hardware and software configuration management
- Risk assessment of computerized systems
- Security
- Virus surveillance and mitigation
- Time and date stamp synchronization and control
- Internet policy
- Electronic signatures
- Personnel responsibilities for computerized systems
- Management of electronic records (backup/restore, copying, archival)
- System retirement and data migration

- Disaster recovery/contingency planning
- Computerized system incident reporting and handling
- CSV/21 CFR Part 11 compliance training
- Software vendor qualification
- Software development standards
- Management of computerized systems documentation
- Quality assurance oversight of computerized systems
- Periodic review of computerized systems validation
- Maintenance of electronic media (such as application disks, etc.)
- Network qualification
- Network administration

10.3.5.2 Training

The firm should have a centralized department and global computerized system, such as a learning management system, to ensure and track comprehensive employee training in a consistent and efficient fashion. An effective training program will be essential to achieving substantial compliance with Part 11 by ensuring that all personnel are trained in the numerous CSV/Part 11 policies and procedures to be issued and in the more general training modules required for Part 11 compliance.

10.3.5.3 Software Vendor Qualification

The firm should develop streamlined options for qualifying software vendors prior to purchase or upgrade of software systems. In addition, the firm must centralize control over purchase decisions to prevent the introduction of inappropriate or incompatible software. IT/IS approval ensures that the software provides the technical features required for Part 11 compliance and is consistent with and can be appropriately integrated into the firm's long-term computing vision.

10.3.5.4 Computerized Systems Validation

The firm must consolidate and unify the corporate CSV strategy. To do so might require eliminating isolated approaches to CSV wherein each department has its own, slightly different CSV procedure or strategy for outsourcing CSV projects. Instead, the firm should have global policies and procedures for CSV that are risk-based and tailored to system type and that provide validation tools and templates for ease of use. To promote a unified approach to CSV within the firm, training in CSV policies must be part of the core curriculum for each employee. The firm may choose to establish a Validation Control Steering Committee composed of representatives from QA, IT/IS, and Management of functional areas to disseminate and promote the new unified CSV strategy, to act as gatekeepers to evaluate proposals for new software system purchases and approve Requests for Capital Expenditures, and to assign and oversee ad hoc validation teams composed of personnel from the User group, QA/Compliance group, and IT/IS group to validate each new software system.

10.3.5.5 Change Control

The firm should have a centralized and comprehensive database system to document and track changes to FDA-related computerized systems, both networked and nonnetworked, and to ensure that change control responsibilities are clearly delegated for all types of computerized systems (including software associated with networked applications, laboratory instruments, other standalone applications, spreadsheets, databases, electronic document systems, computerized manufacturing systems, etc.). The firm may choose to establish a centralized Change Control Steering Committee composed of representatives from QA, IT/IS, Engineering, and Management of functional areas. The Change Control Steering Committee should convene to evaluate change requests for changes to validated systems (i.e., validated processes, validated software, qualified equipment, etc.). Using a risk-based approach to compliance, the Change Control Steering Committee should evaluate computerized system changes deemed to be critical and ensure that QA, IT/IS, and System Owners are appropriately involved in testing, implementing, and documenting the change.

10.3.5.6 Electronic Records Management

The firm must establish a centralized and comprehensive system to securely maintain accurate and complete electronic records from all FDA-related systems within the firm. To do so efficiently requires that all software systems be brought under the purview of the IT/IS department, as stated previously, and that stand-alone software systems are networked whenever possible. The firm must also document and test a disaster recovery plan to ensure availability of all computerized systems and restoration of associated electronic records in the event of a disaster.

As part of this initiative, the firm must also formally address a strategy for making accurate and complete copies of electronic records, the long-term retention and maintenance of electronic records, obsolescence issues, and system retirement. Led by the central IT/IS function, the firm must define and implement, on a corporate-wide basis, electronic records storage technology standards that promote electronic record integration and efficiencies across the firm globally. In addition, ease of storage, security, environmental controls, and retrievability of electronic records over short-term and long-term periods must be considered. The firm must inspect all user group areas to locate and retrieve all copies of application software and source code for storage in centrally maintained, secure archives.

10.3.5.7 Security

The firm should develop and implement a Corporate IT/IS Security Plan that addresses all physical and logical security controls for facilities and systems, including networked and nonnetworked systems. The plan must include strategies to standardize and control all network workstations, since these offer the primary mode of entry into the firm's networks and all resident applications and electronic records. The plan should also include evaluation and security remediation, if necessary, of all remote access entries to all Local Area Networks (LANs) and Wide Area Networks (WANs), including security risk assessment of laptops used to access the network internally and from remote sites.

10.3.5.8 Electronic Signatures Management

The firm must establish a centralized infrastructure for managing electronic signatures as legally binding equivalents of handwritten signatures. This activity, once accomplished, ensures the administration of electronic signatures for any computerized systems in current use or used in the future. Electronic signature requirements of 21 CFR Part 11 apply to any employee, agent, or representative of the firm who electronically signs an FDA-related electronic record. This includes full-time or part-time employees, temporary employees, and contractors or consultants who are granted user access rights and issued electronic signatures for any of the firm's FDA-related software systems. Ideally, Human Resources (HR) leads this initiative as a result of their immediate knowledge of the hiring and departure of employees, agents, and representatives of the firm.

Activities include sending a letter to FDA certifying that electronic signatures in use at the firm now or anytime in the future are intended as the legally binding equivalent of handwritten signatures per 21 CFR Part 11.100 (c); documenting a corporate electronic signature policy and procedure; establishing a comprehensive database system for documenting all employees, agents, or representatives of the firm, to potentially include full-time employees, part-time employees, temporary workers, and contractors or consultants; training all employees, agents, and representatives of the firm in the requirements of the electronic signature policy and procedure; if warranted, collecting signature certification statements from each employee, agent, and representative; and verifying and documenting the verification of the identities of any employee, agent, or representative prior to the issuance of an electronic signature. In addition, the firm should have procedures for deactivating network user ID/password logon access that include written HR procedures to ensure that HR personnel inform all FDA-related computerized system administrators, including network administrators, of the need to deactivate or change system access rights when employees, agents, or representatives leave the firm or change job responsibilities.

10.3.5.9 Corrective and Preventative Action (CAPA)

The firm should have a CAPA program and a global CAPA software system to comprehensively document all FDA-related quality issues at the firm, perform root cause analyses, conduct risk assessments, identify all corrective actions, track completion status of corrective actions, and trend occurrences of issues in order to identify potentially larger, systemic quality system issues or failures. A comprehensive and effective CAPA program is essential to achieving an effective computerized systems compliance program. It ensures that there is a mechanism to appropriately identify, report, track, resolve, and trend complaints, incidents, and quality issues related to validated computerized systems.

10.3.6 Qualify All Networks

An essential part of validating/ensuring the integrity and reliability of any software application is the qualification of the computing environment in which it is used. For networked applications, this means qualifying the network. Qualifying networks on which FDA-related software applications and electronic records reside ensures and documents their consistent, reliable, and secure operation. This one activity alone is a cornerstone of the computer compliance program that provides immediate benefits toward bringing all networked software applications into a defensible state of control.

Basic elements of network qualification include the following:

- Specification of the network and creation of version-controlled network diagrams, approved by IT/IS and QA

- Documentation of written procedures that address requirements for network qualification, maintenance, and control
- Implementation of business processes and systems to consistently follow and document adherence to written procedures in practice

Table 10.1 lists examples of network qualification procedures and activities that should be considered, based on risk. More in-depth references on network qualification are available [9,10].

10.3.7 Use Technology to Facilitate Efficient and Effective Communications between Centers of Knowledge

Rapid knowledge sharing will become increasingly possible as the firm's global computing vision is realized. Senior Management and QA will have real-time knowledge of product quality issues as they occur and be able to take immediate corrective action. This system will bypass the current inefficient, delayed response process of waiting to receive and review periodic, after-the-fact reports. To prepare for this, the firm must take actions such as the following: identify the centers of knowledge; identify who requires access to information from which knowledge centers; determine database integration that might need to occur to facilitate compilation of knowledge; identify data sets and associated metadata necessary for contextual interpretation of data; develop tools for efficient data mining; develop data conversion tools and determine how and if data currently stored in certain formats (e.g., flat files) should be converted to other more integrated and queryable formats; and develop visualization and interpretation tools.

Once a healthy corporate culture for computerized systems compliance is created, individual computerized systems can be validated in an efficient and sustainable manner. In addition, costs of implementing the computerized systems compliance infrastructure can be distributed across

TABLE 10.1   Qualifying Networks

Examples of Topics to Consider in Procedures for Qualified Networks

Network qualification

Network performance monitoring (including network traffic bandwidth, errors, and utilization of disk space for network databases or file systems)

Network security (including inactivity timeouts on network workstations — set at 15 minutes at many firms)

Maintenance of firewall

Maintenance of network hardware

Control and synchronization of time and date stamp on all servers and clients

Virus surveillance and mitigation for the network

Startup and shutdown procedures

Control of access to Internet

Control of user access to local drives on workstations

Administration and control of remote access to the network

Hardware (e.g., routers, switches, hubs, workstations, etc.) configuration management

Software configuration management (to include management of workstation software configuration)

Reporting and handling maintenance events or incidents related to the network hardware and components

Controls on introduction of new software applications to the qualified network

Disaster recovery planning/business continuity

Training of network management personnel

Storage of source code or source application software disks

Periodic testing of uninterruptible power supply (UPS) units and generators

Network data center access control and administration

Controls for transportable media (e.g., floppy disks, CD-Rs, etc.)

Others

Examples of Activities to Consider for Qualified Networks

Write and execute Network Qualification Protocols (with preestablished specifications, testing requirements, preestablished test methods, etc.); review test data; write Network Qualification Summary Report that summarizes or concludes how the testing results compared to the anticipated results (i.e., predefined test specifications); etc.

Write all network procedures.

Write and execute Network Security Plan.

Create maintenance logs.

(continued)

TABLE 10.1   Qualifying Networks (Continued)

Examples of Activities to Consider for Qualified Networks (continued)

Create system to track network-related incidents.

Establish network performance monitoring logs and schedule for reporting metrics.

Create and maintain version-controlled, approved inventory lists of all software applications on the network.

Create and maintain version-controlled, approved inventory lists of all network hardware components.

Implement dynamic configuration management for network hardware and software.

Make periodic back-ups of network configurations.

Follow change control for major network changes.

Establish gatekeeper to control new applications coming onto the network.

Document training of network management personnel.

Establish secure, environmentally controlled archives for off-site storage of source code and application disks.

Synchronize and secure, via technical means where possible, the time and date stamp for all networked servers and workstations.

Establish logs of periodic testing of Uninterruptible Power Supply (UPS) and generators that support data centers.

Qualify software system controlling badge access to data center.

Conduct security audit of entire network and facility (include penetration and social engineering tests).

Establish logs of environmental monitoring of data center.

Document and test detailed disaster recovery plan that addresses contingency plans to protect the network systems, data center, network applications, and electronic records in the event of a disaster.

Document periodic tests of the ability to restore critical electronic records and applications from network backup or archival media stored over long periods of time.

Others

all individual computerized system remediation and validation projects, significantly reducing the costs associated with the implementation of any single or given system.

10.4 VALIDATION OF INDIVIDUAL COMPUTERIZED SYSTEMS

Each computerized system that is integral to the biopharmaceutical manufacturing process — whether it be a complex, custom-configurable data management system that is globally deployed, such as an Enterprise Resource Planning (ERP) system or global clinical Electronic Data Capture system, or a small spreadsheet used to calculate product impurities — must be validated to ensure its consistent and reliable performance over time. In the biopharmaceutical arena, Web-based software systems, data warehousing and data mining systems, robotics, microarray systems, and other currently novel technologies add unique complexities to the validation process. Table 10.2 lists examples of various types of computerized systems that currently are commonly found in pharmaceutical and biopharmaceutical manufacturing environments.

TABLE 10.2 Examples of Computer System Types

Computerized manufacturing systems, such as building management systems (BMS), supervisory control and data acquisition (SCADA) systems, process analytical technology (PAT) systems, manufacturing execution systems (MES), distributed control systems (DCS), etc.

Computerized laboratory instruments, such as chromatography data systems, dissolution software systems, particle monitoring software systems, microarray systems, robotics systems, etc.

Large-scale data and information management systems, such as enterprise resource planning (ERP) systems, laboratory information management systems (LIMS), clinical data management systems (CDMS), etc.

Spreadsheets, such as those used to calculate laboratory results or track and trend quality control (QC) data, environmental monitoring, statistical analysis software, etc.

Databases, such as those used for corrective and preventative action (CAPA), complaint handling, adverse event reporting and handling, scheduling equipment maintenance and calibration, scheduling and tracking employee training, etc.

Document manangement systems, such as Electronic Document Management Systems (EDMS) used for controlling policies and procedures.

The fundamental principles of validating any software system remain independent of system type and serve to fulfill the purpose of obtaining "confirmation by examination and provision of objective evidence that computer system specifications conform to user needs and intended uses, and that all requirements can be consistently fulfilled" [11,12]. CSV simply applies commonsense principles to implementing and using a computerized system. In everyday language, these basic principles include the following:

- Decide what you want. Write it down.
- Look at what you want and ask what risks are associated with the system complexity, with the system type, with the intended use of the system, with the individual wants, and with the associated business process. Are there any risks to product quality, patient safety, or data integrity? If so, what are the sources of these risks? How can these risks be controlled? How can you prove your controls are adequate? Write down this thought process.
- Get organized. Pick persons to be involved and key activities. Do not plan to do any more or any less than what your commonsense risk assessment dictates. Write down your plan.
- Brainstorm. Design the system to get what you want. Write it down.
- Build and test the system. Keep records. Continue reworking your wants and the design until you have built a satisfactory fully assembled product. Revise lists of wants and design when necessary.
- Check the fully assembled system against your wants and the design to verify its consistency and adequacy. Keep records of this check.
- Install and configure the fully assembled system in the firm's computing environment. Run tests to see if the installation worked. Identify and fix any problems. Keep records.
- Run tests to reconfirm that the key functions of the system work in the firm's test computing environment.

Identify and fix any problems that arise in the firm's test environment. Keep records.

- Turn the system over to the users and have them try it out in their production environment. Identify and fix any problems that arise in the firm's end-user production environment. Keep records.
- Release the system to the users for real-life use. Frequently or continuously monitor the system for a certain or defined period of time after release to be sure that it remains stable under normal usage conditions. Keep records.
- Once you feel comfortable that the system is stable, shift to a mode of periodic but regularly scheduled monitoring. Keep records.
- Use the system in a controlled manner. Keep records.
- Maintain the system in a controlled manner. Keep records.
- When you no longer need the system or are ready to upgrade, retire the system and its records in a controlled manner. Keep records.

Translated into validation jargon, the preceding process is described as follows: implement, maintain, and retire any computerized system according to a well-defined and documented System Development Life Cycle (SDLC). There are several possible SDLC approaches, such as the "Waterfall Model," the "Spiral Model," the "Incremental Development Model," and others [12,13]. A typical software life cycle outlined in FDA Guidance, *General Principles of Software Validation*, January 2002 [12], includes the following phases: quality planning, system requirements definition, detailed software requirements specification, software design specification, construction or coding, testing, installation, operation and support, maintenance, and retirement. Another common model is frequently referred to as the "V-Model," which describes the verification framework for system specification and qualification within the SDLC [14]. This model includes the following phases: planning and specification phase (with validation plan, user requirements specification, functional specification, supplier assessments), design phase (with design and configuration specifications, design reviews), system construction phase (with construction and code reviews), testing phase (with unit and integration testing, or monitoring of system supplier for vendor-supplied systems), installation phase (with installation qualification), acceptance testing phase (with operational qualification and performance qualification), validation summary, operation and maintenance phase, and retirement phase. Other models address the same basic concepts with different terminology. For example, some models refer to end-user testing in the production environment as "User Acceptance Testing" while others include it under the term "Performance Qualification."

Any one of these SDLC approaches or uses of terminology is defensible for the system type and the organization — as long as the SDLC selected addresses risks and provides "objective evidence that computer system specifications conform to user needs and intended uses, and that all requirements can be consistently fulfilled" [11,12]. These references [11–13] outline SDLC phases and examples of types of validation activities and "deliverables" (i.e., documents produced as a result of the validation activity) for each phase. The choice of validation activities and deliverables must be tailored to the *type* of computerized system. For example, common sense dictates that larger, more complex computerized systems require a different set of validation activities than those of smaller, single-use systems. Again, the overriding or key consideration is to *make choices based on risk*.

> *Key Concept:* Risk assessment must be superimposed on the entire CSV process to guide the scope and depth of all validation activities and documentation.

This chapter presents some key CSV concepts and an overview of each of the phases in a typical SDLC. As mentioned previously, there are several references available that provide more in-depth information on computerized systems validation and FDA expectations for computerized systems [3,6,12–19].

10.4.1 Risk Assessment and Management

Risk assessment and management must occur throughout the SDLC. At a minimum, the firm should conduct risk assessment following specification of system requirements, as part of vendor assessment, when designing qualification tests and test strategies, when resolving test deviations, when evaluating and implementing changes to validated systems, when responding to computer-related incidents or problems, and when determining data migration and electronic record archival strategies. In all cases, the firm must justify and document risk assessment and risk management.

Risk assessment answers the following questions: What can go wrong with the system that might impact product quality, patient safety, data integrity, or the business? How might these errors occur? What is the likelihood or probability of their occurrence? It begins with an overall assessment of risk associated with the business processes and environment in which the computerized system will be used and continues on through the evaluation of individual features available or lacking in the proposed computerized system. Examples of factors to consider include, but are not limited to, the following: patient populations targeted by the associated biopharmaceutical therapy; type and route of associated biopharmaceutical therapy; relation of computerized output data to product labeling, safety, and efficacy; number of system users; user skill sets and limitations; stability of supporting IT architecture; types of technologies used and their associated vulnerabilities; impact of system failure and maintenance downtime; and availability and effectiveness of system features for security, audit trail, feedback, traceability of data, retrievability of records, and many others. For vendor-supplied systems, such as Off-the-Shelf (OTS) software systems and configurable software packages, the firm must also consider such factors as the robustness of the vendor's SDLC and practices, the known history of system failure rates and types of failures, and the vendor's responsiveness to customer complaints.

Risk management addresses these questions: What can be done to prevent or control risks? What ongoing checks and balances will ensure that controls continue to function properly over time? Risk management strategies include designing and implementing technical system controls to mitigate risks, conducting a level of system testing that is commensurate with severity of risk (e.g., to appropriately challenge key control points), and implementing administrative and procedural process controls following system release that continue to mitigate risks. Some firms choose a risk elimination or avoidance strategy when the risks associated with a new technology are deemed to be excessive. Finally, the level of documentation of "objective evidence" and level of personnel involved in CSV activities should reflect the overall criticality of the system.

Example of Risk Assessment and Risk Management: With a spreadsheet used to calculate product impurities, for example, risk assessment will identify one risk scenario as the possibility of producing incorrect impurities results. This risk will be considered critical since it might lead to product being released into the market with levels of impurities detrimental to patient health. Potential sources of the risk of incorrect results might include incorrect entry into the spreadsheet of source data used to calculate the result or use of an incorrect calculation algorithm in the spreadsheet. The risk mitigation strategy might then include procedural or technical controls to verify data input, verification of correctness of the calculation algorithm, and security controls to protect the algorithm from modification once it is verified as correct. Appropriateness of the algorithm would be verified during design qualification. Technical controls over input verification and security of the algorithm would be challenged during the testing phase. Adherence to written procedures that require a second party to verify data entries and to periodically manually calculate and verify results would be ensured through training and follow-up audits.

A few examples of many references that offer additional guidance on risk assessment and management include FDA's *Guidance on Off-the-Shelf Software Use in Medical Devices* [20], FDA's *Guidance for the Content of Pre-market*

Submissions for Software Contained in Medical Devices [21], the GAMP 4 *Guideline for Risk Assessment* [14], and the international standard ISO 14971-1, *Medical Devices — Risk Management* [22].

10.4.2 Planning Phase/Personnel Responsibilities for CSV

The planning phase of the SDLC most often occurs together with the system specification phase and results in the following: clear assignment of personnel roles, resources, and responsibilities for each task; determination of required material and financial resources; documentation of validation strategy based on risk assessment; determination of expected validation deliverables; expectation for change control of system and documentation; listing of written procedures necessary to support the administration, maintenance, and use of the system; determination of training requirements and schedule for persons that develop, use, and maintain the system; strategy for data conversions if the system is replacing a legacy system; and specification of the overall acceptance criteria for validation. This information is typically documented in a Validation Plan that is a "dynamic controlled document."

> *Key Concept:* All key validation documents, such as the Validation Plan, Requirements Specifications, and Design and Configuration Specifications, should be maintained as dynamic controlled documents, i.e., documents that are versioned, approved, and updated through change control to continually reflect the actual system and system validation.

As stated previously, the Validation Plan should adequately define personnel roles and responsibilities for various phases of the SDLC and define signature responsibilities for each of the validation deliverables. There are at least three primary personnel functions that must be involved in each validation project: the System Owner and the System Users, i.e., the primary persons responsible for the business use of the computerized system; a Quality Representative, such as a Quality Assurance or IT/IS Compliance representative; and a Technical Representative, such as an IT/IS application developer or technology specialist. The CSV responsibilities recommended for each of these three key functional roles are listed in the following sections.

10.4.2.1 System Owner and System Users

The System Owner and System Users are the primary persons responsible for the validation status of their computerized system and for ensuring that all FDA regulations, including 21 CFR Part 11 and FDA predicate rules, and any written procedures applicable to the computerized system are followed. This requires that the System Owner and System Users be actively involved in the validation. Examples of System Owner/User responsibilities include, but are not necessarily limited to, the following: ensuring that user requirements are clearly and unambiguously defined and that appropriate assessments of the risks associated with each intended use of the FDA-related computerized system are performed; reviewing and approving specifications; assisting with vendor selection and assessment, if applicable; developing end-user SOPs for the system; ensuring that all users are trained in the system prior to its use; performing end-user testing of the system; ensuring that the validation summary report accurately and completely reflects the conduct of the validation and that all deviations are appropriately documented and resolved; ensuring that the system is operated and electronic records are maintained in accordance with written procedures; and, eventually, ensuring that the system is retired in accordance with written procedures.

> *Key Concept:* The System Owner and System Users have primary responsibility for the validation status of the software that they use for FDA-related purposes and must actively participate in the validation process.

10.4.2.2 Information Technology (IT)/Information Systems (IS)

IT/IS personnel, such as the designated System Administrator, Database Administrator, or other technical representatives, are responsible for configuring and maintaining the system in accordance with internal policies and procedures, specified system requirements, and FDA regulations. In addition, the System Administrator and technical representatives assist the System Owner with the validation of the system by conducting activities such as the following: specifying technical requirements of the system; assessing technical risks of the system; assisting with vendor selection and assessment, if applicable; assisting with specifying design and configuration; assisting with selecting and customizing the system; implementing technical solutions and system configuration required to comply with specified requirements; conducting IT/IS-related testing; assisting with the resolution of any test deviations; assisting with the preparation of the validation summary report; and assisting with ongoing maintenance and retirement of the system.

10.4.2.3 Quality Assurance and Compliance

QA and IT/IS Compliance personnel shall assist the System Owner with the definition of FDA requirements for the system and the assessment of risks associated with the intended use of a computerized system by providing compliance expertise related to CSV, 21 CFR Part 11, and any FDA predicate regulations applicable to the system. QA and IT/IS Compliance personnel must also ensure that internal policies and procedures are followed. In all cases, QA and IT/IS Compliance personnel must function independent of the activities that they ensure. Examples of QA and IT/IS Compliance activities might include the following: assisting with the definition of FDA-related electronic records created, modified, maintained, archived, retrieved, or distributed by the FDA-related computerized system; assisting with the definition of FDA-critical data entry fields within the FDA-related computerized system; assisting with the definition of signatures required by FDA rules for various system-related events, data fields, and electronic records for the FDA-related computerized system; assisting with the definition of quality control points that should be built into the software configuration design; assisting with vendor selection and assessment; ensuring that the validation documentation accurately and completely reflects the conduct of the validation; and ensuring that all deviations were appropriately documented and resolved. QA and Compliance personnel are also responsible for monitoring FDA-related computerized systems and associated validation documentation on a periodic basis for accuracy, completeness, and compliance with current FDA requirements.

> *Key Concept:* QA/Compliance personnel must be involved in validation in a role that is independent of the preparation of validation deliverables and conduct of the validation activities.

10.4.3 System Specification Phase

The System Specification Phase of the SDLC typically includes the following validation activities: documentation of system requirements specifications, assessment of vendors, initiation of documentation of the traceability matrix, and documentation of design and configuration specifications.

System Users and technical personnel, with the input of Quality/Compliance personnel, as necessary, must document the system requirements specifications defining users' needs and the intended uses of the system. This activity is one of the most critical of the SDLC, since without documented user needs and intended uses, it is impossible to confirm with objective evidence that the system can consistently meet them.

> *Key Concept:* Documentation of user requirements is an essential validation activity since without defined requirements it is difficult to build and then prove through testing that the system will adequately and consistently meet users' needs.

To specify user requirements, users must translate the business environment and business process in which the computerized system will be used into discrete system requirements. To specify technical requirements, technical representatives must translate the computing environment and data-processing flows into discrete system technical requirements. Of course, for FDA-regulated firms, the need to comply with 21 CFR Part 11 is inherent in the business environment. Therefore, Part 11 requirements must be specified for every computerized system used for FDA-related purposes.

Examples of system requirements specifications include, but are not limited to, the following: system inputs; features of data entry fields; system outputs in terms of reports and specific electronic records and associated metadata that will be created, modified, maintained, archived, retrieved, or distributed by the system; record signature requirements; query tools; functions the system will perform; system performance requirements; internal and external interfaces for software, hardware, and personnel; how users will interact with the system (e.g., security requirements, training requirements, etc.); error detection, reporting, and handling; computing operating environment (e.g., operating system, hardware platform, etc.); and ranges, limits, boundary values, and defaults for data fields and processing events.

Requirements must be specified such that they are unique, detailed, unambiguous, and directly traceable to system design. Vague or nonspecific requirements lead to imprecise system design and ultimately can result in a system that does not satisfy user needs. For example, a requirement simply specified as "The system must provide a computer-generated audit trail" does not provide the detail required to clarify how the audit trail is to be implemented. The likely result is that the software will, indeed, have an audit trail, but that the IT/IS personnel responsible for system configuration, in the absence of more information, will not know for which data fields or data flows the audit trail should be activated. After release of the system for use, users (and the FDA) might be shocked to discover that modifications of critical data were not captured in an audit trail because the audit trail was never turned on for that field.

> *Key Concept:* System requirements must be specified in a detailed and unambiguous way in order for the resulting system to conform to user needs and intended system uses.

Risk assessment must be integrated into requirements specifications. Each requirement should be assigned a criticality ranking based on its importance to the overall reliability, functionality, and integrity of the computerized system. The criticality ranking of requirements may be used to guide the selection of systems (e.g., in the case of vendor-supplied systems) and to guide the level of validation testing of the computerized system. The following risk matrix describes criticality rankings:

H = High criticality — A requirement with an associated risk that, if not met, has a predictably significant negative impact on product, patients, data, or business, having significant medium- to long-term negative impact and potentially catastrophic consequences. Requirements with high-criticality rankings are considered *essential* requirements (i.e., "must-haves").

M = Medium criticality — A requirement with an associated risk that, if not met, has moderate negative impact on product, patients, data, or business, having short- to medium-term detrimental effects. Requirements of medium criticality might be desired requirements that are not essential for core system functionality but that might enhance the overall performance or security of the system.

L = Low criticality — A requirement with an associated risk that, if not met, has a minor negative impact on product, patients, data, or business, having no long-term detrimental effects. Requirements of low criticality might be desired requirements that are not essential for core system functionality but that might improve by a lesser degree than medium-criticality requirements the overall performance or security of the system.

Example: In the detailed requirements specification, users should specify the types of electronic records (i.e., core electronic records and associated metadata) that will be created, modified, maintained, archived, retrieved, or distributed by the system. This list should include electronic records required by FDA predicate rules as well as electronic records not required by FDA regulations but that satisfy business needs. The list should also identify the data entry fields required to create these records. Using risk assessment, users then assign a criticality ranking to each electronic record and data entry field. These criticality rankings subsequently guide decisions regarding turning on computer-generated audit trail features when configuring software for use. For example, the users might decide that fields ranked with low criticality do not require audit trails, whereas fields with medium criticality require "silent audit" — i.e., the audit trails run without being visible to the user — and that fields ranked as highly critical, such as those capturing critical data in fulfillment of an FDA predicate rule, would require "active audit" — i.e., wherein the user is prompted to enter a reason prior to saving a modification or deletion of a data entry.

To avoid inappropriate risk assessments, or those that overlook significant risks, it is recommended that the risk assignments for both requirements and corresponding test scripts be determined through the collective input of System Owner and Users, IT/IS, and Quality/Compliance personnel.

Risk assessment decisions for system requirements must be documented. One option is to document these directly in the requirements specifications documents. Another format for doing so is in the Traceability Matrix. This document should be initiated following definition of system requirements and filled in as subsequent validation activities are performed. The Traceability Matrix typically links, in tabular form, each requirement and its assigned criticality ranking to its design specification, test scripts, and testing documentation. Once completed, this document shows that system requirements have been appropriately designed and that there is verifiable test evidence that they have been satisfied. The Traceability Matrix provides a comprehensive overview of the validation process that facilitates design reviews, facilitates Quality and Compliance audits of the system and validation documentation, allows ready retrievability of validation documentation that pertains to any given requirement, and facilitates change control and configuration management during the system maintenance phase.

> *Key Concept:* The Traceability Matrix provides a bird's-eye view of the approach and adequacy of the validation of a given computerized system.

Once requirements are defined and assigned their respective criticality rankings, the firm can begin the design and development process. Firms can choose to design and develop the software in-house or to purchase the primary software code from a vendor. It is becoming increasingly rare for pharmaceutical firms to develop custom or "bespoke" code in-house since many software solutions are available from external vendors, and development costs are frequently lower. If the firm chooses to purchase components of the computerized system from a vendor, the system requirements specifications should be incorporated into the Request for Proposal or equivalent document. The vendor's ability to meet the defined requirements, especially critical requirements, must be a deciding factor in determining whether to purchase the specific vendor's system or an alternative system. In addition, the pharmaceutical manufacturer must conduct an assessment of the vendor's quality practices and controls prior to purchasing the component. The Parenteral Drug Association's (PDA) Technical Report No. 32, *Auditing of Suppliers Providing Computer Products and Services for Regulated Pharmaceutical Operations* [23], provides a detailed approach to conducting and documenting these assessments. The level of detail of the vendor assessment should be commensurate with the overall system criticality.

The documentation of detailed system design and configuration specifications is necessary to properly construct and configure the system. Design and configuration specifications documents translate system requirements specifications into physical (i.e., computer hardware and equipment) and logical (i.e., software) representations of the system to be implemented. Typical elements in these documents include, but are not limited to, the following: software code design, including logical structure, controls, processing steps, and algorithms; data structures and data flows; definitions of variables; errors, alarms, and messages; software configuration (e.g., security profile configuration, audit trail configuration, system menu features and availability, etc.); supporting software; software interfaces; communication links; hardware design and configuration (i.e., assembly); equipment design and configuration; and network configuration design.

At the end of the design and configuration specification process, a design review should be conducted to confirm that the proposed design and configuration are correct, accurate, complete, consistent with the predefined requirements and intended use, and testable.

10.4.4 System Development Phase

During the system development phase of the SDLC, the computerized system components are constructed and tested, modules are assembled and tested, and the system is then fully assembled and tested. The types of testing conducted during development include unit testing, integration testing, and system-level testing, which are discussed in more detail in available references [12,14]. Software source code is also reviewed during this phase to evaluate its conformance with coding standards and the corresponding detailed design specifications document. Firms that purchase vendor-supplied systems would verify the adequacy of the vendor's development practices, including its testing and code and design review practices, during the vendor assessment.

10.4.5 Implementation and Testing Phase

Once the computerized system is successfully developed and tested from unit testing through system-level testing, it is released by the developers (to the firm from the vendor for vendor-supplied systems) for installation and qualification.

The goal of this phase of the SDLC is to obtain objective evidence, traceable to written specifications, that provides verification that the system is properly installed, the system operates throughout specified operating ranges, and the system is capable of performing or controlling the activities of the business processes it is required to perform or control while operating in its specified operating environment and will continue to do so under conditions of normal usage. In general, technical personnel perform installation and operational qualification, whereas users — who are trained in sufficiently detailed written procedures that define system use in the business environment — should execute tests of the system's ability to perform or control processes in the business production environment.

> *Key Concept:* User acceptance testing should be performed in the production environment by users trained in written procedures that define use of the system for FDA-related purposes.

As for all other phases of the SDLC, risk assessment must guide the scope and depth of qualification testing of the system. A somewhat common misperception of those outside the CSV field is the belief that qualification testing must repeat tests of each and every hardware and software feature. This is not realistic and would not provide returns commensurate with costs. The goal of all qualification testing is to obtain a "level of confidence" through the testing and collection of "objective evidence" that specified requirements implemented through the computerized system can be consistently fulfilled [12]. In general, the extensiveness of testing and the documentation of test results of an individual system requirement should be commensurate with the risk assigned to the requirement.

Qualification tests might include the following: verification tests (i.e., positive tests that demonstrate that the expected outcome is achieved); challenge tests (i.e., positive/range/boundary/negative testing) that prove the system responds properly to challenges (e.g., with error messages or denial of operation sequence); and stress, volume, load, or capacity tests that demonstrate the range or limits of system performance in the operating environment. Tests should be specified prior to the execution of the testing and include the predefined acceptance criteria for each.

Testers must document testing following good documentation practices, e.g., using indelible ink and making legible and attributable corrections when necessary. At the outset of testing, testers should document the test environment in a manner that is unambiguous and provides sufficient detail that creates a clear link between the description of the test environment and the individual test cases. This allows for future reconstruction of scenarios that produced a certain outcome and is most important or even vital when analyzing the causes of unexpected negative outcomes. Testers then document test results as they execute the tests, and a second party verifies these results. It is generally not sufficient to document the results of test sequences with only notations of "pass" or "fail" on the test sheet. Where common sense dictates, the firm must also substantiate test outcome with documented evidence (e.g., by creating a screen shot at the end of a test sequence or upon triggering computer-generated error messages, etc.).

> *Key concept:* Test results should be documented as testing occurs, substantiated with documented evidence, and verified by a second party.

Testers must document and resolve deviations of the actual test outcome from the expected outcome. Deviations should be addressed in accordance with a risk assessment approach that ensures that the system will not be released for FDA-related use until all deviations are defined and ranked by criticality, the impacts on data and the system are evaluated, and effective corrective actions are implemented in priority order. Attempts should be made to resolve system flaws revealed by test deviations in the following priority order: by implementing technical fixes, where possible; by disabling problematic features where technical fixes are not possible; and by implementing rigorous procedural controls (e.g., written procedures and training) for deviations for which technical fixes and disabling are not possible — with the caveat that the system must not be released for FDA-related use until all deviations determined to be critical are corrected through technical, rather than procedural, fixes.

> *Key Concept:* The system must not be released for FDA-related use until all test deviations are resolved adequately in accordance with risk.

Following the successful completion of qualification testing, and adequate resolution of deviations, the system may be released for FDA-related use. There should be a period of frequent or continuous post-go-live performance monitoring of the system that is commensurate with the overall system criticality and inherent risks. For large, complex systems, this might warrant preparation and execution of a protocol to monitor the day-to-day use of the system for predetermined parameters, with defined specifications measured at predefined intervals over a sufficient period of time (e.g., 6 months to 1 year following release into production environment for critical global systems). After the firm has obtained objective evidence that the system performs appropriately under the rigors of everyday use, monitoring can be done on a more periodic basis.

> *Key Concept:* There should be a period of frequent or continuous post-go-live performance monitoring of the system that is commensurate with risk.

10.4.5.1 Validation Summary Report

Once all aspects of the Validation Plan have been successfully executed, a Validation Summary Report should be developed and submitted to Quality Assurance/Compliance personnel and Management. This document should summarize all validation activities and deliverables set forth in the Validation Plan and provide a concluding statement of the outcome of the validation project. Most importantly, this report, or equivalent documents, should provide a summary of deviations that occurred during testing that includes a full listing of all deviations, an assessment of the criticality of each, the impact of each on data and the system, a full description of corrective actions taken and of the adequacy of the resolution of each, and, where applicable, the justification for releasing the system with these deviations and selected corrective actions or workarounds, where applicable. The Validation Summary Report represents a valuable tool for documenting and assessing the robustness of both the CSV project and the FDA-related computerized system.

10.4.5.2   System Maintenance Phase

The firm must have written procedures that govern the ongoing maintenance of the system. Some of the procedures will be specific for the system, while others, such as those procedures listed in Section 10.3, would apply more generally to all computerized systems. Examples of system-specific procedures might include, but are not necessarily limited to, those addressing the following: use of the system for FDA-related purposes; supervisory review of the system's FDA-related electronic records and necessary metadata (such as audit trails); end-user administration and control of the system (including requests to grant or revoke user access, security within user work areas, end-user training on system use, reporting errors and incidents, requesting changes to the system, etc.); and technical administration, support, and maintenance of the system (including security rights administration, performance monitoring, change control, configuration management, electronic records management, disaster recovery, etc.).

During this phase, in order not to jeopardize the "validation status" of the computerized system, all changes to software, hardware, instruments, equipment, and documentation must adhere to risk-based change control and configuration management procedures. QA/Compliance personnel should periodically review the validation documentation and system change control and configuration management documentation to ensure that the system is being maintained in a controlled manner according to these procedures. In addition, QA/Compliance should routinely review incident logs to determine whether system-related incidents are being adequately resolved and whether there is a pattern of system-related incidents that might indicate potentially larger, systemic quality system issues or failures.

> *Key Concept:* Just as reviews of product complaint logs and product adverse-event records provide insight to the quality of a product released to market, reviews of computerized system change control logs and computerized system incident logs provide insight to the ongoing "health," i.e., robustness and control, of a computerized system.

10.4.5.3   System Retirement Phase

If users determine over time that the system is no longer needed or should be replaced, they must ensure that the system is formally retired in a manner that ensures that the system is effectively removed from user access and that FDA-related electronic records from the system — and any necessary contextual information such as metadata and related systems documentation — are maintained in a readily retrievable manner throughout the records retention period set by applicable FDA predicate rules. The firm should have written procedures that set forth general requirements for this process.

The personnel functional roles and responsibilities for system retirement generally correspond to those assigned during the early phases of the particular system's SDLC and are, at least in part, based on system criticality. Risk assessment must also be applied to system retirement activities to ensure that they are commensurate with the criticality of the system and its associated electronic records. Typically, a retirement plan should be developed that describes the detailed steps for retirement of specific systems, especially critical systems. The retirement plan includes such elements as a system overview and summary of the system's history; the plan for storage and retrieval of the system's electronic records and associated metadata, including plans for data migration and conversion to new systems or formats and/or plans for maintenance of necessary hardware/software to retrieve records; roles and responsibilities for organization, review, and storage of systems documentation (such as user manuals, validation documentation, system configuration documentation, etc.); and the plan for the physical and logical removal of the system from user access. The successful execution of the retirement plan should be summarized, along with any deviations and their resolutions, and reported to management.

10.5 CONCLUSION

Validation of a computerized system ensures that it operates reliably and consistently over time to the satisfaction of users, management, regulators, and ultimately patients who are treated with biopharmaceuticals produced through processes that require the direct or indirect use of the computerized system. When performed using a risk-based approach and in a culture that fosters commitment to computerized system compliance, CSV adds value to the product and process that is commensurate with cost. Moreover, a sound CSV program encourages the introduction of new and exciting technologies with the ultimate promise of safer, more effective, and more affordable medicines.

DEFINITIONS

Change Control — The process of ensuring that a computerized system remains validated following a change. It includes assessing the impact of the change and performing appropriate activities to ensure that the system remains in a validated state.

Coding Standards — Written procedures describing coding (i.e., programming) style conventions specifying rules governing the use of individual constructs provided by the programming language, and naming, formatting, and documentation requirements that prevent programming errors, control complexity and promote understandability of source code.

Computerized System — An organized set of hardware, software, networks, equipment or instruments, and supporting procedures and documentation that is used to create, modify, maintain, archive, retrieve, or transmit, in digital form, information related to the performance of one or more business functions. A computerized system might be a stand-alone unit or consist of several interconnected units. Computerized systems include, but are not necessarily limited to, desktop systems, client/server systems, software-driven instruments or equipment, and Web-based systems.

Computerized Systems Validation — Confirmation by examination and provision of objective evidence that computerized system specifications conform to user needs and intended uses and that all requirements can be consistently fulfilled.

Configurable Software Packages — Software systems that permit users to develop their own applications by configuring/amending predefined software modules.

Configuration Control — An element of configuration management consisting of the evaluation, coordination, approval or disapproval, and implementation of changes to configuration items after formal establishment of their configuration identification.

Configuration Specification — Specification of the configuration parameters of the system in its intended, fully configured operational environment, i.e., in the production environment.

Design — The process of defining the architecture, components, interfaces, and other characteristics of a system or component of the system.

Design Qualification (DQ) — The documented verification that the proposed design of facilities, systems, and equipment is suitable for the intended purpose.

Design Specification — Specification of the design of the architecture, components, interfaces, and others characteristics of a system or system component.

Disaster Recovery Plan — A written plan to ensure that systems can be re-created from backup data in the event that primary system hardware, software, and supporting facilities are unavailable or destroyed or when supporting personnel are unavailable.

Electronic Record — Any combination of text, graphics, data, audio, pictorial, or other information representation in digital form that is created, modified, maintained, archived, retrieved, or distributed by a computer system.

Electronic Signature — A computer data compilation of any symbol or series of symbols executed, adopted, or authorized by an individual to be the legally binding equivalent of the individual's handwritten signature.

FDA-Related Computerized System — Computerized system that creates, modifies, maintains, archives, retrieves, or distributes electronic records in fulfillment of any of the requirements of any U.S. Food and Drug Administration (FDA) regulation or that are intended for submission to the FDA under the requirements of the United States Federal Food, Drug, and Cosmetic Act and the Public Health Service Act, even if such electronic records are not specifically identified in FDA regulations.

Handwritten Signature — The scripted name or legal mark of an individual handwritten by that individual and executed or adopted with the present intention to authenticate a writing in a permanent form. The act of signing with a writing or marking instrument such as a pen or stylus is preserved. The scripted name or legal mark, while conventionally applied to paper, may also be applied to other devices that capture the name or mark.

Installation Qualification (IQ) — The documented verification that the computerized system components are delivered as designed and specified and that all key aspects of hardware and software installation adhere to appropriate specifications and manufacturer's requirements.

Integration Testing — An orderly progression of testing in which system components (hardware, software elements, materials, procedures, etc.) are combined and tested, to evaluate whether system components interact as expected, until the entire system has been integrated and tested.

Metadata — Electronic data ancillary but essential to the reconstruction of the creation or handling of the electronic records for which the computerized system is primarily used. Examples of metadata include electronic audit trails, electronic data libraries, system configuration files, etc.

Off-the-Shelf Software (OTS) — A generally available software component used by a pharmaceutical manufacturer for which the pharmaceutical manufacturer cannot claim complete software life cycle control.

Operational Qualification (OQ) — The documented verification that the computerized system operates as specified throughout representative or anticipated operating ranges.

Performance Qualification (PQ) — The documented verification that the computerized system is capable of performing or controlling the activities of the processes it is required to perform or control, as specified, throughout all anticipated operating ranges while operating in its normal operating environment (i.e., in the production environment).

Predicate Rule Requirements — Requirements set forth in the United States Federal Food, Drug, and Cosmetic Act, the Public Health Service Act, or any U.S. Food and Drug Administration (FDA) regulation.

Production Use — Using the system in the fully configured operational environment to support FDA-related activities.

Raw Data — Any worksheets, records, memoranda, notes, or exact copies thereof that are the result of original observations and activities and which are necessary for the reconstruction and evaluation of a work project, process, study report, or other FDA-regulated activity. Raw data may be hard/paper copy or electronic but should be known and defined in system procedures. Copies of electronic records must be accurate and complete, i.e., contain all associated metadata.

Reliability — The ability of a computerized system or component to perform its required functions under stated conditions for a specified period of time.

Structural Testing — Verification that program code, databases, and configurable system components were developed and configured using good software engineering practices and in accordance with design specifications.

System Development Life Cycle (SDLC) — A methodology that encompasses activities for a computerized system to be selected, designed, developed, implemented, maintained, and eventually retired.

Unit Testing — The testing of individual or a limited number of functions within the system in isolation. Paths through the code might be tested, including calculations. It includes stress testing of input fields (e.g., boundary testing, invalid data entry). Unit testing is generally conducted to verify the implementation of the design for one or a limited number of software elements (i.e., a unit or module).

REFERENCES

1. U.S. Food and Drug Administration, Guide to Inspection of Computerized Systems in Drug Processing (The Blue Book), Washington, February 1983.

2. U.S. Food and Drug Administration's Electronic Freedom of Information Reading Room, Warning Letters and Responses, URL: http://www.fda.gov/foi/warning.htm.

3. Title 21, Code of Federal Regulations, Part 11, Electronic Records; Electronic Signatures; Final Rule, 62 Federal Register 13430, March 1997.

4. Petition submitted to FDA by Pharmaceutical Research and Manufacturers of America, November 30, 1999, available at www.fda.gov.

5. U.S. Food and Drug Administration, Pharmaceutical Current Good Manufacturing Practices (cGMPs) for the 21st Century: A Risk-Based Approach, URL: http://www.fda.gov/cder/gmp/index.htm; a two-year initiative launched on August 21, 2002.

6. U.S. Food and Drug Administration, Guidance for Industry, Part 11, Electronic Records; Electronic Signatures — Scope and Application, August 2003.

7. Health Insurance Portability and Accountability Act of 1996, Public Law 104-191, One Hundred and Fourth Congress, Washington, D.C., April 21, 1996.

8. Sarbanes-Oxley Act of 2002, One Hundred and Seventh Congress, Washington, D.C., January 23, 2002.

9. Quinn, T., The Hollis Group C3Q™ Methodology for Qualifying Network Infrastructure, available at www.hollisgroup.com.

10. Huber, L., Best Practices: Network Quality Package, Vol. 2.1, August 5, 2003, available at www.networkcompliance.com.

11. U.S. Food and Drug Administration, Draft Guidance for Industry, 21 CFR Part 11; Electronic Records; Electronic Signatures — Glossary of Terms, August 2001 (withdrawn).

12. U.S. Food and Drug Administration, General Principles of Software Validation; Final Guidance for Industry and FDA Staff, Center for Devices and Radiological Health, January 2002.

13. U.S. Food and Drug Administration, Glossary of Computerized System and Software Development Terminology, Division of Field Investigations, Office of Regional Operations, Office of Regulatory Affairs, August 1995.

14. Good Automated Manufacturing Practice (GAMP) Guide for Validation of Automated Systems in Pharmaceutical Manufacture, version 4.0, GAMP Forum, International Society for Pharmaceutical Engineering (ISPE), Tampa, FL, December 2001.

15. Technical Report No. 18, Validation of computer-related systems, *PDA J. Pharm. Sci. Technol.*, 49, January–February 1995.

16. International Committee on Harmonisation (ICH) Tripartite Guideline E6, Good Clinical Practice: Consolidated Guideline, 62 Federal Register 25691, May 1997.

17. U.S. Food and Drug Administration, Draft Guidance for Industry: Computerized Systems Used in Clinical Trials, Revision 1, September 2004.

18. Technical Report No. 31, Validation and Qualification of Computerized Laboratory Data Acquisition Systems, *PDA J. Pharm. Sci. Technol.*, 53, June 1999.

19. U.S. Food and Drug Administration, Guidance for Industry, ICH Q7A Good Manufacturing Practice Guidance for Active Pharmaceutical Ingredients, Center for Drug Evaluation and Research, Center for Biologics Evaluation and Research, August 2001.

20. U.S. Food and Drug Administration, Guidance for Industry, FDA Reviewers and Compliance on Off-the-Shelf Software Use in Medical Devices, Center for Devices and Radiological Health, September 1999.

21. U.S. Food and Drug Administration, Guidance for the Content of Pre-Market Submissions for Software Contained in Medical Devices, Center for Devices and Radiological Health, May 1998.

22. ISO 14971-1:1998, Medical Devices — Risk Management — Part 1: Application of Risk Analysis, International Organization for Standardization, 1998.

23. Technical Report No. 32, Auditing of Suppliers Providing Computer Products and Services for Regulated Pharmaceutical Operations, PDA Committee, October 1999.

11

Process Optimization and Characterization Studies for Purification of an *E. coli*-Expressed Protein Product

ANURAG S. RATHORE

CONTENTS

11.1 INTRODUCTION

Use of recombinant proteins as human therapeutics has increased over the past several years. These proteins are often obtained from fermentation of microorganisms, such as *E. coli*. Following initial release of the crude product from the host cell by homogenization, the resulting solution contains species such as other bacterial host cell proteins (HCPs), nucleic acids (DNA and RNA), endotoxin, and other host cell impurities [1,2]. The challenge often in process development is to design a process that can purify the protein of interest from these impurities, to be consistent with current Good Manufacturing Practices (cGMP), and to ensure product safety [3,4]. Unless DNA and HCPs are cleared during processing and reduced to acceptable levels (typically ng/mg for HCPs and pg/mg for DNA), the product is unlikely to be used for clinical or commercial purposes [1,5]. These issues, combined with the presence of other product-related impurities that have very similar physicochemical properties to the product, make purification of the target molecule a challenge.

In view of these issues, designing an optimal purification process is often a complicated and multiphase procedure that involves a careful consideration of the numerous factors that may impact the quality (safety) and quantity (yield) of the final product [6–11]. Another key output of process development studies at small scale is to ensure the robustness of each process step prior to its transfer to a manufacturing facility [12–15]. This is often achieved by performing the so-called process characterization studies.

In this chapter, an approach is presented to efficiently and successfully perform process development studies to result in an "optimal" and a "robust" process. This is achieved through presentation of a case study of process development performed for a chromatographic step used to purify a protein product expressed in *E. coli* [11,15]. The focus of this chapter is to differentiate between process "optimization" and "characterization" and to emphasize careful planning and execution of the small-scale studies that often precede a successful attempt at process validation. Chapters 3 and 4 have addressed the topics of process characterization and scale-down modeling in greater detail.

11.2 AN APPROACH TO PROCESS DEVELOPMENT

This section describes an approach to develop a purification process. The overall philosophy is illustrated in Figure 11.1. The input to this effort is a process that had not been optimized and has been used to make early clinical supplies. The output is a robust and characterized process that could be successfully scaled up for manufacturing Phase III and commercial supplies. It is seen that process development following this approach is performed in two steps, namely process optimization and process characterization. The objectives of these two steps are an optimal and a robust process, respectively.

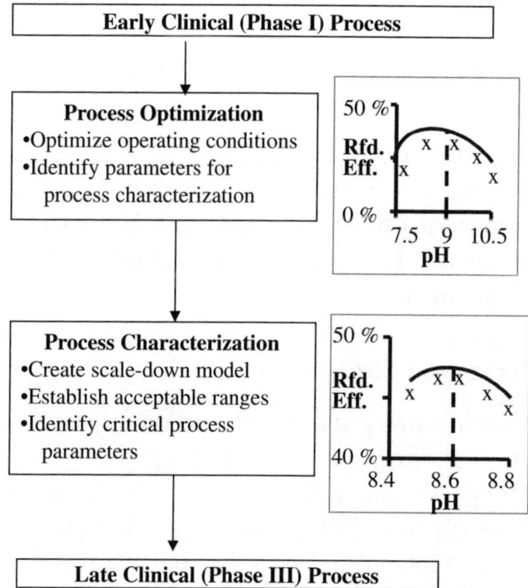

Figure 11.1 Illustration of an approach for process development.

In this discussion, acceptable range (AR) is defined as the range in which the process parameter can vary without having an unacceptable impact on the performance criteria for the process step, such as quality of the product, clearance of an impurity/additive, or recovery of the process step. AR is typically determined from small-scale studies in the laboratory. Operating range (OR) is defined as the range in which a process parameter varies from lot to lot. OR is generally the range that is included in the batch records for the manufacturing process. In this study, critical process parameters (CPP) are defined as those parameters for which AR < 2 × OR.

11.2.1 Process Optimization Studies

As illustrated in Figure 11.1, the two key objectives for these studies are as follows:

- Optimize operating parameters for the chromatographic steps.
- Identify "key" process parameters that require further characterization.

In order to achieve this, experiments are performed such that each parameter is varied over a wide range and its effect on the step yield and elution pool purity is examined. For example, as illustrated in Figure 11.1, pH for the refold step is varied between 7.5 to 10.5 units.

11.2.2 Process Characterization Studies

In these studies, experiments are performed and each parameter is varied over a narrow range, determined by the variation typically seen at large scale, and its effect on the step yield and pool purity is examined. For example, as illustrated in Figure 11.1, pH for the refold step is varied between 8.6 ± 0.2 units to allow for 8.6 ± 0.1 pH unit variation at large scale.

As mentioned previously, selection of "key" parameters for process characterization is performed based on data obtained from process optimization studies. Depending on the abundance and type of data available, some kind of a risk assessment analysis might be valuable. Hazard Analysis and Critical Control Points (HACCP), Failure Mode and Effects Analysis (FMEA), and cause-and-effect diagrams are some of the tools that could be used effectively for this purpose [16].

The key objectives for characterization studies are as follows:

- Create scale-down model for performing process characterization studies.
- Establish acceptable ranges for all "key" process parameters.
- Generate list of "critical" process parameters (CPP) for use during process validation.

It should be noted that while characterization studies result in a more optimal process, robustness and not optimization is the focus for these experiments. It is also evident from Figure 11.1 that in contrast to process optimization, characterization is performed on fewer process parameters (deliverable from process optimization studies) and experiments test a relatively narrow variation in process parameter (determined by variation seen at large scale). Further, as the outputs of the characterization studies feed into the validation protocol in the form of the CPP, it is critical that these studies are performed using a "scale-down" model of the process and analytical methods that have undergone appropriate qualification.

11.3 EXPERIMENTAL

11.3.1 Process Chromatography Procedures

A general flowchart for the process, which was used to produce early clinical supplies, is shown in Figure 11.2. Recombinant *E. coli* were grown, and the protein subunit was produced as insoluble inclusion bodies within the cells. The inclusion bodies were isolated by repeated homogenization and centrifugation and the protein subunit was solubilized with urea and refolded. The refold solution was filtered and directly loaded onto a cation exchange (CE) column for removal of endotoxin, misfolded monomer, and aggregates of the product. This is followed by an anion exchange (AE) column for further removal of endotoxin, host cell protein (HCP), misfolded monomer, and aggregated forms of the product. Two intermediate ultrafiltration/diafiltration (UF/DF) steps were utilized for concentrating protein and for buffer exchange. Finally, 0.2-mm filtration was performed, and the resulting bulk protein solution was stored frozen at −70°C. A detailed description of the process can be found elsewhere [11,15].

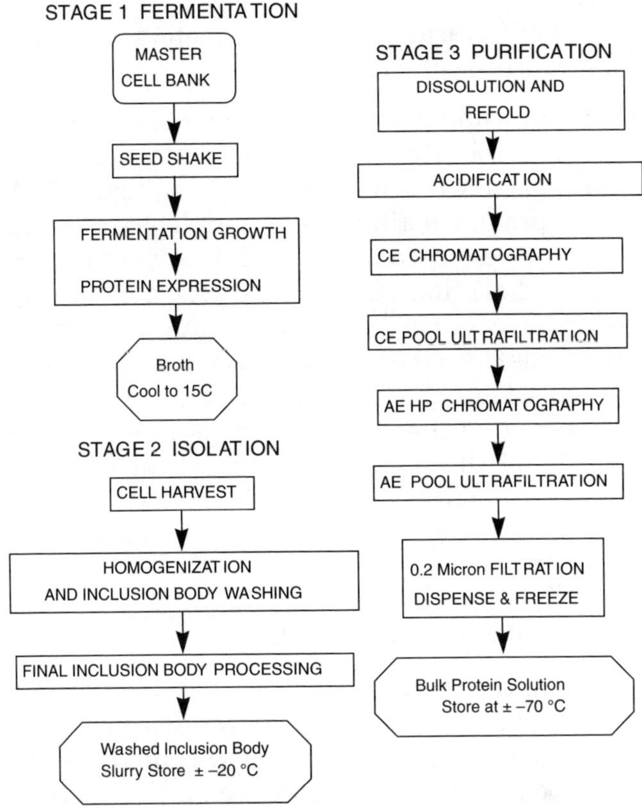

Figure 11.2 Overall process flowchart. (Adapted from Rathore, A.S., Chromatographic process development for purification of a recombinant *E. coli*-expressed protein, in *Scale-Up and Optimization in Preparative Chromatography*, Rathore, A.S. and Velayudhan, A., Eds., Marcel Dekker, 2002, pp. 317–338. With permission.)

Experiments were performed at room temperature using 10-ml columns. Figure 11.3 illustrates the column dimensions, buffers, procedures, linear flow velocities, gradient slopes, and other operating conditions for the Q column. The two columns were run and the resulting fractions were analyzed by a variety of analytical tools, which are described in the following section.

11.3.2 In-Process Analytical Methods

Several different analytical methods were used during development and characterization of the purification process. These included RP-HPLC, SE-HPLC, AE-HPLC, CE-HPLC, and UV absorbance at 280 nm (A280).

11.3.2.1 Ultraviolet Spectroscopy at A280

Since proteins show significant absorbance at 280 nm, their concentration can be estimated based on the UV absorbance at 280 nm in the absence of other A280-absorbing species. The extinction coefficient for this product is 0.98 $(mg/ml)^{-1}$ $(cm)^{-1}$.

11.3.2.2 Size-Exclusion HPLC (SE HPLC)

This method separated the product homodimer from monomeric, truncated, and aggregated forms. The method used a TosoHaas G2000SWxl column (30 cm × 7.8 cm) with 100 mM sodium phosphate, dibasic, and 350 mM ammonium sulfate, pH 7.0, as the mobile phase with detection at 280 nm.

11.3.2.3 Anion-Exchange HPLC (AE HPLC)

This method resolves product from various impurities, such as endotoxin, HCP, aggregate forms, and some product-related impurities based on charge differences. The method used a TosoHaas TSK-Q5PW column (7.5 mm × 75 mm) with 50 mM Tris buffer, pH 8.8, and bound protein was eluted with a linear NaCl gradient with detection at 280 nm.

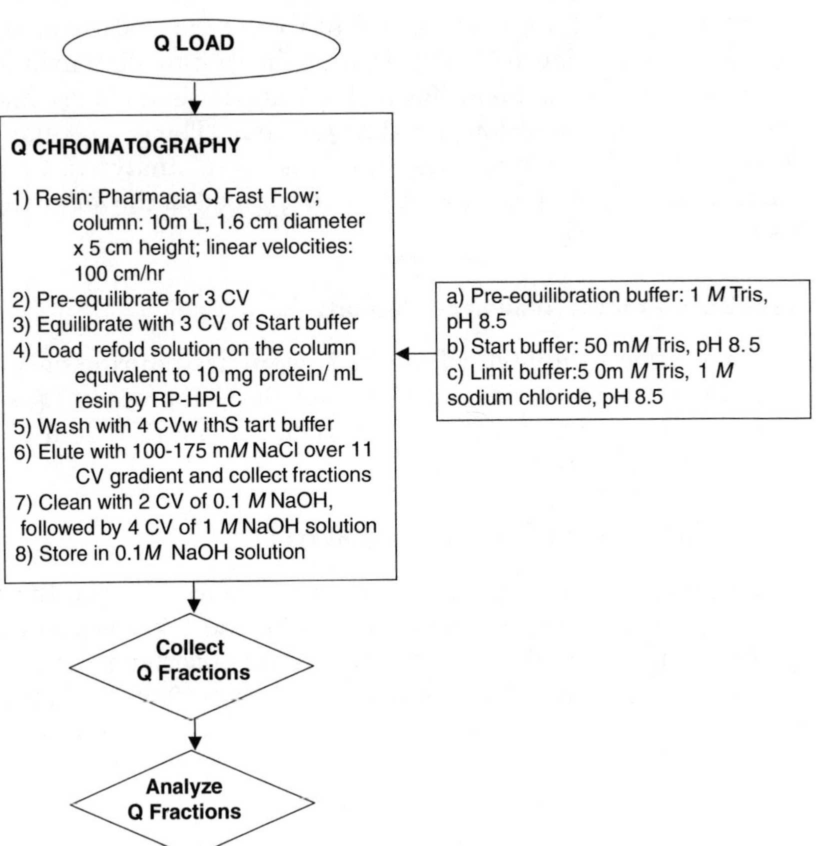

Figure 11.3 Operating procedure for the Q column. (Adapted from Rathore, A.S., Chromatographic process development for purification of a recombinant *E. coli*-expressed protein, in *Scale-Up and Optimization in Preparative Chromatography*, Rathore, A.S. and Velayudhan, A., Eds., Marcel Dekker, 2002, pp. 317–338. With permission.)

11.3.2.4 Cation-Exchange HPLC (CE HPLC)

This method separated product from various impurities, such as endotoxin, host cell proteins (HCP), aggregates, and product-related impurities. The analysis used a Dionex ProPac WCX-10 column (4 mm × 250 mm) with 50 mM sodium acetate, pH 5.25, as the mobile phase, and bound protein was eluted with a linear NaCl gradient with detection at 280 nm.

11.3.2.5 Reversed-Phase HPLC (RP-HPLC) of Reduced Samples

RP-HPLC of reduced samples was used as a quantitative measure of the total amount of product present. The samples were reduced and denatured by treatment with a solubilizing solution (0.4 M DTT, 4% SDS, and 0.8 M Tris; 900 µl sample plus 100 µl solubilizing solution) and analyzed on a Vydac C4 column (#214TP54, 4.6 mm $\times$ 150 mm, 5 mm particle size) at room temperature. A gradient of acetonitrile/water in the presence of 0.1% trifluoroacetic acid was used for performing the separation with detection at 210 nm.

11.4 PROCESS OPTIMIZATION STUDIES

The objective of these studies was to result in an "optimal" process that is suitable for manufacturing the product at large scale. This was achieved by following a multistep approach. First, parameters were identified for each unit operation for which process optimization studies will be performed. This selection is typically based on our scientific understanding of the unit operation and its role in the process and prior experience with the unit operation during manufacture of preclinical supplies. Second, experiments were performed and each process parameter was varied over a wide range and its effect on the step yield and pool purity was recorded. Third, data were analyzed and optimal operating conditions for each unit operation were chosen.

Resin selection plays a central role in performance of a chromatography column. Hence, an extensive resin screening was performed using an approach that was published recently [10]. Nine resins — Pharmacia Q Fast Flow®, Pharmacia Q High Performance®, Pharmacia DEAE Fast Flow®, Whatman QA52, Whatman Q, Whatman DE53, Bio-Rad High Q, Bio-Rad DEAE, and TosoHaas Q650M — were screened for the AE column. Two parameters, product recovery and pool purity, were used to evaluate resin performance. Product recovery was defined as the sum of product peak areas (in mAU) in the pooled fractions per milliliter of injected sample. Pool purity was defined as the purity of the total pool formed by combining the fractions that meet the pooling criteria. The optimal resin found for the AE column was the Pharmacia Q-Sepharose High Performance® resin [10,11].

Once the resin had been chosen, it was decided to evaluate the effect of pH, conductivity, protein loading, flow velocity, load concentration, temperature, bed height, and gradient slope on performance of the column [11]. In the following, some of the results obtained from these experiments are presented for the second chromatographic step, i.e., the Q column.

The Q column is primarily involved in removal of HCP, aggregates, and product-related impurities. Separations were performed following the procedure illustrated in Figure 11.3, and clearance of the different host cell impurities is shown in Table 11.1. It is seen that the Q column plays an important role in reducing the HCP levels to acceptable levels.

Figure 11.4 and Figure 11.5 show purity (on y-axis) of the various Q column fractions (on x-axis) for a typical run as determined by analysis by SE-HPLC and AE-HPLC, respectively [11]. The shaded areas show the pooled fractions. As seen in Figure 11.4, the Q column removes the aggregated form, the monomer, and the truncations from the dimer. The pooling criterion for the development studies was that the

TABLE 11.1 Clearance of Host Cell Impurities by Q Column*

Process Stream	Endotoxin** (EU/mg product)	HCP** (ng/mg product)
Q Load	<1	106
Q Pool	<1	<25

* Adapted from Reference 15.
**Numbers are an average of 5 different pilot scale lots.

purity of a pooled fraction should be >85% by CE-HPLC or >95% by AE-HPLC. The Q pool and the Q load samples were analyzed by RP-HPLC for measuring the quantity of the product and, thus, the step yields were calculated.

As mentioned previously, the effects of pH, conductivity, protein loading, flow velocity, temperature, bed height, and gradient slope on performance of the Q column were evaluated. Some of the results are shown in Table 11.2. Experiments were conducted at loading/elution flow velocities of 50/50, 100/100, and 200/200 cm/hr. It was observed that recovery and pool purity of the Q column show a significant dependence on the flow velocity. As seen in Table 11.2, as the flow velocity was increased from 50 to 100 cm/hr, the recovery fell from 54 to 49 mAU/ml and pool purity from 91 to 87%. A further increase in the flow velocity to 200 cm/hr caused a sharp deterioration in the quality of separation, and none of the fractions met the pooling criteria. In order to get optimized separation, it was decided to perform the separation at loading and elution flow velocity of 50 cm/hr.

Experiments were also conducted to explore the range of protein loading (3–10 mg protein/ml resin) and gradient slope (100–175, 80–200, and 50–220 mM NaCl over 11 CV). As seen

TABLE 11.2 Optimization of Chromatographic Conditions for Q Column (Pharmacia Q HP resin)*

	Flow Velocity, cm/hr			Protein Loading, mg/mL		Gradient Slope, mM NaCl/CV		
	50	100	200**	3	10	100–175	80–200	50–220
Recovery, mAU/mL (by CE HPLC)	54	49	0	49	44	100***	84***	71***
Pool purity, % (by CE HPLC)	91	87	0	87	87	98***	98***	98***

* Adapted from Reference 15. The shaded areas denote conditions chosen as optimal for step operation.

**None of the fractions met the pooling criteria.

***Analysis was done by AE-HPLC.

in Table 11.2, it was observed that the increase in protein loading from 3–10 mg/ml was accompanied by a slight loss in recovery (from 49–44 mAU/ml). However, the recovery exhibited a sharp decrease upon increasing the gradient slope (from 100–71 mAU/ml). As a result, protein loading of 9 mg protein/ml resin and gradient of 100–175 mM NaCl over 11 CV were chosen as final operating conditions.

Further, experiments were performed to scout pH range 8.0–9.5. It was observed that the selectivity between the various components decreased at pH 8.0 in comparison to pH 8.5. Also, at pH 9.0 some precipitation of the product was observed indicating that the protein was not stable at this pH. Based on these results, pH 8.5 was chosen as the pH for operating the Q column. Effects of load conductivity and bed height on Q column performance were also investigated, and these parameters were not found to have any significant effect within the ranges studied.

Based on these results, pH of the Q load, pH of the equilibration and elution buffers, and gradient slope were chosen as parameters that would require further characterization. Since this was an ion-exchange polishing step, load conductivity was also included for further investigation to ensure robustness of this process step. Flow velocity, despite being shown to significantly affect the recovery, was not identified for process characterization as the chosen operating velocity of 50 cm/hr was well below 100 cm/hr, which was shown to deliver acceptable column performance.

11.5 PROCESS CHARACTERIZATION STUDIES

It follows from Figure 11.4 and Figure 11.5 that the resulting Q pool has all the impurities reduced to 2% level. The criteria for pooling the fractions for the Q column for the process characterization studies were changed to 0.80 mg/ml protein concentration by A280 and 90% purity of the fraction by AE-HPLC.

Table 11.3 summarizes the results obtained during characterization studies of the Q Sepharose HP Column. Based on historical ranges, we defined the column performance to

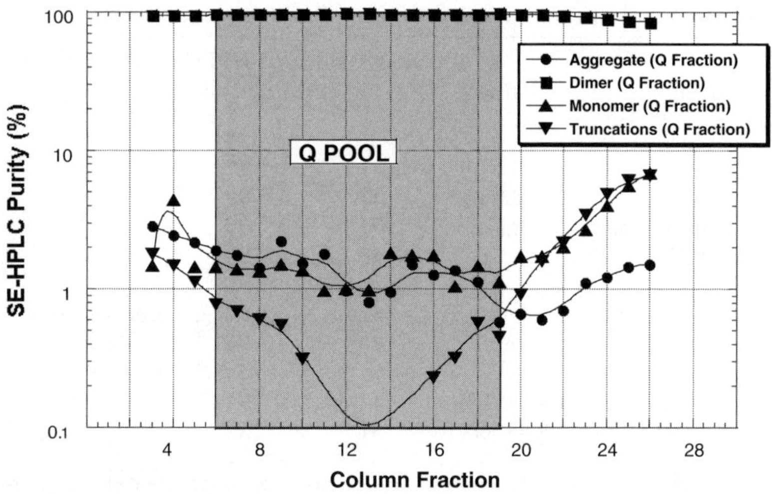

Figure 11.4   Purity of Q column fractions by SE-HPLC.

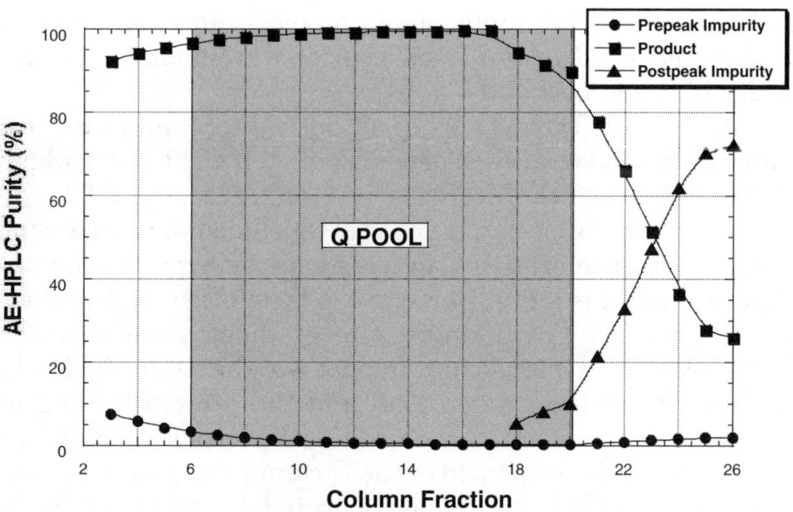

Figure 11.5   Purity of Q column fractions by AE-HPLC.

TABLE 11.3 Summary of Q Column Characterization*

Variable	Value	Step Yield %	AE-HPLC Purity, %	Acceptable Range
PH of Q load	8.7	4l9	94	**
	8.5	51	92	
	8.3	39	92	
pH of equilibration and elution buffer	8.7	51	92	**
	8.3	43	93	
Conductivity of Q load	Control	51	92	Control to Control +10%
	+10%	47	95	
Gradient slope (mM NaCl/ # of CVs)	100–175/9	44	94	**
	100–175/11	51	92	

* Adapted from Reference 15. Column performance is unacceptable if changing the parameter leads to a >15% change in Q column step yield or a >5% change in Q Pool purity.

**Need reevaluation after the operating ranges in the manufacturing plant are known.

be unacceptable if changing a parameter led to a >15% change in the step yield of the Q column or a >5% change in the purity of the Q pool.

As seen in Table 11.3, pH of both the column load and buffers led to a significant decrease in step yield, particularly at low pH. Since the decrease in step yield at pH 8.3 was >15%, the column performance was concluded to be unacceptable. Importance of pH in an ion-exchange separation when high resolution is a requirement has been observed by others as well [12,14]. Furthermore, the gradient slope was also found to have a significant impact on the step yield. The conductivity of the column load and the protein loading on the column, however, were found to have only a marginal effect both on the step yield of the Q column and on the purity of the Q pool. This too is corroborated by other published studies [12].

Based on the results obtained from process characterization, pH of Q column load, pH of equilibration and elution buffer, and gradient slope were identified as CPP. As mentioned earlier in Section 11.2, these parameters will be monitored during process validation runs at scale.

11.6 SUMMARY

This chapter presents an approach to efficiently and successfully perform process development studies to result in an "optimal" and a "robust" process. The approach for process development of the Q column step, as summarized in Figure 11.6, is a two-step process.

First, process optimization studies are performed to evaluate the effect of process parameters that have been chosen for that unit operation. This is achieved by varying each process parameter in a wide range to allow for identification of optimal operating conditions for the unit operation, as well as identification of "key" parameters that would require further process characterization. As seen in Figure 11.6, these

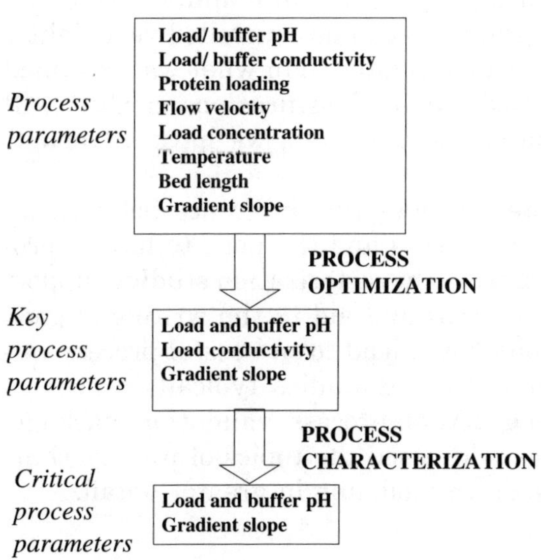

Figure 11.6 Illustration of process development approach.

studies identified three parameters for further characterization from a total of eight that were examined. At the end of this step, we have an "optimal" process.

Second, process characterization studies are performed to evaluate the effect of "key" parameters that have been identified during process optimization. This is achieved by varying each process parameter in a relatively narrow range, based on the operating range for that parameter. The final result is establishment of the acceptable ranges for the different parameters and identification of "critical" process parameters (CPP). This information is then specified in the process validation protocol, and monitoring and control of these critical parameters is demonstrated at full scale during process validation. As seen in Figure 11.6, out of the three "key" parameters identified by the process optimization studies, two of them — namely, load/buffer pH and gradient slope — were identified as "critical" process parameters. It is expected that these parameters will need to be further examined after their operating ranges at the manufacturing site are known. If these parameters can be controlled very tightly at full scale (operating range tighter than what was assumed for small-scale analysis), their classification as CPP will be reexamined. At the end of this step, we have a "robust" process.

I hope this chapter clarifies the difference between an "optimal" and a "robust" process and the need to have a process that is both. The process characterization studies support the robustness of the process and aid in the writing of good validation protocols that would lead to successful process validation. Documentation of these studies typically serves as strong support for the actual process validation package. Chapters 3 and 4 have addressed the topics of process characterization and scale-down modeling in greater detail.

ACKNOWLEDGMENT

The work presented here is a compilation of previously published studies [11,15,17] and was performed at Pharmacia Corporation, Chesterfield, MO.

REFERENCES

1. O'Keefe, D.O., DePhillips, P., and Will, M.L., Identification of an *Escherichia-coli* protein impurity in preparations of a recombinant pharmaceutical, *Pharm. Res.*, 10, 975–979, 1993.

2. Wilson, M.J., Haggart, C.L., Gallagher, S.P., and Walsh, D., Removal of tightly bound endotoxin from biological products, *J. Biotechnol.*, 88, 67–75, 2001.

3. Briggs, J. and Panfili, P.R., Quantitation of DNA and protein impurities in biopharmaceuticals, *Anal. Chem.*, 63, 850–859, 1991.

4. Rathore, A.S., Sobacke, S.E., Kocot, T.J., Morgan, D.R., Dufield, R.L., and Mozier, N.M., Immunological methods of analysis for residual host cell proteins and DNA in process streams from a purification of an *E. coli* expressed product, *J. Pharm. Biomed. Anal.*, 32, 1199–1211, 2003.

5. de Oliveira, J.E., Soares, C.R.J., Peroni, C.N., Gimbo, E., Camargo, I.M.C., Morganti, L., Bellini, M.H., Affonso, R., Arkaten, R.R., Bartolini, P., Ribela, M.T.C.P., High-yield purification of biosynthetic human growth hormone secreted in the *Escherichia coli* periplasmic space, *J. Chromatogr. A*, 852, 441–450, 1999.

6. Sofer G. and Hagel, L., Purification design, optimization and scale-up, in *Handbook of Process Chromatography — A Guide to Optimization, Scale-up and Validation*, Academic Press, New York, 1997, pp. 27–113.

7. Wisniewski, R., Boschetti, E., and Jungbauer, A., Process design considerations for large-scale chromatography of biomolecules, in *Biotechnology and Biopharmaceutical Manufacturing, Processing, and Preservation*, Avis, K.E. and Wu, V.L., Eds., Interpharm, Buffalo Grove, 1996, pp. 61–198.

8. Sofer G. and Mason, C., From R&R to production: Designing a chromatographic purification scheme, *Bio/Technology*, 5, 239–244, 1987.

9. Chung, B.H., Choi, Y.J., Yoon, S.H., Lee, S.Y., and Lee, Y.I.J., Process development for production of recombinant human insulin-like growth factor-I in *Escherichia coli*, *Ind. Microbiol. Biotech.*, 24, 94–99, 2000.

10. Rathore, A.S., Resin screening to optimize chromatographic separations, *LC-GC*, June, 2–15, 2001.

11. Rathore, A.S., Chromatographic process development for purification of a recombinant *E. coli* expressed protein, in *Scale-up and Optimization in Preparative Chromatography*, Rathore, A.S. and Velayudhan, A., Eds., Marcel Dekker, 317–338, 2002.

12. Kelley, B.D., Jennings, P., Wright, R., and Briasco, C., Demonstrating process robustness for chromatographic purification of a recombinant protein, *BioPharm*, October, 36–47, 1997.

13. Martin-Moe, S., Ellis, J., Coan, M., Victor, R., Savage, J., Bogren, N., Leng, B., Lee, C., Burnett, M., and Montgomery, P., Validation of critical process input parameters in the production of protein pharmaceutical products: A strategy for validating new processes or revalidating existing processes, *PDA J. Pharm. Sci. Tech.*, July/August, 315–319, 2000.

14. Seely, R.J., Hutchins, H.V., Luscher, M.P., Sniff, K.S., and Hassler, R., Defining critical variables in well-characterized biotechnology processes, *BioPharm*, April, 33–36, 1999.

15. Rathore, A.S., Process characterization of the chromatographic steps in the purification process of a recombinant *Escherichia coli* expressed protein, *Biotechnol. Appl. Biochem.*, 37, 51–61, 2003.

16. Seely, R., Munyakazi, L., and Haury, J., Statistical tools for setting in process acceptance criteria, *BioPharm*, 14, 28–34, 2001.

17. Rathore, A.S. and Velayudhan, A., Guidelines for optimization and scale-up in preparative chromatography, *Biopharm*, January, 34–42, 2003.

12

Validation of the ZEVALIN® Purification Process — A Case Study

LYNN CONLEY, JOHN MCPHERSON, AND
JÖRG THÖMMES

CONTENTS

12.1 INTRODUCTION AND SCOPE

In this chapter, a case study is presented that describes validation of a purification process for a therapeutic monoclonal antibody. ZEVALIN is a radiolabeled monoclonal antibody for the treatment of several types of non-Hodgkin's lymphoma. The monoclonal antibody is expressed and secreted by Chinese hamster ovary (CHO) cells. The treatment dosage is substantially lower than that of unlabeled antibody treatments because only a small amount of radiolabeled antibody is needed to irradiate and destroy tumor cells. Since ZEVALIN is such a low-dosage drug, only a few production lots were required to satisfy product needs for phase I/II and phase III clinical trials. This posed substantial challenges for process validation due to the fact that only very few data points from manufacturing-scale campaigns were available to design a process validation. The intention of this chapter is to describe an approach to deal with the challenge of setting acceptance criteria for process validation based on limited manufacturing-scale experience. In this regard, the scenario outlined subsequently may be considered a typical one for low-dosage biopharmaceuticals.

One of the most recent definitions of process validation is found in ICH Q7A, which defines process validation as "documented evidence that the process, operated within established parameters, can perform effectively and reproducibly to produce an intermediate or active pharmaceutical ingredient (API) meeting its predetermined specifications and quality attributes" [1]. Various regulatory documents refer to concepts of process validation and provide guidance for process validation [1–3]. Validation should extend to those operations determined to be critical to the quality and purity of the API [1]. Among the quality attributes that should be considered are chemical purity, qualitative and quantitative impurity profiles, physical characteristics, and microbial quality [3]. The critical process parameters are those that are most likely to affect the quality attributes. They should be determined by sound scientific judgment and should typically be based on research, scale-up, or manufacturing experience [1]. Critical process parameters should be controlled and monitored during process validation studies. Process validation studies should confirm that the impurity profile for each API is comparable to or better than historical data and, where applicable, comparable to or better than the profile determined during process development or for batches used for pivotal clinical and toxicological studies. In this chapter, we will discuss the strategy used to validate the ZEVALIN purification process. The validation of the purification process encompassed a broad range of activities such as removal of host impurities (protein and DNA), non-host-related impurities (Protein A, insulin, methotrexate, urea, endotoxin, and bioburden), chromatographic adsorbent reuse lifetime, filter chemical compatibility and extractable studies, viral evaluation and characterization of the purification process, and establishment of in-process hold times.

The ZEVALIN purification process starts from harvested cell culture fluid (HCCF) and concludes with purified bulk drug substance (BDS). Validation of process steps converting the bulk drug substance to the drug product is not addressed in this chapter. The ZEVALIN purification process from HCCF to BDS consists of seven purification operations, which include three chromatography steps, two ultrafiltration and diafiltration steps, one viral nanofiltration step, and one low-pH inactivation. Figure 12.1 schematically outlines the process. The first purification step is Protein A affinity chromatography, which removes most of the process-related impurities, host cell protein, DNA, and cell culture media components. This step is followed by the tangential-flow ultrafiltration/diafiltration (TFF) step to concentrate and buffer exchange the intermediate product in preparation for anion exchange chromatography. This step primarily removes DNA. The next operation, hydrophobic interaction chromatography, removes aggregated antibody and serves as a polishing step for HCP and DNA removal. The final step comprises tangential flow ultrafiltration/diafiltration to concentrate and buffer exchange the product into the BDS formulation buffer. The in-process intermediate products pools are 0.2-μm filtered at each step of the process to control microbial burden.

12.2 CHARACTERIZATION STUDIES

12.2.1 Outline and Definitions

During the development of the ZEVALIN purification process, critical process parameters were identified and operating ranges resulting in optimal purity and yield were established. Generally, operational parameters are defined as controllable input (independent) variables that define how the process is to be run. These parameters and their operating ranges are

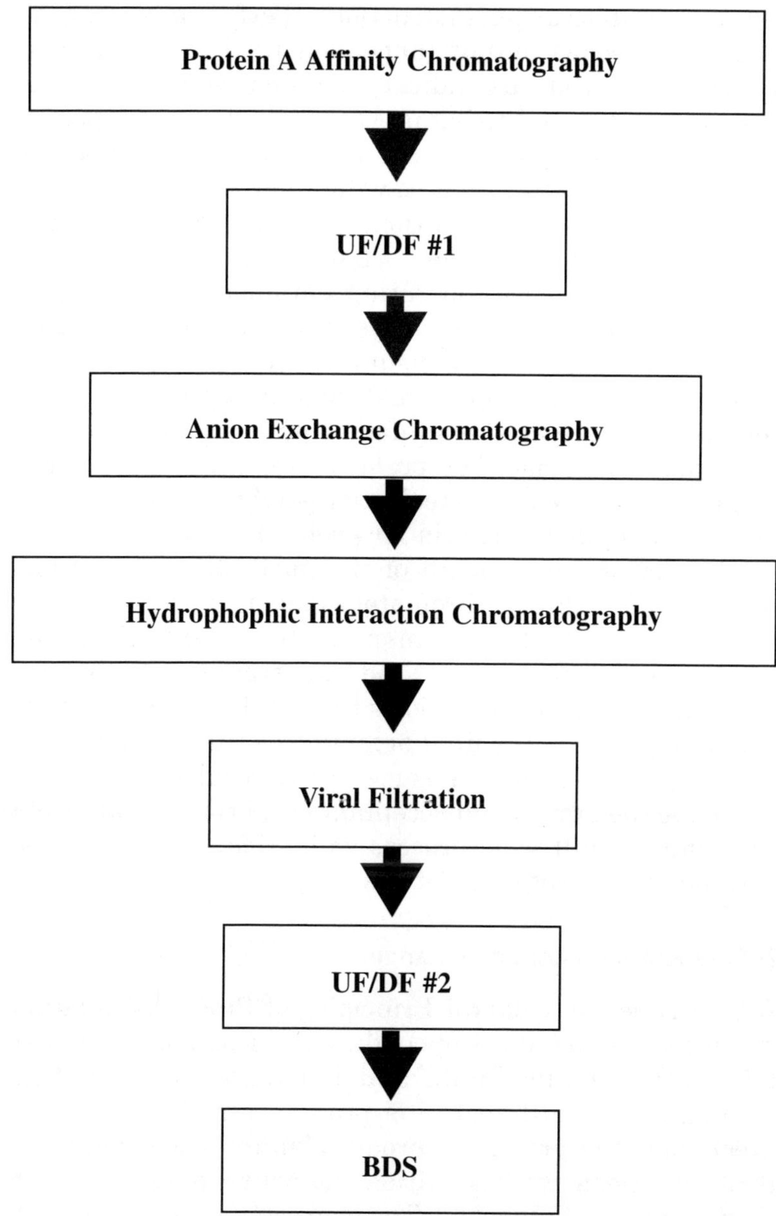

Figure 12.1 The Zevalin purification process.

stated in manufacturing instructions. Performance parameters are defined as output (dependent) variables (such as yield and purity) that are indicators of how well a unit operation functioned [4,5]. During process validations, the performance parameters have to meet predetermined acceptance criteria for a prospective process validation. In preparation of the ZEVALIN process validation, a small-scale study was performed to characterize the variability of the performance parameters when critical operating parameters were tested at the center of and slightly beyond the normal operating range. This was intended to ensure that the process was not operated at the edge of failure. Additionally, it provided a data set for assessing potential manufacturing excursions from the normal operating range. The performance parameter ranges from this small-scale characterization study were used to set provisional acceptance criteria for preliminary full-scale process validation studies for all of the purification operations from Protein A affinity chromatography to viral filtration. Pursuing this concept, agreement of the results from the preliminary full-scale process validation studies with the provisional acceptance criteria allows the provisional acceptance criteria to be used as the final acceptance criteria for process validation protocols. In case some of the results were found to be outside the provisional acceptance criteria, the data from the preliminary full-scale process validation studies may be used to set the acceptance criteria.

12.2.2 Operating Parameter Ranges

FDA Guidelines on General Principles of Process Validation define *worst case* as "a set of conditions encompassing upper and lower processing limits and circumstances including those within standard operating procedures, which pose the greatest chance of process or product failure when compared to ideal conditions. Such conditions do not necessarily induce product or process failure" [2]. The characterization study was designed considering FDA definitions of *worst case*, in which the upper and lower operating ranges were evaluated. Similar to the approach outlined by Smith et al. [6], three sets of experiments were performed: one at the set point or center of the operating range, as well as one each at the upper and lower operating limit. Each step in the purification process, from the Protein A affinity chromatography to viral filtration, was evaluated in this manner. The upper operating limit from each step was predicted to have the lowest yield and was defined as worst-case conditions based on previous development data. The lower maximum operating range was predicted to have the highest yield and was defined as best case in terms of yield. All of the upper limit experiments for each process step were "forward linked," resulting in the worst-case process run as discussed by Gardner et al. [5]. Lower-limit experiments and center points were treated in a similar fashion. Table 12.1 summarizes the normalized critical operating parameters evaluated in the small-scale study.

12.2.3 Small-Scale Characterization Study Results

Yield and purity were evaluated as two relevant performance parameter categories. The step yield under best, worst, and set point case conditions shown in Figure 12.2 shows that for both Protein A and UF/DF#1, only minor variations (4%) were found. The three other steps followed the expected trend with the worst-case conditions resulting in the lowest yield. Six assays were performed to determine purity, with four assays evaluating product-related impurities and two assays evaluating process-related impurities. In this context, product-related impurities are defined as molecular variants of the desired product that do not have properties comparable to the desired product with respect to activity, efficacy, and safety. Process-related impurities are defined as substances that may be derived from cell culture, cell substrates, or downstream processing [7]. The product-related assays chosen were SDS-PAGE and Size Exclusion HPLC, both assessing molecular weight variants; cation exchange HPLC, assessing charge variants; and a competitive binding assay, assessing binding activity. The SDS-PAGE and Size Exclusion HPLC assays also detected process-related impurities in the harvested cell

TABLE 12.1 Normalized Critical Operating Parameters of the Zevalin Purification Process

Protein A	Worst Case	Set Point Parameters	Best Case
Fluid velocity	$1.05 \times X$ cm/hr	X cm/hr	$0.95 \times X$ cm/hr
pH	$X - 0.2$	X	$X + 0.2$
Loading capacity	$1.2 \times X$ mg/ml	X	$0.56 \times X$ mg/ml

Viral Inactivation	Extreme #1	Typical Parameters	Extreme #2
pH	$X - 0.15$	X	$X + 0.15$
Time	$X + 8$ hr	X hr	$X - 15$ hr

UF/DF #1 – UF	Extreme #1	Typical Parameters	Extreme #2
UF cross-flow	$X - 20$ l/m²/hr	X l/m²/hr	$X + 20$ l/m²/hr
TMP	$X + 3$ psi	X psi	$X - 3$ psi
Mass/surface area	$0.75 \times X$/m²	X g/m²	$1.25 \times X$ g/m²
Concentration	$0.75 \times X$ mg/ml	X mg/ml	$1.25 \times X$ mg/ml
NaCl adjustment	$X - 50$ mM	X mM	$X + 50$ mM
DV	$1.1 \times X$	X	$0.9 \times X$
DF cross-flow	$X - 20$ l/m²/hr	X l/m²/hr	$X + 20$ l/m²/hr
TMP	$X + 1.5$ psi	7 psi	$X - 1.5$ psi

Anion Exchange	Extreme #1	Typical Parameters	Extreme #2
Fluid velocity	$1.1X$ cm/hr	X cm/hr	$0.9X$ cm/hr
pH	$X + 0.1$	X	$X - 0.1$
Loading capacity	$1.5 \times X$ mg/ml	X mg/ml	$0.56 \times X$ mg/ml

HIC	Extreme #1	Typical Parameters	Extreme #2
Fluid velocity	$1.1 \times X$ cm/hr	X cm/hr	$0.9 \times X$ cm/hr
pH	$X - 0.1$	X	$X + 0.01$
Loading buffer	$X + 50$ mM	X mM	$X - 50$ mM
Equil/wash buffer	$X - 50$ mM	X mM	$X + 50$ mM
Loading capacity	$1.44 \times X$ mg/ml	X mg/ml	$0.5 \times X$ mg/ml

Viral Filtration	Extreme #1	Typica Parameters	Extreme #2
Concentration	$2 \times X$ mg/ml	X mg/ml	$0.5 \times X$ mg/ml
Filtration pressure	$X + 0.2$ psi	X psi	$X - 0.2$ psi
Mass/surface area	$1.66 \times X$ mg/cm²	X mg/cm²	$0.5 \times X$ mg/cm²

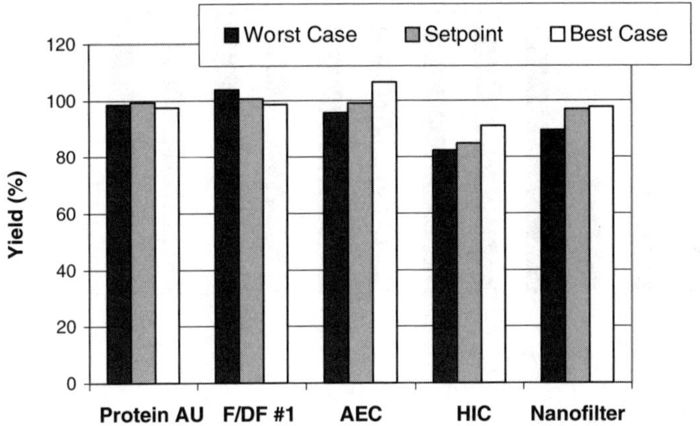

Figure 12.2   Characterization study results evaluating yield for best-case, set point, and worst-case conditions for each process step.

culture fluid and Protein A eluate. When the ZEVALIN purity after the different purification operations was measured using SDS-PAGE, CIEX-HPLC, and binding activity, best, worst, and set point case conditions resulted in similar results at each step. The data variability observed was within the expected precision of the assay. Therefore, these performance parameters were not included in the full-scale process validation protocols. As shown in Figure 12.3, the Size Exclusion HPLC (SEC) assay results from the small-scale characterization studies varied greater than the expected precision of the assay, and therefore this performance parameter was included in each purification process step validation protocol. Host cell DNA and host cell proteins (HCP) were chosen as process-related impurities and monitored throughout the small-scale characterization. For all purification operations, trends could be observed; therefore, these performance parameters were moved forward into the full-scale studies. The acceptance criteria for most in-process product pools for DNA and HCP concentration during the full-scale process validation protocol were based on four standard deviations from the mean of the characterization study. Four standard deviations were used

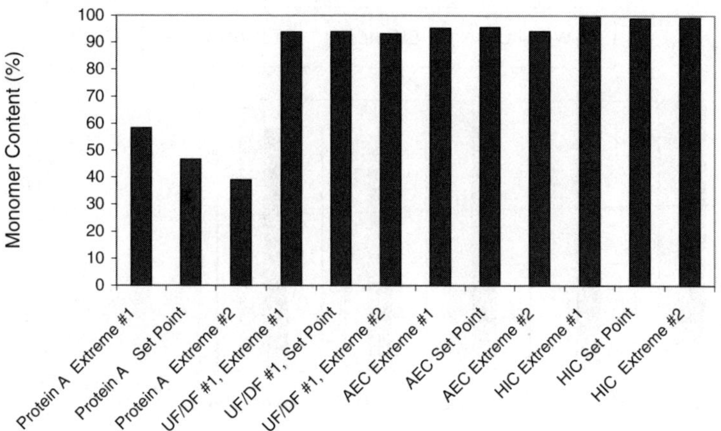

Figure 12.3 Characterization study results evaluating the monomer content for best-case, set point, and worst-case conditions for each process step.

to encompass all the process variation based on the small sample size of three purifications runs.

The acceptance criteria for monomer content in the Protein A eluate were based on 2.5 standard deviations of the mean for the characterization study and preliminary full-scale runs. The combined data set was used since a broad range of results was observed in the characterization study. Due to the increased number of samples available for this parameter, the acceptance criteria could be set using 2.5 standard deviations of the mean.

Characterization studies were also performed for removal of Protein A, insulin, urea, and endotoxin for chromatography steps, endotoxin inactivation, in-process hold times, and filter chemical compatibility. These preliminary studies provided an understanding of the expected process performance ranges under certain operating conditions and resulted in a data set to define predetermined acceptance criteria for prospective process validation protocols at both full and small scale.

12.2.4 Small-Scale Process Validation Studies

Process validation studies were performed at either full or small scale depending on the purpose of the study. Small-scale process validation studies, generally performed prior to full scale, were conducted to demonstrate the capability of the process when challenged with contaminants or process extremes in terms of extended reuse or hold times for in-process product, buffers, filters, and chromatography absorbents. The small-scale process validation studies were intended to complement the full-scale studies by providing additional understanding of the purification process. Small-scale process validation studies for ZEVALIN can be placed into two categories: contaminant spiking studies (virus, endotoxin, and urea) and extended-time or reuse studies (chromatographic adsorbent reuse lifetime studies, filter chemical compatibility and extractables studies, product stability hold time, and solution hold times). Contaminants are defined as any adventitiously introduced materials (e.g., chemical, biochemical, and microbial species) not intended to be part of the manufacturing process of the drug product or drug substance [7]. The spiking studies were performed using small-scale systems since introducing contaminants at full scale is undesirable for worker safety and would affect the quality of the product. In spiking studies, each contaminant was spiked into the in-process product at ≤10% concentration since a higher spike could affect the process step's ability to perform its intended function. The spiked process steps were performed using representative operating process parameters, and the processes were evaluated for their ability to remove or inactivate the contaminant.

The extended-time or reuse process validation studies were performed to demonstrate in-process product and buffer stability, as well as to ensure that the filters and adsorbents can be reused for several cycles. Scale-down was qualified to ensure that results from small-scale studies reliably predicted the performance of full-scale systems. Qualification of small-scale chromatography, TFF, and filtration systems is discussed in the next section of this chapter.

12.2.5 Qualification of Scale-Down Models

12.2.5.1 Introduction

As a typical example of small-scale validation work, systems used for viral clearance studies will be used to demonstrate the concept of scale-down models. In order to show how such models are qualified as representative of the full-scale manufacturing process, viral clearance studies for hydrophobic interaction chromatography (HIC) and nanofiltration will serve as an example from ZEVALIN process validation.

Prior to initiation of the viral clearance studies, blank and mock runs were performed for both chromatography and filtration steps. The blank runs (runs performed without a viral spike) qualified the scale-down model as being representative of the full-scale manufacturing process. In addition, mock runs (runs spiked with 5% [v/v] viral storage solution but no virus) were performed to demonstrate that the viral storage solution does not have a negative effect on the starting material or the performance of the small-scale model. Upon completion of the runs, samples were analyzed to determine product recovery, and the results were compared to data established during development and characterization of the purification process. The samples from these runs were also analyzed for purity by SEC-HPLC (monomer content) and SDS-PAGE. These results were compared with either development or manufacturing standards.

12.2.5.2 Hydrophobic Interaction Chromatography

Scale-down of chromatography operations typically is achieved by keeping certain critical parameters constant. These are bed height and fluid velocity (which determine the residence time in the column) as well as the ratio of process fluid volume to column volume in each step. This ensures that the column load (in milligrams of product per milliliter of adsorbent) as well as the equilibration, wash, and elution volumes (in column volumes) are kept constant across scales. Typically, scale-down is achieved by reducing the column diameter and thereby reducing the absolute column volume and amount of product consumed. The comparability of the packing quality of the column is usually measured by the height equivalent of a theoretical plate (HETP). During the small-scale studies, comparability was attained by ensuring that the specifications for this parameter are met at both scales. In addition, the chromatography runs were performed using released raw materials and components and using product load pools from full-scale production lots.

Table 12.2 shows the process parameters used during the HIC study. By keeping both bed height and fluid velocity constant, an identical residence time was achieved over a scaling factor of 1700. The column loading was maintained and column packing integrity was demonstrated by HETP values of less than 0.1 cm.

The overall product recovery, SEC-HPLC analysis (monomer content), and SDS-PAGE were chosen as performance parameters to evaluate whether the small-scale performance was within the full-scale manufacturing ranges. Table 12.3 summarizes step yield and purity comparison by monomer content and SDS-PAGE. The yield obtained during the small scale, blank, and mock runs (98–99%) was within two standard deviations of the full scale (92 ± 10%). The proportion of monomeric antibody (96%) was within two standard deviations of the commercial scale (98 ± 2). The SDS-PAGE results were comparable at both scales.

TABLE 12.2   Hydrophobic Interaction Chromatography Operational Parameters

Parameter	Scaled Down	Commercial
Scale-down factor	1700	NA
MAb load amount	7.8 mg/ml	≤7.8 mg/ml
Load and wash fluid velocity	100 cm/hr	100 cm/hr
Bed height	15 cm	15–16 cm
MAb load concentration	1.5 mg/ml	≤1.5 mg/ml
Temperature	17–26°C	15–26°C

TABLE 12.3 Performance Parameters of the Hydrophobic Interaction Chromatography at Small and Commercial Scale

	Yield	Monomer Content	SDS-PAGE
Commercial scale	92 ± 11%	98.8 ± 0.4%	Compares to reference
Blank runs/ mock spiked runs	91%	98–99%	Compares to reference

As a final proof of comparability, representative chromatograms of blank and mock small-scale runs were compared to full-scale chromatograms (Figure 12.4). The chromatograms can be regarded as comparable with the exception of the absolute values of the absorption at 280 nm, which is shown on the abscissa. The absorption at 280 nm is influenced by the concentration of absorbing species in the fluid as well as by the optical path length of the detection unit, which is higher in a commercial-scale chromatography unit in order to allow preparative volumetric flow. Hence, the absolute absorption values of the commercial-scale chromatograms cannot be expected to be identical.

12.2.5.3 Nanofiltration

Scale-down of the nanofiltration step was accomplished by maintaining the ratio of protein load per membrane surface area, the proportion of wash buffer to surface area, operating temperature, and the load pressure. Parameters relevant to the scale-down of nanofiltration and parameters considered critical to the operation of the process are shown in Table 12.4.

The product recovery, SEC-HPLC analysis, and SDS-PAGE were chosen as performance parameters. Table 12.5 summarizes the step yield, proportion of monomeric antibody, and SDS-PAGE purity results. The product recovery obtained from the small-scale, blank, and mock runs (99–100%) corresponded to the expected yield at commercial scale (>95%). The proportion of monomeric antibody for the blank run (100%) was comparable to commercial scale (99%). The monomer content measured after the mock run (96%) was slightly

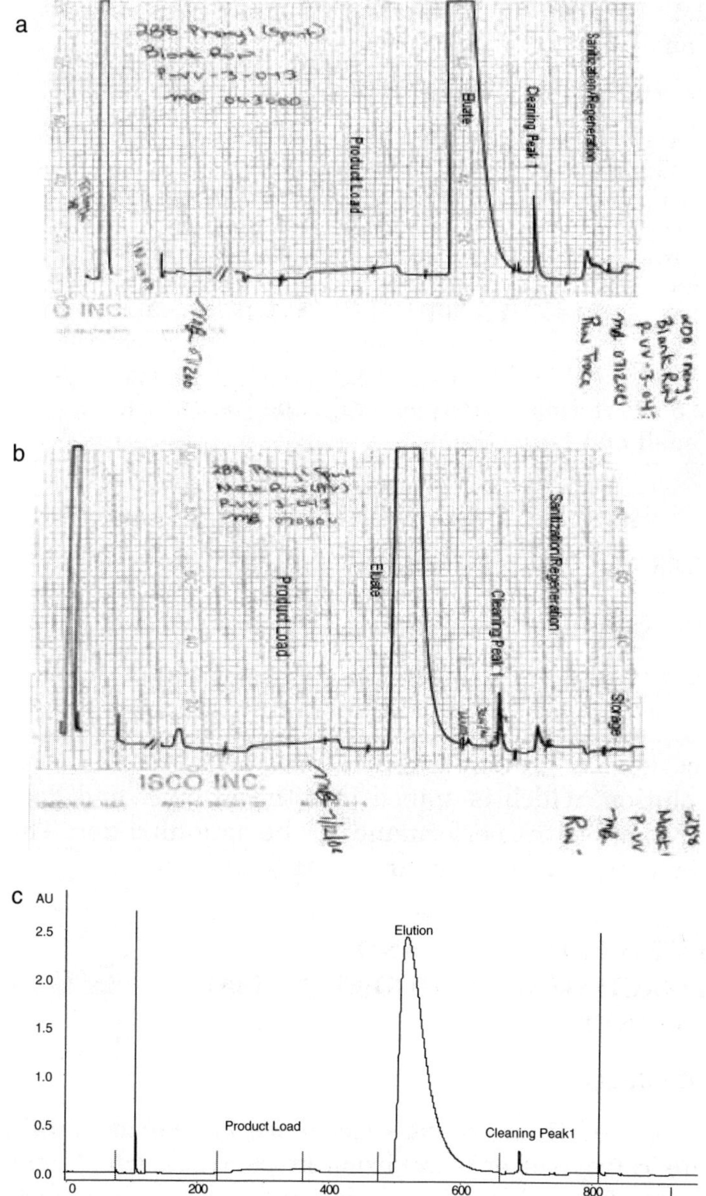

Figure 12.4 Comparison of blank (a) and mock (b) small-scale chromatograms with commercial-scale (c) chromatograms of the hydrophobic interaction chromatography step.

TABLE 12.4 Nanofiltration Operational Parameters
at Small and Commercial Scale

Parameter	Scaled Down	Commercial
Membrane area	10 cm^2	16,000 cm^2
Scale-down factor	1600	NA
Equilibration buffer	Identical	Identical
MAb load concentration	0.80–0.82 mg/ml	<0.7 mg/ml
Load pressure	15 ± 1 psi	<15 psi
Mass/surface area	10 mg/cm^2	≤10 mg/cm^2
Temperature	15–26°C	15–26°C

TABLE 12.5 Performance Parameters of the Nanofiltration
Step at Small and Large Scale

	Step Yield	Monomer Content	SDS-PAGE
Commercial Scale	>95%	99%	NA
Blank runs/ mock spiked runs	99–100%	95[a]–100%	Compares to reference

[a] Mock run.

reduced because a protein stabilizer was added to the viral
storage solution, which is spiked into the product and does
not appear to affect the performance of the nanofiltration. The
SDS-PAGE results were comparable at both scales.

12.3 PROCESS EVALUATION AND CHARACTERIZATION STUDIES OF VIRAL CLEARANCE

12.3.1 Introduction

Cell lines derived from rodent species are known to contain
endogenous retrovirus or retrovirus-like particles, which may
be infectious (C-particles) or noninfectious (cytoplasmic A-
and R-particles) [8]. The potential risk of viral presence in
the ZEVALIN producer cell line was assessed by quantifying
the amount of retrovirus in the HCCF. Transmission electron

microscopy (TEM) performed on harvested cell culture fluid shows less than 1.3×10^5 retrovirus-like particles per milliliter from an "end of production" sample. The current "Points to Consider in the Manufacturing and Testing of Monoclonal Product for Human Use" states that negative TEM results should result in the assumption that the virus titer is equivalent to the lowest limit of detection (1×10^6 particles/ml). The number of retrovirus-like particles per milliliter observed in the "end of production" was less than the detection limit of the assay, and this specific sample defines the viral load of the process material. In light of this known virus load, the capability of a purification process to clear viruses has to be demonstrated. Small-scale clearance studies were performed concurrent to ZEVALIN manufacturing for this purpose. The objective of the viral clearance studies was to ensure the capability of inactivating and removing not only noninfectious endogenous retrovirus, but also a broad spectrum of virus classes, members of which could potentially contaminate the process materials. Viruses for the clearance studies were chosen to resemble agents that can enter the manufacturing processes via a number of routes and may therefore be present in the harvested cell culture fluid (HCCF). These viruses exhibit a wide range of physicochemical properties, providing a robust challenge to the ability of the purification process to clear potential infectious virus.

The following model viruses were chosen:

- Xenotropic murine leukemia virus (MuLV) — Specific model retrovirus for the noninfectious retrovirus-like particles seen in CHO cells, RNA virus, 80–110 nm, low physicochemical resistance, model virus used to evaluate product viral safety
- Pseudorabies virus (PRV) — Nonspecific model virus, enveloped double-stranded DNA virus, 150–250 nm, medium physicochemical resistance, model virus used to characterize the robustness of the process
- Reovirus type 3 (Reo-3) — Nonspecific model virus, nonenveloped double-stranded RNA virus, 60–80 nm,

medium physicochemical resistance, model virus used to characterize the robustness of the process

- Porcine parvovirus (PPV) — Nonspecific model virus, nonenveloped DNA virus, 16–26 nm, high physico-chemical resistance, model virus used to characterize the robustness of the process

The ZEVALIN purification process was designed to provide both viral inactivation and viral removal capabilities. Four steps in the manufacturing process were chosen for the viral challenge studies: the low-pH hold step immediately following affinity chromatography, the anion exchange and hydrophobic interaction chromatography steps, and the nanofiltration step. The model viruses used to assess the clearance capability of each operation were selected based on the potential contribution of that step to the overall clearance for that class of virus. Therefore, not all steps were challenged with all viruses. Process intermediates were evaluated for cytotoxicity and viral interference for each of the test systems, resulting in recommendations for appropriate dilutions for testing. Additionally, studies to evaluate the potential for inactivation of the chosen model viruses by sanitizing solutions used on Protein A, anion exchange, and hydrophobic interaction chromatography adsorbents were performed.

Viral clearance studies were performed in duplicate using scaled-down replicas of the commercial purification process. As discussed in the previous chapter, the relevant scale-down and critical operation parameters were conserved to ensure that the small-scale viral clearance studies were representative of the commercial process. All of the in-process intermediates used in these viral clearance studies were taken from commercial manufacturing product pools.

A 5% virus spike was added to the starting material before performing each chromatography and nanofiltration operation. A 10% spike was added to the starting material for the low-pH inactivation and the evaluation of the sanitization agents.

Virus reduction factors, R, for an individual inactivation or removal step were calculated as follows:

$$R = \log_{10}(v_1 c_1/v_2 c_2) \text{ or } \log_{10}(v_1 c_1) - \log_{10}(v_2 c_2) \text{ [9]} \quad (12.1)$$

where

> R is the reduction factor
> v_1 is the volume of the starting material
> c_1 is the concentration of the virus in the starting material
> v_2 is the volume of the postprocessing material
> c_2 is the concentration of the virus in the postprocessing material

Guidelines [12] also state that 95% confidence limits (interval) for reduction factors should be calculated whenever possible in clearance studies for "relevant" and specific "model" viruses. The confidence interval should be calculated for the reduction factor as follows:

$$CV = \pm\sqrt{S^2 + A^2} \quad (12.2)$$

where S^2 is the confidence interval for the starting material and A^2 is the postprocessing confidence interval.

12.3.2 Virus Inactivation

12.3.2.1 Low-pH Treatment Subsequent to PROSEP A Column Chromatography

Low-pH treatment of product at pH <4.0 is recognized as an effective, robust inactivation step of enveloped viruses. The data from this study demonstrate that over a 60-minute time course, the titers of PRV and MuLV in the low-pH-treated process intermediate showed very fast inactivation kinetics, as evidenced by a marked reduction already at the first time point of $T = 5$ minutes. Complete inactivation was obtained in these studies. All values reported as less than quantifiable indicate that no active virus was detected, and theoretical titers were reported based on the application of a Poisson distribution of the sample results. The MuLV viral load at time zero was determined using the media control sample, which contains an identical amount of spiked virus in virus growth media and shows whether the starting material has an effect on the reducing the virus titer.

The reduction factors obtained for PRV were on average $\geq 5.12 \pm 0.12$ logs. The mean reduction factor obtained for MuLV was $\geq 5.63 \pm 0.43$. The results from this study confirm that low-pH treatment is an effective, robust step for inactivating enveloped viruses. Figure 12.5 summarizes the kinetics of the MuLV and PRV inactivation.

12.3.3 Virus Removal

12.3.3.1 Nanofiltration

The nanofilter used (DV50, Pall) has a membrane that is capable of removing viruses of 50 nm or greater in size. The average reduction factors obtained for the viruses evaluated in this study were $\geq 3.20 \pm 0.50$ for MuLV and $\geq 4.36 \pm 0.36$ for Reo-3, thus demonstrating that the nanofiltration step can be considered a robust and effective virus clearance step within the ZEVALIN purification process.

12.3.3.2 Chromatographic Viral Reduction

Chromatographic methods using various stationary phases can provide effective virus reduction; however, any measured reduction may be specific to the virus tested. For more generic viral clearance, a combination of orthogonal chromatography steps is considered to provide a general barrier even for unknown viruses.

All of the three chromatography steps employed in the ZEVALIN purification process may contribute to viral clearance. Protein A chromatography, however, was not evaluated for its ability to remove virus. Since antibodies adsorbed to Protein A affinity adsorbents are eluted by lowering the pH, it is difficult to differentiate whether any viral clearance observed is due to inactivation at low pH or due to removal by Protein A chromatography. Therefore, only anion exchange and hydrophobic interaction were evaluated as an orthogonal combination of chromatography steps during the small-scale virus clearance study. The adsorbents from the small-scale

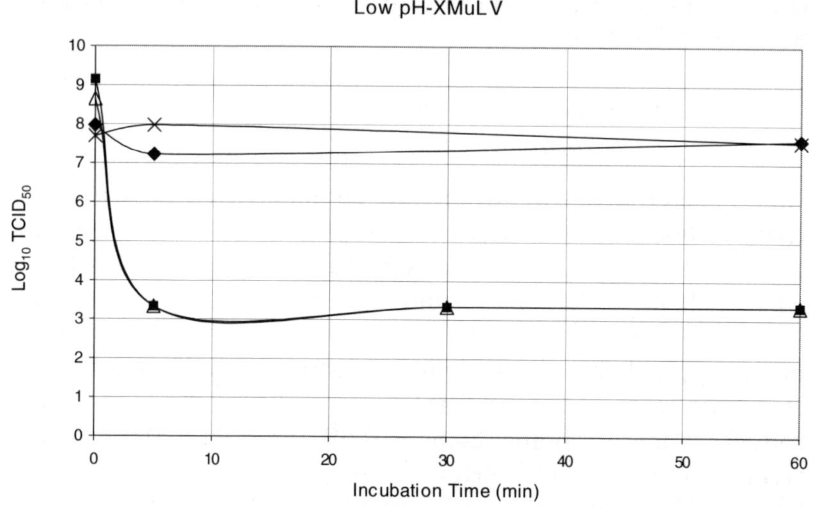

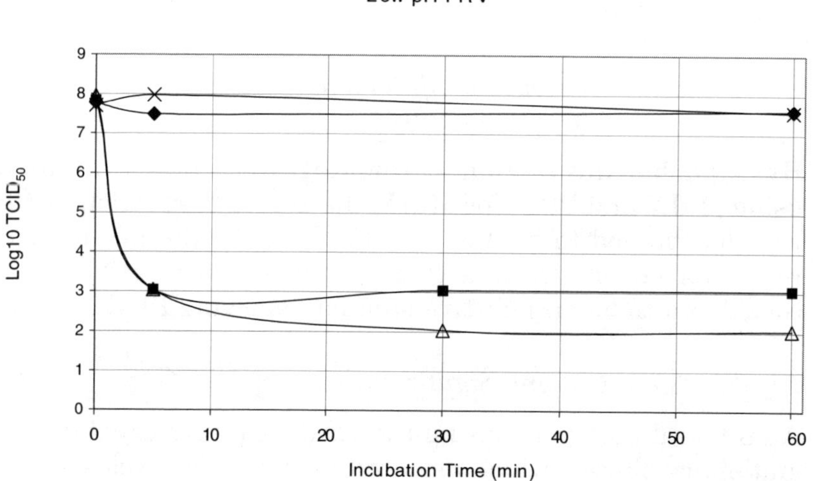

Figure 12.5   Low pH kinetics of inactivation for XMuLV and PRV.

chromatographic adsorbent use life validations were used in the viral clearance studies. At the end of these studies, the anion exchange adsorbent had been used for 10 cycles and the hydrophobic interaction chromatography adsorbent had been used for 14 cycles.

12.3.3.2.1 Anion Exchange Chromatography

Anion exchange chromatography demonstrated to be an effective method for removing the complete panel of viruses. The average reduction obtained for MuLV, PPV, and Reo-3 was ≥4.78 ± 0.49, 5.84 ± 0.86, and 4.04 ± 0.32, respectively. The studies performed with PRV resulted in a situation that is not untypical for virus clearance studies. Between the two runs performed, considerable variability was found, with reduction factors being ≥4.84 ± 0.09 and 3.11 ± 0.86, respectively. Since the reduction varied by more than one log between both experiments, which exceeds variability of the assay for determining the virus titer, the lowest calculated reduction factor is used as a measure of clearance across this processing step.

12.3.3.2.2 Hydrophobic Interaction Chromatography

Hydrophobic interaction chromatography was evaluated using MuLV and PPV. For MuLV, the average reduction factor was determined to be 4.65 ± 0.82. For PPV, the mean virus reduction factor was less than 1 log; therefore, HIC is not considered to be an effective step for removing PPV.

12.3.3.2.3 Column Sanitization

An integral part of ensuring the viral clearance capability of stationary phases, which are used in successive cycles, is the ability to demonstrate adequate cleaning. Therefore, the sanitizing solutions used for the anion exchange and hydrophobic interaction chromatography adsorbents (1 N NaOH) and the Protein A affinity adsorbent (30% ethanol/0.5 M acetic acid) were assessed for their inactivation potential with respect to the panel of challenge viruses. Under manufacturing conditions, these adsorbents are exposed to the sanitizing solutions between 6 and 16 hours. To model worst-case conditions, data were collected for each virus over a maximum exposure period of 5.75 hours. For the enveloped viruses, limited time course studies were also performed to collect additional data at earlier time points.

For Reo-3, PRV, and MuLV, marked decreases in titers were observed at the first time point assessed after exposure to the sanitizing agents. The average reduction factors for 1 N sodium hydroxide were 5.25 ± 0.91 for Reo-3, 5.75 ± 0.60 for PPV, 6.25 ± 0.69 for PRV, and 6.04 ± 0.53 for MuLV. The average reduction factors for the 30% ethanol/0.5 M acetic acid were <1 for PPV, 6.18 ± 0.56 for PRV, and 5.66 ± 0.48 for MuLV. Since the Reo-3 reduction factors (5.04 ± 0.46 and 6.26 ± 0.73) varied by more than one log, the lowest calculated reduction factor, 5.04 ± 0.46, was used as a measure of clearance. Viral inactivation results obtained with the sanitizing agents provide assurance that enveloped viruses still adsorbed to the stationary phase at the completion of the process step will be inactivated. Figure 12.6 presents two examples of the kinetics of inactivation for XmuLV and Reo-3 with sodium hydroxide.

12.3.4 Summary

The individual viral reduction factors for the process steps evaluated in the viral clearance study are summed to calculate the overall reduction viral reduction factors for the process. All of the process steps evaluated are considered to use orthogonal mechanism for clearing viruses and are considered additive in calculating the overall viral reduction factors. All four process steps evaluated are effective at clearing MuLV, the specific model virus, which is used to calculate the estimated particles per dose. The other three nonspecific model viruses — PRV, Reo-3, and PPV viruses — were used to characterize the robustness of process. The process steps characterized using PRV, Reo-3, and PPV showed varying degrees of effectiveness at clearing these nonspecific model viruses. PRV is effectively inactivated during the low inactivation step and was only removed with moderate efficiency during the

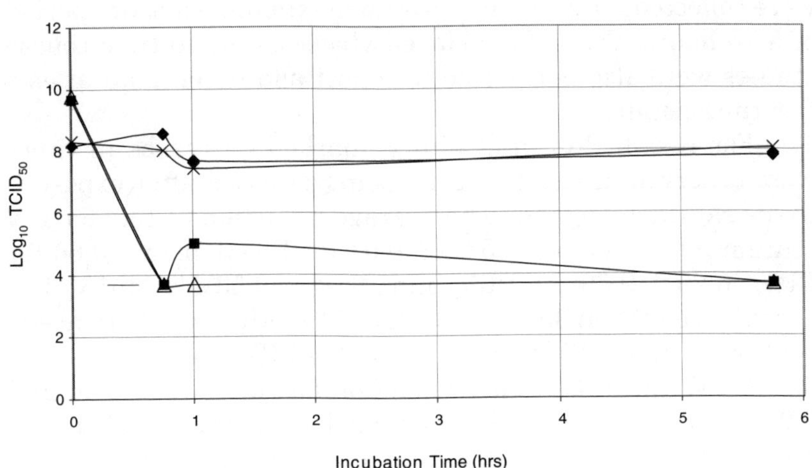

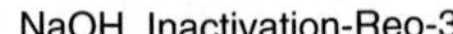

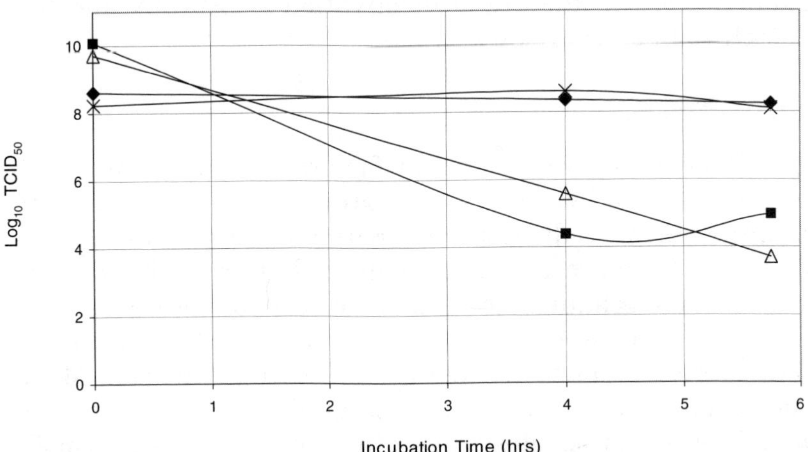

Figure 12.6 Sodium hydroxide inactivation kinetics for XMuLV and Reo-3.

anion exchange chromatography step. Reo-3 was effectively removed at both the anion exchange chromatography and viral filtration steps. PPV was effectively removed during the anion exchange chromatography step, and no removal was achieved at the hydrophobic interaction chromatography step.

The average of duplicate runs was used in determining the individual reduction factors for each virus and process step, except PRV for the anion exchange chromatography step and Reo-3 for the 30% ethanol/0.5 M acetic acid. The lowest value of the duplicate runs was used for the PRV, anion exchange reduction factor, and Reo-3 for the 30% ethanol/0.5 M acetic acid. The duplicate runs had reduction factors that varied by more than one log, which is the limit of variation between valid test results. All other individual reduction factors were within one log for the duplicate runs. Process steps that have a reduction factor <1 were not considered to be additive and were not included in the calculation of overall clearance. The overall viral clearance factors for each of the challenge viruses are summarized in Table 12.6.

TABLE 12.6   Overall Viral Clearance (log 10)

	MuLV	PRV	Reo-3	PPV
Low pH treatment subsequent to Protein A column chromatography	≥5.63 ± 0.43	≥5.12 ± 0.12	—	—
Anion exchange chromatography	≥4.78 ± 0.49	3.11 ± 0.86	≥4.04 ± 0.32	5.84 ± 0.86
Hydrophobic interaction chromatography	≥4.65 ± 0.82	—	—	<1
Viral filtration	≥3.20 ± 0.50	—	≥4.36 ± 0.36	—
Overall	≥18.26 ± 1.16	>8.23 ± 0.87	≥8.40 ± 0.48	5.84 ± 0.86

Note: — = not tested as part of this clearance study.

Viral clearance studies summarized here demonstrate that the ZEVALIN purification process provides overall reduction factors of $\log_{10} \geq 18.26 \pm 1.16$ for MuLV, $\geq 8.23 \pm 0.87$ for PRV, $\geq 8.40 \pm 0.48$ for Reo-3, and 5.84 ± 0.86 for PPV.

12.3.5 Estimating the Viral Load for the Process

The potential risk of viral presence in the producer cell line was assessed by quantifying the amount of retrovirus in the harvested cell culture fluid (HCCF). Transmission electron microscopy (TEM) performed using HCCF samples from a representative manufacturing run showed $<1.3 \times 10^5$ retrovirus-like particles per milliliter from the "end of production" sample. The current "Points to Consider in the Manufacturing and Testing of Monoclonal Product for Human Use" [10] states that negative TEM results should be interpreted such that an equivalent titer to the lowest limit of detection is assumed (1×10^6). The capability of the ZEVALIN purification process to eliminate substantially more virus than is estimated to be in a single-dose equivalent of HCCF was therefore estimated assuming 1×10^6 retrovirus-like particles per milliliter. As shown in Table 12.6, the calculated clearance factor for the specific model retrovirus MuLV is $>10^{18.26}$. The volume of harvested cell culture fluid (HCCF) needed to produce a dose of product was determined to be 67 ml/dose. Therefore, the estimated number of particles per dose is

$$\frac{\text{Viral particles in HCCF for a single dose}}{\text{Viral clearance factor}}$$

$$= \frac{(\leq 1 \times 10^6 \text{ particles/ml}) \times (67 \text{ ml/dose})}{>10^{18.26}}$$

$$= 3.7 \times 10^{-11} \text{ particles/dose}$$

Therefore, the final product can be estimated to contain less than one retrovirus-like particle per 27 billion doses, thus providing substantial assurance of the viral safety of the ZEVALIN antibody from retrovirus infections. Additionally, the overall viral clearance factors obtained for PRV, Reo-3, and PPV demonstrate that the process is robust for inactivation/removal of viruses that cover a range of physico-chemical characteristics including large and small RNA and DNA viruses, as well as enveloped and nonenveloped viruses.

12.4 CHROMATOGRAPHIC ADSORBENT USE LIFE

To qualify the repeated use of each adsorbent for purification of the ZEVALIN antibody, the performance of each resin was evaluated at small scale for multiple cycles of use. The Protein A affinity, anion exchange, and hydrophobic interaction chromatography processes were scaled down according to the concept previously discussed. Each stationary phase was evaluated over a specified number of cycles.

The purpose of the lifetime studies is to demonstrate that throughout multiple cycles of use the chromatographic performance is consistent. Process performance is evaluated by measuring the clearance of process impurities, the effectiveness of regeneration steps to prevent carryover of impurities, and product recovery. In combination, these process performance parameters are used to determine the limit for maximum adsorbent reuse.

Shown subsequently is an example of one chromatographic lifetime study for the anion exchange chromatography step.

The second chromatographic step in the ZEVALIN purification process uses a strong anion exchange resin. The anion exchange chromatography step is designed to reduce host cell DNA and potential viral contaminants. Product flows through the column while impurities are removed by adsorption. UF/DF #1 product from full-scale manufacturing lots was processed over a small-scale anion exchange chromatography for 10 cycles of use. Table 12.7 describes the operational parameters used for the small-scale process compared to commercial scale. The main process impurity (host cell DNA) was measured before and after processing, and the overall DNA clearance factor was used as the performance criterion. Figure 12.7 shows the DNA removal for the anion exchange chromatography step at small scale and compares the data with

TABLE 12.7 Anion Exchange Chromatography Operational Parameters

Parameter	Scaled Down	Commercial
Scale-down factor	119	NA
Column bed height	15–16 cm	15–16 cm
Load and wash flow rate	100 cm/hr	≤100 cm/hr
Load pH	7.7 ± 0.2	7.7 ± 0.2
Antibody load	11.7 mg/ml	≤11.7 mg/ml
Temperature	Ambient	Ambient
HETP	<0.1 cm	<0.1 cm

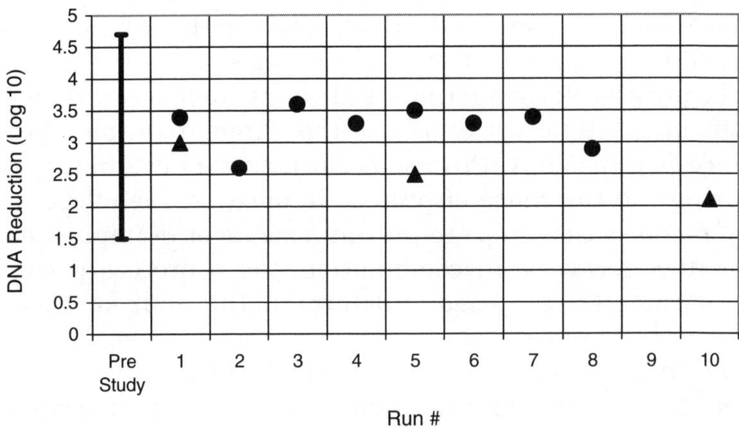

Figure 12.7 Anion exchange resin lifetime host DNA clearance results from small-scale (▲) and full-scale manufacturing (●). The prestudy bar represents the variation of ±4 standard deviations from the characterization study.

full-scale manufacturing. Additionally, the expected range of DNA clearance from the characterization study is shown and demonstrates that both small- and full-scale results met the expected range.

Product recovery over the 10 cycles of reuse for the anion exchange chromatography is shown in Figure 12.8 and is compared with full-scale manufacturing results. The product recovery was consistent for the 10 cycles evaluated (98.9% ±

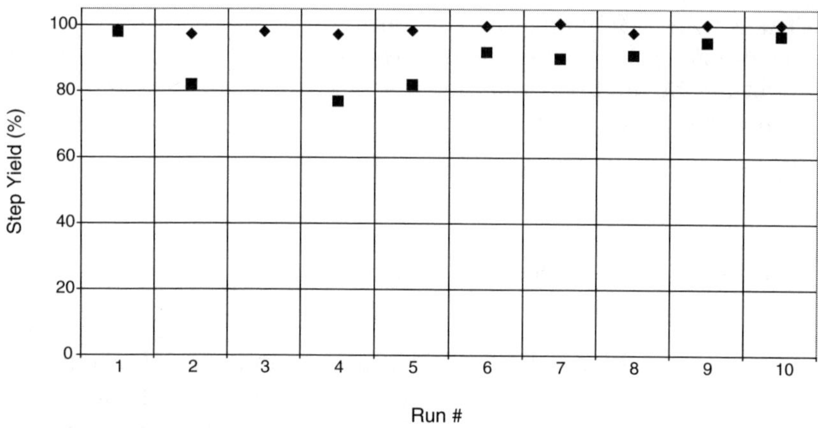

Figure 12.8 Anion exchange resin recovery results from small-scale (♦) and full-scale manufacturing (■).

1.3%) and lies within the same range as the manufacturing scale. Besides consistent performance, a second element of an adsorbent reuse study is to ensure that cleaning and regeneration procedures show consistent efficiency and minimize impurity carryover between cycles. Cleaning efficiency was verified by the absence of DNA and HCP buildup on the anion exchange adsorbent and was measured by comparing HCP and DNA pool concentrations for a new adsorbent to data obtained after several cycles of chromatography had been completed. No upward trend in these data was observed. In addition, three blank cycles were performed at equal intervals during the resin's lifetime (after the first, fifth, and tenth cycle). In a blank cycle, a complete chromatography operation is performed with the exception that during the load phase the product is replaced by a buffer. Inserting such blank cycles in between true chromatography runs ensures that impurities, which might accumulate during the stationary phase, do not leach off the column during the wash step. The results are summarized in Table 12.8.

The concentration of DNA and HCP in the blank cycle effluents was below the limit of quantification for each sample. In addition, the levels of DNA in the anion exchange

TABLE 12.8 HCP and DNA Results for Blank Cycles during the Adsorbent Lifetime Evaluation Study for the Anion Exchange Step

Cycle Number	pg DNA/ml	ng HCP/ml
Cycle 1	<20	<15.6
Cycle 5	<20	<15.6
Cycle 10	<20	<15.6

chromatography product exhibited no trend over 10 cycles. As a result of these studies, the maximum reuse lifetime of the anion exchange chromatography resin was set at nine cycles (nine product lots).

12.5 FULL-SCALE PROCESS VALIDATIONS

12.5.1 Process-Related Impurity Removal

In the 1997 "Points to Consider in the Manufacturing and Testing of Monoclonal Antibodies for Human Use" [10], it is suggested that, whenever possible, contaminants or additives (antibiotics, other media components, host cell proteins, chromatography reagents, preservatives, or components that may be leached from the affinity chromatography columns, such as Protein A) should be found to be below detectable levels in the bulk drug substance using a highly sensitive analytical method. The aforementioned additives are process-related impurities as defined by ICH, which are substances that may be derived from cell culture, cell substrates, or downstream processing [7]. In the same FDA document, it is suggested that the DNA concentration in the final product should, whenever possible, be no more than the 100 pg of cellular DNA per dose. This requirement is based on recommendations from a WHO study group in 1987 [11]. In 1996 [12], the WHO reassessed the potential risk presented by residual cellular DNA and revised its recommendation up to 10 ng per dose. A dose is defined as the amount of drug given over a 24-hour period. It is anticipated that the FDA will revise this guideline in the next updated version. ICH Q7a also suggests that process validation studies should confirm that the impurity profile for each API is comparable to or better than historical data and, where applicable, comparable to or better than the profile determined during process development or for batches used for pivotal clinical and toxicological studies [3].

The goal of the full-scale manufacturing validation of the ZEVALIN purification process was to demonstrate that impurities are consistently reduced to safety levels recommended by regulatory guidelines. Only those process steps that significantly contributed to the removal of impurities during the development and the characterization studies were evaluated during the validation. The process impurity range shown in this section is from the first nine production lots, which are representative of the commercial manufacturing process. Data from the conformance lots were included in the process validation.

12.5.1.1 Host Cell Protein and DNA

During the full-scale manufacturing validation, it was demonstrated that the ZEVALIN purification process is able to consistently remove Chinese hamster ovary host cell–derived proteins (HCP) and DNA. HCP was evaluated in the HCCF, the Protein A affinity pool after UF/DF #1, the hydrophobic interaction chromatography pool, and the bulk drug substance.

HCP concentration was monitored using an ELISA-based assay that employs anti-HCP antibodies and electro-chemiluminescence detection.

Figure 12.9 shows the HCP results of samples taken at the four points in the purification process discussed previously. The majority of the HCP is removed during the Protein A step with at least a 100-fold reduction. The HCP is removed to <10 µg/mg after the HIC step and <800 ng/mg in the BDS.

Samples from the same in-process points were also analyzed for DNA content using the Threshold Total DNA Assay. Analysis of the data shows that the purification process can reduce the host cell DNA from an average of 3.1×10^7 pg DNA

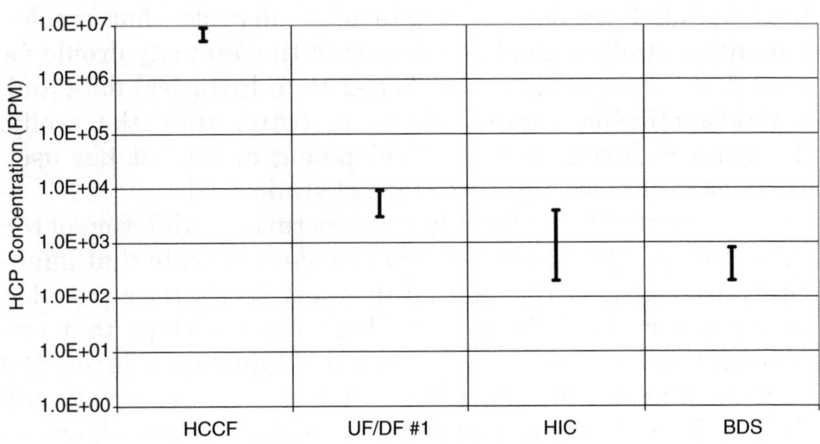

Figure 12.9 HCP ranges for each process step during commercial manufacturing.

per mg of antibody to <2.3 pg DNA per milligram of antibody. Figure 12.10 shows the DNA concentration measured at four points in the purification process. The bar at each process step shows DNA range observed during commercial manufacturing.

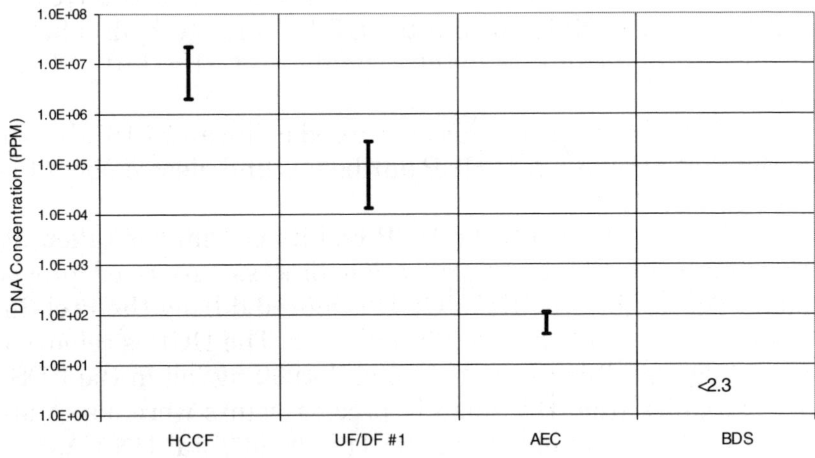

Figure 12.10 DNA concentration ranges observed for all steps of commercial manufacturing.

The purification process provides a consistent and effective removal of host cell DNA and HCP. The purification process is sufficiently robust to limit host cell DNA to ≤2.3 pg/mg of ZEVALIN, which corresponds to a maximum value of 4.6 pg DNA per dose for a 70-kg person. This value is well below the WHO recommended upper limit of 10 ng of DNA per dose.

12.5.2 Removal of Non-Host-Related Impurities

12.5.2.1 Human Recombinant Insulin and Methotrexate

Human recombinant insulin and methotrexate are components that are added to the cell culture media for ZEVALIN production or seed cell culture. The insulin concentrations measured in the harvested cell culture fluid were 200–1200 µg/ml. During process validation, it was demonstrated that insulin was removed during the Protein A chromatography step to less-than-quantifiable levels for all lots tested. Methotrexate is added to the cell culture media to maintain selective pressure on the integrated and amplified ZEVALIN antibody genes during the continuous culture stage of the cell culture process. As the culture volume is expanded from 1-liter spinner flasks to initiate a production run, methotrexate supplementation is discontinued, and this results in a dilution of the methotrexate in the expanded volume. The culture volume expansion is initiated from several 1-liter spinner flasks and expanded through several seed bioreactors to the 2000-liter production bioreactor. Therefore, the concentration of methotrexate in the harvested cell culture fluid is calculated to be approximately 92 pg/ml, which is considerably less than the limit of quantification for the methotrexate assay. During process validation, measuring methotraxate concentration in the HCCF confirmed that methotraxate was below the LOQ of the assay.

12.5.2.2 Urea

Urea is commonly used as a column regeneration buffer for industrial chromatography. Both the Protein A affinity chromatography and hydrophobic interaction chromatography (HIC) steps of the ZEVALIN purification process use 4 M urea for column regeneration after each cycle of product processing. The chaotropic property of urea (disrupts hydrogen bonds) aids in the removal of process residuals from the column. By the same mechanism of action, concentrated urea is known to denature proteins, and therefore its removal from the column is necessary prior to product processing. Following its use, and prior to product loading of the next cycle, urea is displaced from either column by extensive wash with several buffers. An important goal of process validation therefore is to demonstrate that the large-volume washes effectively reduce urea to less-than-quantifiable levels prior to product load.

In the small-scale chromatography resin use lifetime validations for Protein A and hydrophobic interaction chromatography, urea was measured in "blank" cycles (see previous) performed at intervals over the intended resin use lifetime. Protein A was tested after cycles 1, 40, and 75 and hydrophobic interaction chromatography was tested after cycles 1, 5, 10, and 14. In all of the blank cycles, less-than-quantifiable levels of urea were found. Urea was also measured in the bulk drug substance at commercial scale, and less-than-quantifiable levels were found for all nine lots.

In addition to column lifetime studies and testing of the bulk drug substance, the second ultrafiltration and diafiltration step was evaluated for its capability to remove urea. The function of this step is to concentrate and buffer exchange the product into its final formulation buffer. Since urea is a small molecule — significantly smaller than the nominal molecular weight cutoff of the tangential-flow filtration membrane — urea can be expected to pass through the membrane into the permeate, while the product is retained. In a small-scale validation, the UF/DF #2 load material was spiked with 100 mM urea, and the UF/DF process was performed using representative

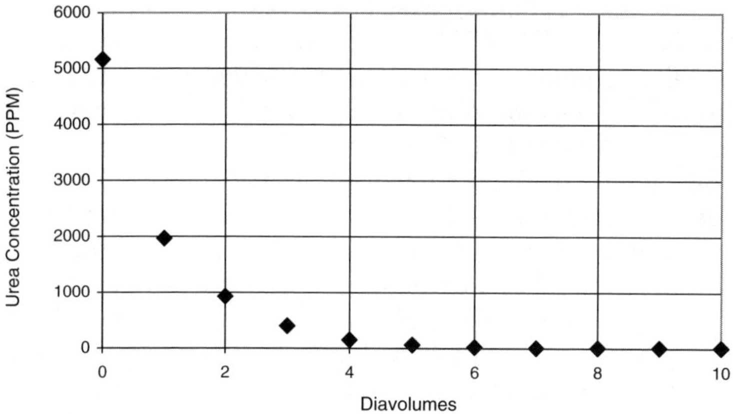

Figure 12.11   Removal of urea during ultrafilteration/diafiltration #2.

operating parameters of the full-scale commercial manufacturing process. The membrane surface-area-to-mass ratio, cross-flow velocity, diafiltration protein concentration, diavolumes exchanged, and sanitization and equilibration parameters were the same as in the commercial process. The validation was performed in triplicate, and in all three runs <6.4 µg/ml of urea was measured after 8 out of 10 diavolumes of diafiltration buffer were exchanged. Figure 12.11 shows the decrease in urea concentration during one of the three runs.

12.5.2.3 Endotoxins

Since endotoxins are pyrogenic substances, they can lead to symptoms such as fever in humans. Therefore, endotoxin limits, such as less than five endotoxin units per kilogram of body weight, have been developed for drugs for human use [13]. Endotoxins are lipopolysaccharides from the cell wall of gram-negative bacteria, which are highly negatively charged and form multimeric complexes depending on the solution conditions. A purification process should have the capability of removing and inactivating endotoxins, as well as demonstrate that it consistently produces a product well below specified safety levels. A threefold approach was taken to control endotoxin levels during the ZEVALIN manufacturing process. As a first measure, endotoxin inactivation procedures were introduced to the process for depyrogenating the chromatography systems and adsorbents before use. Second, steps capable of removing endotoxin were identified. Both approaches were performed using small-scale models since a purposeful contamination of product and equipment was not feasible. The third approach was to demonstrate that the removal and inactivation procedures were effective at commercial scale by monitoring all in-process product pools as well as the final product for endotoxin. The harvested cell culture fluid (HCCF) was the only in-process product pool to contain low levels of endotoxin (<0.25–2.7 EU/ml). All the other in-process product pools and the bulk drug substances contained less-than-quantifiable levels of endotoxin, demonstrating that the product was safe in terms of endotoxins.

12.5.2.3.1 Small-Scale Endotoxin Removal Studies

Protein A was shown to be the principal removal step for endotoxin during characterization studies and was validated using a small-scale model that was representative of the commercial process. The in-process intermediates used in the spiking study were taken from commercial manufacturing. The HCCF was spiked with approximately 200 EU/ml endotoxin, and the Protein A chromatography was performed using the spiked load. Samples from all the Protein A chromatography fractions were analyzed for endotoxin. The validation was performed in triplicate. Table 12.9 presents the results from the Protein A chromatography endotoxin spiking study.

The results of the endotoxin spiking study demonstrate that the flow-through and wash effluent fractions contained >95% of the endotoxin. No endotoxin was detected in the cleaning, regeneration, and storage solutions. The Protein A eluates from all three runs contained less-than-detectable amounts of endotoxin with an approximate 2000-fold reduction in endotoxin. These data demonstrate that the endotoxin

TABLE 12.9 Removal of Endotoxin during the Small-Scale Spiking Study

	Measured Endotoxin (EU/ml)		
	Run #1	Run #2	Run #3
Spiked HCCF	180.2	292.9	210.4
Flow-through and wash effluent	143.1	241.4	180.3
Elution	<1.0[a]	<0.5[a]	<0.5[a]
Cleaning effluent	<0.25[a]	<0.25[a]	<0.5[a]
Regeneration effluent	<0.25[a]	<0.25[a]	<0.5[a]
Storage effluent	<0.25[a]	<0.25[a]	<0.5[a]

[a] Less than the limit of detection of the assay.

flows through the column and is washed away with complete clearance of endotoxin by the Protein A chromatography.

12.5.2.3.2 Endotoxin Inactivation by 1 N Sodium Hydroxide

The purpose of this study was to demonstrate the effectiveness of sodium hydroxide as an endotoxin-inactivating agent. Sodium hydroxide (1 N) is used as a sanitizing and endotoxin-inactivating agent in the anion exchange and hydrophobic interaction chromatography steps. The chromatography columns are incubated with 1 N sodium hydroxide for at least 6 hours before use. In this study, approximately 200 EU/ml of endotoxin was spiked into a 1 N sodium hydroxide solution, and samples were taken at 0, 1, 4, and 5.75 hours incubation time. The samples were immediately neutralized with sodium phosphate and acetic acid. A positive control of 200 EU/ml of endotoxin was spiked into LAL water and used to determine the starting amount of spiked endotoxin. The negative control was LAL water. All of the samples were tested using kinetic quantitative chromogenic LAL analysis. Table 12.10 presents the results of the study.

The positive control showed an average endotoxin content of 178 EU/ml. The inactivation samples showed approximately a 50% reduction at $T = 0$ with average endotoxin

TABLE 12.10   Endotoxin Inactivation by
1 *N* NaOH

Sample	Endotoxin Concentration (EU/ml)		
	Run #1	Run #2	Run #3
$T = 0$	101.90	90.43	109.30
$T = 1$ hour	49.22	82.97	101.50
$T = 4$ hours	13.00	19.51	16.79
$T = 5.75$ hours	4.66	4.01	4.22
Positive control	142.2	205.4	186.2
Negative control	<0.5	<0.5	<0.5

content of 103 EU/ml and a 41-fold reduction by $T = 5.75$ with average endotoxin content of 4.3 EU/ml.

Since the Protein A chromatography removes endotoxin from HCCF to below the limit of detection (<0.4808 EU/mg), endotoxin measured in the chromatography loads during the subsequent chromatography steps can be expected to also be below the limit of detection. Therefore, a potential endotoxin contamination of load material during the anion exchange and hydrophobic interaction chromatography resins will be very low. In the unlikely case that the low residual levels (less than limit of detection) of endotoxin bind to the resins of subsequent chromatography operations, the 1 *N* sodium hydroxide endotoxin inactivation data in Table 12.10 provide assurance that these low endotoxin levels can be reduced by an additional 41-fold.

12.5.2.4   Protein A

Protein A is coupled to a stationary phase resulting in an affinity chromatography matrix. During the chromatography, Protein A can potentially leach from the matrix into the eluate. Protein A is an immunomodulator and can elicit secondary immunological phenomena [14]. An important goal of process validation therefore is to demonstrate that the bulk drug substance contains less-than-quantifiable levels of Protein A. The bulk drug substance was the only process step tested for Protein A content due to assay sensitivity issues with in-process samples. Less-than-quantifiable levels were observed in all the bulk drug substance samples.

12.5.3 Monomer Content

The monomer content was monitored through the purification process using the size exclusion HPLC assay. The size exclusion HPLC recognizes product-related impurities, antibody fragments, and aggregates as well as process-related impurities. The monomer content was evaluated in the Protein A eluate, Protein A eluate pool after UF/DF #1, anion exchange chromatography pool, hydrophobic interaction pool, and bulk drug substance. Analysis of the data shows that the purification process can consistently produce a product >98% monomer in the bulk drug substance. Figure 12.12 show the monomer results at five points in the process.

12.5.4 In-Process Hold Times

The ZEVALIN purification process was designed to be a continuous process with no long-term in-process hold points. Process intermediates are filtered through steam-sterilized 0.2-µm filters into steam-sterilized stainless steel tanks prior to further processing. Occasionally, the in-process product pools

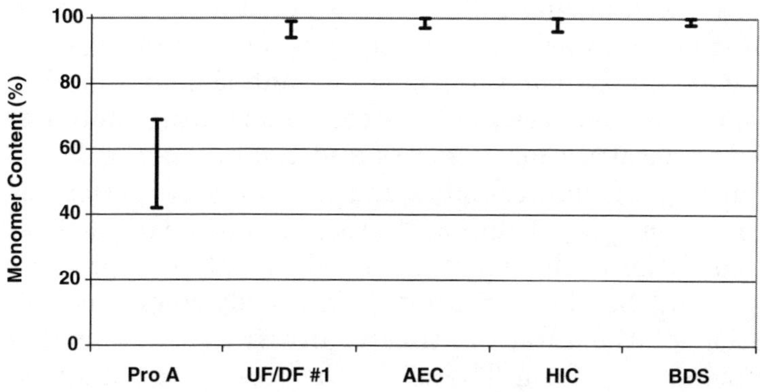

Figure 12.12 Range of monomer content observed during commercial manufacturing.

may need to be stored between purification steps for longer periods of time. To add flexibility to manufacturing operations and accommodate any unforeseen delays to the production schedule, extended hold times were validated to show that no adverse effect on the quality of the product is found. Hold time validation encompasses two aspects: product stability as well as the assurance that the product pool remains clean and relatively free of bioburden and endotoxin over the hold time in a specific type of vessel. Process intermediates were purposely held beyond the typical time for processing during full-scale manufacturing to establish an upper hold time process limit. Samples were taken from the hold vessel after filtration and at the end of the hold step and tested for bioburden and endotoxin. The test results were below in-process action limits for bioburden and endotoxin for all process samples, thus demonstrating that the product pool showed no increase in bioburden and endotoxin. The bulk drug substances met release specifications, which included a full panel of stability-indicating assays demonstrating that the product was stable during the hold period of 48 hours at ambient temperature.

In addition, a small-scale stability validation was performed to demonstrate that the product could be held for 14 days in stainless steel vessels and provided supportive data that the in-process product pools were stable if extended storage were required. In this study, samples of in-process product pools were taken during full-scale manufacturing and transferred to small stainless steel containers. The containers and closures were constructed of the same materials as the full-scale in-process hold vessels. The containers were stored at ambient temperature for 48 hours and then at 2–8°C for 12 additional days. Stability-indicating assays were performed for samples removed at different storage times. Given these storage conditions, the most likely chemical and physical changes would be the formation of antibody aggregates or degradation of the intact antibody into fragments smaller than its monomeric form. Therefore, the most relevant stability-indicating tests to be utilized in this study were the ones that determined the percentage of monomeric IgG or the amount of aggregation and degradation. In addition, determination of the total protein content was also utilized to account for any protein loss due to precipitation or absorption to storage surfaces. No appreciable change was observed with any of the samples assayed at the various time points. Analysis of these samples demonstrated that the in-process product pools are stable at ambient temperature for 48 hours and at 2–8°C for an additional 12 days.

12.6 FILTER COMPATIBILITY AND EXTRACTABLES

12.6.1 Compatibility

The ZEVALIN purification process utilizes various types of filters with different nominal pore sizes for filtering in-process product and process solutions. These filters can be categorized into three functional groups: prefilters, sterilizing-grade filters, and a nanofilter. The prefilters were used in the process to remove large particulates and have a nominal pore size of ≥ 0.45 µm. They are installed in front of chromatography columns and sterilizing-grade filters to provide protection from fouling of chromatography absorbent or premature plugging of the filters. The sterilizing-grade filters are used to remove microorganisms and have nominal pores sizes of $0.1–0.22$ µm. The nanofilter is used to remove viruses ≥ 50 nm in size. The filters used in the ZEVALIN purification process were evaluated for compatibly with product and process solutions. The filter compatibility study encompassed two main aspects. The first aspect was that the product or process solutions should not adversely affect the ability of the filter to perform its intended function. The second aspect was that the filtration process should not impact the quality of the solution. The ability of the filter to perform its intended function can be quantitatively measured by evaluating membrane performance characteristics, permeability (flow rate), and integrity (bubble point or forward flow diffusion test). These tests were performed in water before and after soaking the filter in product or process solutions. The filters were exposed to the solutions and agitated for a greater length of time than normal operating conditions and at temperatures in the upper normal operating range. The permeability at a constant pressure and temperature is related to the thickness and the porosity of the membrane. Flow rate increases after filter exposure can indicate that the porosity or the thickness of the membrane has changed. This may suggest that in-process product or process solutions may have adversely affected the membrane. The filter integrity tests performed for the compatibility studies were either the bubble point or the forward flow diffusion test. The integrity tests were performed according to the manufacturer's recommended procedure for each filter. The bubble test is performed by wetting the filter with an appropriate fluid and then applying gas pressure to the filter. The pressure at which the first flow of bubbles emerges from the filter defines the bubble point. The bubble point measurement relates to the effective diameter of the largest pores present in a membrane, which, along with membrane thickness and pore tortuosity, directly influences the retention properties of the membrane [15]. The bubble point is inversely related to the largest pore size at a constant temperature for a given wetting fluid and test gas. The higher the bubble point pressure, the tighter the membrane structure, which indicates the smaller pore sizes. The forward diffusion flow test is performed by wetting the filter with appropriate buffer, applying pressure below the bubble point, and measuring the gas flow through the filter. The forward flow test is not directly related to pore size and is associated with the thickness of the membrane, total porosity, and test gas diffusivity across the membrane [15]. Filter manufacturers have empirically correlated integrity tests to the filter's ability to remove *Brevundimonas diminuta* (a small bacteria) for the 0.22- and 0.1-µm filters and to the ability of the nanofilter to remove viruses ≥50 nm. The acceptance criteria for integrity and permeability tests were based on the manufacturer's recommendation for each filter type.

The filtered manufacturing solutions were assessed for quality by comparing attributes of each tested solution pre- and postfiltration. The attributes evaluated to assess quality included the following: pH and conductivity for the buffers, monomer content or SDS-PAGE, pH and conductivity for the product, and pH and osmolality for cell culture media. The studies evaluating membrane performance characteristics were performed using 47-mm discs or small-scale cartridges with the same type of membranes used in the manufacturing process. The manufacturing solutions used in the study were selected to represent process extremes (pH, solvent strength, solute level) to provide suitable challenge to each type of filter. In close collaboration with the filter manufacturers, it was determined which solutions were to be used as process extremes. A characterization was performed to determine the expected variability to the quality attributes and was used to set acceptance criteria.

Shown subsequently is an example of a compatibility study for the 0.22-µm filter for the HIC in-process product pool. The HIC eluate is normally filtered at ambient temperature (15–26°C) in ≤2 hours at commercial scale. During the compatibility study, HIC eluate and the small-scale cartridges were agitated and statically soaked at 26.9°C for 12 hours. Three filters from three different lots were used for this study. Table 12.11 shows the results for one of the three filters evaluated as an example of a typical set of compatibility results obtained for a specific filter. The forward flow diffusion and permeability measurements were within the manufacturer's recommendations (≤20 cc/min for the forward flow test and 10% increase in flow from the pre- and postfiltration).

TABLE **12.11** Typical Set of Compatibility Test Results for the Example of a 0.22-µm Filter for the HIC In-Process Product Pool

	Prefiltration	Postfiltration
Forward flow diffusion test, cc/min	11.8	15.0
Permeability flow rate, cc/min	1250	1180
% Monomer	100	100
pH	6.8	6.8
Conductivity, mS/cm	41.3	40.9

These membrane performance characteristics results demonstrated that the filter was integral before and after product exposure. All the quality attributes were within expected variation for monomer, conductivity, and pH, thus demonstrating that the filtration process did not affect the quality of the product.

12.6.2 Extractables

Filters have the potential of releasing toxic substances into the process stream. It is important that an assessment of these potentially released substances from filter membranes and their support structure be performed to ensure product safety. Most filter membranes and their support structure are constructed of polymers and plastics. The appropriate methodology for evaluating the safety of filter components is based on plastics toxicity testing. A series of plastic toxicity tests are described in USP <88> Biological Reactivity Test, *in vivo* using USP Class VI test methods. In USP Class VI testing, model solvents are used to exhaustively extract potential extractables. The five solvents are 0.9% saline, 5% ethanol in saline, polyethylene glycol 400, vegetable oil, and a pharmaceutical solution if compatible. The filters are exposed to the solvents for an extended period of time at elevated temperatures. For the filters used in the ZEVALIN process, exposure to the solvents was chosen as either 24 hours at 70°C or 60 minutes at 121°C. The extracts are injected into mice and rabbits and observed for signs of toxicity and skin reactivity for 72 hours. In addition, discs of filter housing material attached to the filters were implanted into the paravertebral muscles of rabbits for 7 days and observed for signs of hemorrhage, film, and encapsulation. All of the filters used in the ZEVALIN manufacturing process were determined to be nontoxic as evaluated for biosafety in accordance with USP Class VI testing of plastics. The USP Class VI testing of the filters is considered a worst-case challenge because the solvent and testing conditions are exaggerated with longer process times and higher temperatures than normal operating conditions. These extraction procedures were intended to generate a greater concentration of potential released substances from the filter than may have leached into process streams during normal operating conditions. Extractables are defined as compounds that may be released into a solution at exhaustive contact, while leachables are defined as compounds that migrate into a solution under normal conditions of use. Leachables are considered a subset of extractables. It should be noted that a toxicity test does not identify or quantify the concentration of extractables.

Most filter manufacturers take an analogous approach using different extraction procedures to generate extractables using the model solvent approach [15–17]. The product concentration compared with concentration of extractables is usually 100 to 10,000 times greater than the maximum extractables levels [15]. The ability to directly isolate, identify, and quantify these substances in the presence of product or process solutions is very limited. Product and most process solutions will interfere with these types of assays. Therefore, a model solvent approach uses extraction procedures that are more conducive to identifying and quantifying potential extractables.

Frequently, filter components are extracted using reflux or Soxhlet extraction at high temperatures. In Soxhlet extraction, a solvent (typically water or an alcohol) is continuously distilled over the material to maximize the concentration of extractables in a given volume of solvent [15,16]. Another extraction procedure more commonly used for complete filter devices (due to device size) is a static soak for an extended period of time using a minimum volume of solvent at or slightly above the normal operating temperature. A combination of different solvents may be used to model the extractables for a given process solution. After the extracted material is obtained, various analytical methods can be used to quantify and identify extracted substances. The most common method for quantifying extractables is the gravimetric non-volatile residues (NVR) test in which the weight of residual extractables is determined. In this analytical test, an aliquot of extracted solution is evaporated to dryness and the residue is weight. Solution with a significant amount of salts will be dried with the extractables and will give an overestimation of the extractables. TOC is also frequently used in conjunction with NVR to quantify organic substances. The analytical techniques used to identify extracted substances are Fourier transform infrared spectrometry (FTIR), reversed-phase HPLC (RPHPLC), gas chromatography, (GC) gas chromatography–mass spectrometry (GC–MS), and gel permeation chromatography with refractive index (GPC) [14,17]. Each analytical assay has its limitation, and those limitations are well described by Stone et al. [15] and Reif et al. [17].

The objective of the ZEVALIN filter extractable study was to demonstrate that contact of filters with product or process solutions does not result in unique extractables, which could compromise biosafety. The manufacturers of all filters had already shown that filter extractables are nontoxic by USP Class VI testing, and known extractables had been identified using model solvents. Each filter manufacturer uses specific extraction and analytical test methods already developed for evaluating their filter extractables. Therefore, the filter manufacturers were contracted to perform the filter extractable studies with oversight of the validation from IDEC Pharmaceuticals. The filter study design used a worst-case scenario for the model solvent, emulating the product or process solution, filtration time, process temperature, and sterilization procedure. One filter type was selected to represent all possible pore sizes for the same material of construction. The process solutions selected for the study represented process extremes (pH, solvent strength, solute level) to provide suitable challenge to each type of filter. The chemistry of the filter was taken into consideration in determining the appropriate worst-case model solvent to be used. All product and process solutions for the ZEVALIN purification process could be divided into five model solvents: water for all aqueous solutions and product, dilute HCL pH $\leq$1.5–2 for acidic solutions, dilute ammonium hydroxide pH $\geq$13 for all basic solution, 25% dimethylformamide for urea, and 20% ethanol for ethanol-containing solutions. The time and temperature used for static soak of the filter were at the upper end or above the normal operating range for the process. If the filter was normally steam-sterilized or autoclaved before use, the filter was wetted and autoclaved. The filter was not flushed prior to the static soak, and a minimum volume of solvent was employed to result in the highest amount of extractables.

The analytical techniques used to quantify extractables were NVR and TOC, and the analytical techniques to identify the extractables were FTIR and reversed-phase HPLC, depending on the preference of the manufacturer. The study results demonstrated that extractable levels were very low for all filters tested, and only known extractables were identified. These results complement the USP Class VI testing results and show that the type and amount of potential substances leached from filter do not impact the quality of the product.

Shown subsequently is an example of a filter extractable study for the 0.22-µm filter used to filter an acidic solution. The normal processing time was 30 minutes at ambient temperature (15–26°C). Three filter devices for each model solvent from three different lots were used in this extractable study. Unflushed filters were exposed to a static soak in water or dilute HCl pH 2.0 at 45°C for 72 hours. A control sample was run in conjunction with each model solvent tested that contained the model solvent with no filter.

The analytical methods used to quantify and identify the extractables were gravimetric nonvolatile residues (NVR), total organic carbon (TOC), reversed-phase chromatography (RPHPLC), and Fourier transform infrared spectrometry (FTIR). The average NVR was 3.5 mg with a range of 2.4–4.1 mg for the filter devices extracted in water. The average NVR was 5.0 mg with a range of 4.3–5.9 mg for the filter devices extracted in HCl pH 2.0. The average TOC content was 2.5 mg with a range of 2.1–2.9 mg for filter devices extracted in water. The average TOC content was 2.8 mg with a range of 2.4–3.2 mg for filter devices extracted in HCl pH 2.0.

The RPHPLC analysis of the water and HCl pH 2.0 extract at 214 nm and 254 nm showed no peaks greater than 10 mAU with no extractables being identified. The position of the peaks in the chromatograms indicated that the substances were inorganic compounds (salt) or highly polar, water-soluble compounds (methanol, acetone). FTIR was used to characterize the NVR of both water and HCl pH 2.0 extraction residues. FTIR is an excellent technique for analyzing polymeric and oligomer solutes. Characterization of NVR was accomplished by comparing the FTIR spectra of experimentally derived samples with FTIR spectra of known filter components. The particular regions of interest are the aliphatic region (C–H bonding, ~3000 cm^{-1}), the ester region (C=O bonding, ~1750 cm^{-1}), and the ester and ether regions (C–O–C bonding, ~1500 cm^{-1} and ~1000 cm^{-1}).

The FTIR analysis showed that the water and HCl residues contained a hydrophilic polyacrylate material, a known component of the filter membrane. Figure 12.13 and Figure 12.14 show FTIR spectra of the aqueous and HCl pH 2.0 extracts as well as the reference hydrophilic polyacrylate material residue. Both spectra appear to be remarkably similar. In addition, the residues from the HCl pH 2.0 extraction indicate the presence of silica (reference spectrum shown in Figure 12.13). Silica is not a filter extractable and was identified as a breakdown product of the borosilicate glassware used in the low-pH extraction.

12.7 CONCLUSIONS

One of the objectives of this chapter was to describe an approach to deal with the challenge of setting acceptance criteria for process validation based on limited manufacturing-scale experience. This challenge was addressed by performing characterization studies. Characterization studies are defined as preliminary studies that provide an understanding of the expected process performance ranges under certain operating conditions. The data from the characterization study were used to define predetermined acceptance criteria for process validation. The example we used for characterizing the chromatography steps was based on forward-linking a set of critical operating parameters at each process extreme and at the targeted center point. The acceptance criteria for most of the performance parameters in chromatography process validation protocols were based on four

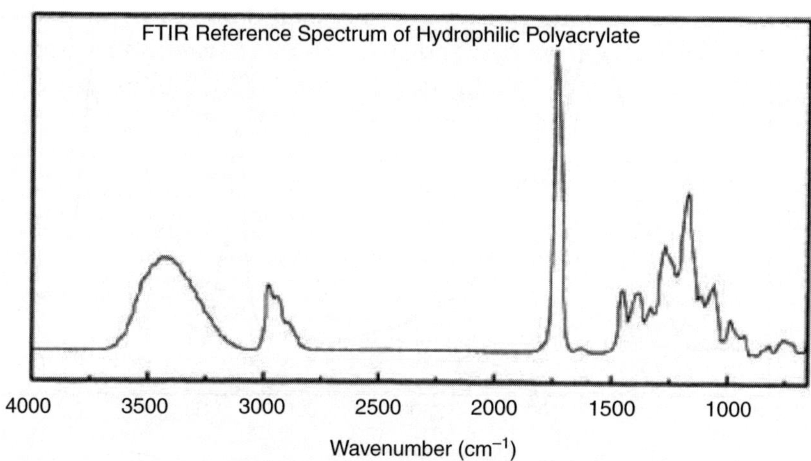

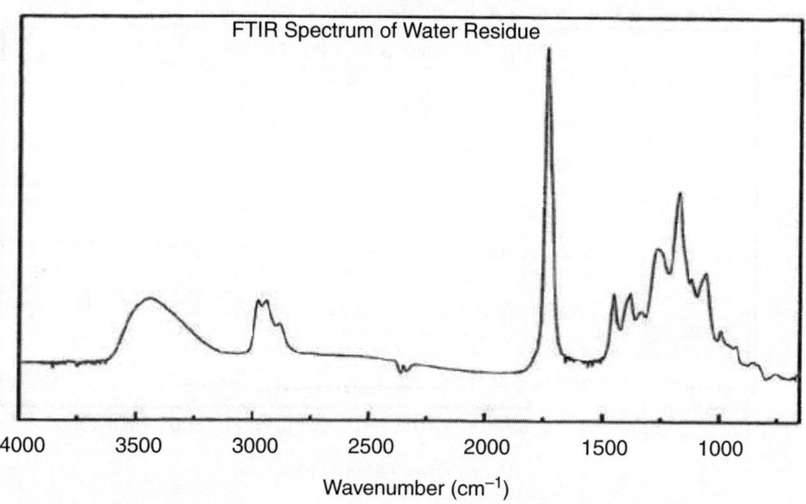

Figure 12.13 FTIR spectra of water extraction residue and hydrophilic polyacrylate references standard.

standard deviations of the data from the characterization study. Four standard deviations were used in an attempt to encompass all of the process variation because a small number of runs (three) were performed. Ideally, it would be preferred to base the acceptance criteria on a sufficiently larger

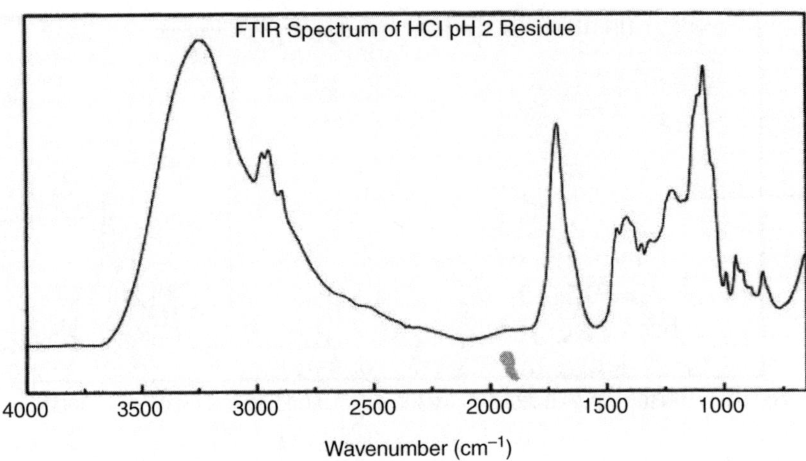

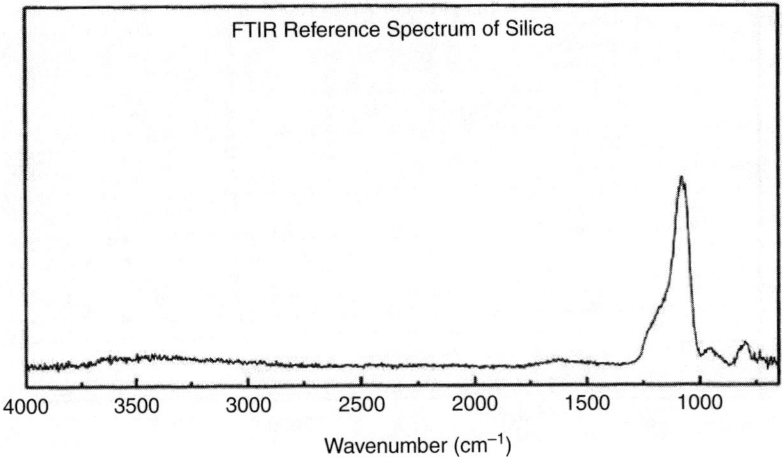

Figure 12.14 FTIR spectra of HCl pH 2 extraction buffer residue and silica references standard.

sample size to provide some degree of confidence in the established limits that would encompass the normal variation in fewer standard deviations. A subset of the performance parameters from the process validation studies is continually monitored in-process, and action limits were established to ensure process consistency. These parameters are continually reevaluated as further manufacturing experience is gained. This reevaluation will allow revision of the action limits and acceptance criteria of future validations as a larger data set is obtained.

The ZEVALIN purification process has been shown to effectively and consistently produce a product that meets its predetermined specifications and quality attributes. The validation of the purification process was accomplished by using a combination of full- and small-scale studies that encompassed a broad range of activities. Full-scale process validation studies demonstrated the consistency and reliability of the purification process under normal operating conditions. Small-scale process validation studies demonstrated the capability of the process at extreme operating conditions. The small-scale models for the chromatography and nanofiltration steps were qualified as being representative of the manufacturing process prior to or concurrent with each validation. Small-scale studies demonstrated that the process is capable of removing and inactivating a broad range of viruses as well as other impurities and contaminants to safe levels. The small-scale process validation studies complemented the full-scale studies by providing additional understanding of the purification process.

In the current development of newer processes, process validation issues are taken into consideration much earlier in development of the purification process by use of a design of experiment methodology. Design of experiment (DOE) is a statistically based methodology in which several operational parameters can be evaluated at the same time using two levels, one at high level and one at low level. Significant operational parameters and their interactions affecting a process step can be identified, and a model predicting the response or output of a performance parameter can be developed. The design of experiment can be set up to provide a high degree of statistical confidence in the predicted outcome of performance parameters. The DOE can be used to find and predict the range of operational parameters that will provide the optimal performance parameters in terms of yield and purity. The 95% prediction interval from the model developed by the DOE can be used to define acceptance criteria in process validation. Characterization studies evaluating both the high and low maximum process operating ranges at small scale or pilot scale are an acceptable means to verify the DOE model such that it can be used to set acceptance criteria for full-scale validations.

REFERENCES

1. ICH Guideline Q7A Step 4, Good Manufacturing Practice for Active Pharmaceutical Ingredients, Nov. 2000.

2. U.S. Food and Drug Administration, Guideline on General Principles of Process Validation, May 1987.

3. U.S. Food and Drug Administration, Manufacturing, Processing or Holding Active Pharmaceutical Ingredients, March 1998.

4. Seely, R., Tomusiak, M., and Kuhn, R., in *Biopharmaceutical Process Validation*, Sofer, G. and Zabriske, D., Eds., Marcel Decker, 2000, p. 130.

5. Gardner, A., Smith, T., Gerber, R., and Zabriskie, D., Worst case approach to validating operation ranges, in *Validation of Biopharmaceuticals Manufacturing Processes*, ACS Symp. Ser. No. 698, Kelly, B. and Ramelmeir, A., Eds., ACS Books, Washington, D.C., 1998, pp. 69–79.

6. Smith, T., Wilson, E., Scott, R., Misczak, J., Bodek, J., and Zabriskie, D., Establishment of operating ranges in a purification process for a monoclonal antibody, in *Validation of Biopharmaceuticals Manufacturing Processes*, ACS Symp. Ser. No. 698, Kelly, B. and Ramelmeier, A., Eds., ACS Books, Washington, D.C., pp. 80–92.

7. ICH Guideline Q6A Step 4, Specifications: Test Procedures and Acceptance Criteria for Biotechnological/Biological Products, March 1999.

8. ICH Q5A Step 4 Consensus Guideline, Quality of Biotechnological Products: Viral Safety Evaluation of Biotechnology Products Derived from Cell Lines of Human or Animal Origin, CPMP/ICH/295/95.

9. Darling, A., Validation of biopharmaceutical purification process for viral clearance evaluation, *Mol. Biotechnol.*, May 2002.

10. Center for Biologics Evaluation and Research, Points to Consider in the Manufacturing and Testing of Monoclonal Antibody Products for Human Use, Rockville, MD, 1997.

11. Acceptability of cell substances for production of biologicals, World Heath Organization Tech. Report Ser. 747, 1987.

12. Griffiths, E., WHO Expert Committee on Biological Standardization: Highlights of the meeting of October 1996, *Biologicals*, 25, 359–362, 1997.

13. Sofer, G. and Hagel, L., *Handbook of Process Chromatography: A Guide to Optimization Scale-Up and Validation*, Academic Press, p. 159.

14. Gagnon, P., *Purification Tools for Monoclonal Antibodies*, Validated Biosystems, Tucson, AZ, 1996, pp. 174–175.

15. Technical Report No. 26, Sterilizing Filtration of Liquids, *PDA J. Pharm. Sci. Technol.*, 52 (suppl.).

16. Stone, T., Goel, V., and Loszcak, J., Methodology for analysis of filter extractables: A model solvent approach, *Pharm. Technol.*, 18, 116–130, 1994.

17. Reif, O., Solkner, P., and Rupp, J., Analysis and evaluation of filter cartridge extractables for validation in pharmaceutical downstream processing, *Pharm. Technol.*, 50, 399–410, 1996.

18. Weitzmen, C., The use of model solvents for evaluating extractables from filters used to process pharmaceutical products, *Pharm. Technol.*, 10, 72–99, 1997.

13

Process Validation of a Multivalent Bacterial Vaccine: A Novel Matrix Approach

NARAHARI S. PUJAR, MARSHALL G. GAYTON,
WAYNE K. HERBER,
CHITRANANDA ABEYGUNAWARDANA,
MICHAEL L. DEKLEVA, P. K. YEGNESWARAN,
AND ANN L. LEE

CONTENTS

13.1 INTRODUCTION

The goal of any process validation is to ensure process consistency and robustness so that each lot of product manufactured is of the same purity, potency, and overall quality as every other lot. The concept of process validation has been reviewed extensively in other chapters of this book, so we will limit our discussions by simply stating the definition in the 1987 FDA Guideline on General Principles of Process Validation[1]:

> Process validation is establishing documented evidence which provides a high degree of assurance that a specific process will consistently produce a product meeting predetermined specifications and quality characteristics.

At Merck, this has meant that the process is thoroughly characterized at laboratory and pilot scale, through both a detailed understanding of individual unit operations and the interactions between the unit operations in their final sequence. The formal process validation exercise is then performed at full scale under predetermined process parameter ranges, with the objective of demonstrating that the process and the product meet predetermined quality attributes. The validation study at full scale usually involves at least three full-scale lots.

13.2 WORST-CASE CHALLENGES

Before arriving at the specifics of the current study, it is instructive to review approaches to process validation that are different from the conventional 3X approach. One such example is the concept of worst-case challenges. This concept is tightly linked with the goal of ensuring that process variable ranges are robust and can produce a consistent output in the face of typical variability in factors relating to process, equipment, raw material, or personnel. In the case of equipment cleaning, validation studies are generally performed under worst-case conditions of process cleaning parameters such as post-use hold time, cleaning agent exposure time, and the number of water rinses. For example, the soiled equipment could be held for 72 hours, a duration longer than what is anticipated during routine operations. Similarly, instead of three full water-for-injection rinses during routine operation, cleaning validation could be performed with one or two water rinses. Once the process is shown to consistently perform well during a "fractional" cycle, confidence is established in the robustness and consistency of the full cycle for routine cleaning. The same approach can be taken for process validation, although in this case, the challenge is often done at laboratory or pilot scale where many more processing permutations can be challenged more cost-effectively. The critical principle to remember is that if parameters controlled at the outer limits of control ranges make product of acceptable quality, then product manufactured within those control points will also meet quality goals.

13.3 FAMILY AND MATRIX APPROACHES TO PROCESS VALIDATION

A variation of a worst-case challenge is encountered when dealing with multiple validation studies within a group of studies. For example, when validating a cleaning cycle for a piece of equipment used for multiple soils, one approach to validation might be to independently develop cleaning processes for the removal of each soil and validate each of these processes. Another preferred approach would be to perform studies to assess the relative ease with which each soil can be removed in a small-scale probe study. Then, the most stubborn of the soils can be selected to represent the others in the development and validation of a worst-case cleaning process. The same cycle can then be used for the other soils.

Similar to the aforementioned situation, albeit with a much greater complexity, is the case of multivalent products where the processes used to manufacture the different products are common (e.g., multivalent and combination vaccines). If a multivalent vaccine is composed of several different antigen components, one approach to process validation might be to validate each antigen independent of all others. In a practical sense, this would mean that in addition to extensive process characterization, the formal process validation study would be performed by making at least three lots of each antigen under predefined conditions and demonstrating that the product meets predefined specifications.

An alternate streamlined approach to independent validation of each antigen might be to: (1) treat the different antigens as a product family, (2) look for similarities within the family, and perhaps group them, and (3) choose one representative from each group to validate. A worst-case approach analogous to the aforementioned cleaning example could be used if applicable, but since manufacturing processes are significantly more complicated than cleaning cycles, a straightforward definition of a "worst case" is not always possible. In the simplest of multivalent products, consider a two-valent product, where both components are made using the exact or very similar processes. One might envision a formal process validation study, where two lots of each of the two components are manufactured, resulting in a total of four lots. While the total number of lots is less than the six required in a conventional process validation, the common process is actually tested over *four* lots, while still evaluating the consistency of the two components. Such an approach is facilitated when the final product can be fully analytically characterized. When extrapolated to larger valences, such as the 23-valent case study in this chapter, it becomes very apparent why this approach should be seriously considered. The key to development of such an approach is to have a thorough understanding of the process and of the process variables that are truly critical to product potency, purity, and stability as well as the similarities and differences between the different components.

While the FDA does not currently have a formal policy on the use of "matrix" or "family" approaches to process validation, opinions by agency employees have been published that leave room for such approaches on a case-by-case basis when a technically sound rationale can be presented.[2–9] To define these terms, a *matrix approach* generally refers to a plan to conduct process validation on different strengths of the same product. The term *family approach*, alternatively, has been used to describe a plan to conduct process validation on different but similar products. In this study, a novel matrix approach was recently applied to the validation of a new process for Pneumovax®23, a 23-valent polysaccharide-based pneumococcal vaccine. The slightly different use of the term *matrix approach* is due to the design of the study being rationalized by an actual matrix of key process parameters, physicochemical properties for the different components, and the number of validation lots represented for each of them in the study. This approach is discussed in more detail the next section.

13.4 CASE STUDY: MATRIX VALIDATION OF PNEUMOVAX®23, A 23-VALENT POLYSACCHARIDE-BASED PNEUMOCOCCAL VACCINE

Pneumovax®23 is a vaccine against adult pneumococcal disease caused by *Streptococcus pneumoniae*. The vaccine consists of a mixture of highly purified capsular polysaccharides from the 23 most prevalent or invasive pneumococcal types of *Streptococcus pneumoniae*. The 23 serotypes account for 85–90% of clinical pneumococcal isolates in the United States.[10] The 23-valent vaccine is manufactured by individually fermenting each different bacterial serotype, isolating its capsular polysaccharide, and mixing the 23 polysaccharides in the final formulation. The original 23-valent vaccine was licensed by Merck in 1983. Over the past few years, a new manufacturing process was developed and a state-of-the-art manufacturing facility was built to take advantage of modern process technologies, as well as to meet evolving regulatory expectations (e.g., removal of animal-derived raw materials).

Regulatory licensure of the new process and facility for the manufacture of the bulk polysaccharides required process validation. In order to demonstrate process validation in the conventional sense, each of the 23 polysaccharides would be required to be manufactured in triplicate for a total of at least 69 lots. This not only presents an impractical situation, it may be unwarranted if the processes for the manufacture of each of the 23 polysaccharides are similar and the manufacturing facility is common. This is indeed the case, and this commonality of the process and the facility allowed the development of a matrix approach to process validation. The "matrix validation" plan was developed by taking into account the similarities in the processes for the 23 polysaccharides, while ensuring adequate representation of the differences in the processes and the underlying physicochemical characteristics. This resulted in a reduced number of total validation lots. In addition, the plan also resulted in the common aspects of the process being tested over a large number of lots, significantly greater than the $n = 3$ required in conventional process validation.

13.4.1 Process Development

The concept of matrix validation was built into the process development effort, right from program inception. For example, a key objective of process development was to develop a *common* process for the fermentation and purification of the 23 capsular polysaccharides. Early identification of a common process was also essential for the parallel construction of the manufacturing facility, one that could eventually accommodate the final process of all the polysaccharides. Based on existing process and analytical information from the current licensed process, those serotypes that were considered challenging were evaluated early during process development to enable the definition of the common unit operations and their worst-case operating conditions. Subsequent development defined the specific process for each of the 23 serotypes.

Three phases of new process development were completed — laboratory, pilot, and full scale — prior to the manufacture of the full-scale validation lots. The laboratory-scale work was performed at less than one hundredth of the full manufacturing scale. Pilot scale was one tenth of the full manufacturing scale. Scale-down versions of the manufacturing process equipment were used at pilot scale to simulate the proposed full-scale manufacturing process more closely than was possible using the laboratory equipment and greatly minimized risks to scale-up. Finally, full-scale engineering lots were also carried out in the new manufacturing facility as a final test of equipment readiness, to finalize manufacturing procedures and documentation, to initiate cleaning validation studies, and to uncover any unexpected scale-up issues. Data from pilot-scale lots and the full-scale engineering lots also provided additional support to the formal full-scale process validation effort.

The final manufacturing process for the fermentation and purification of 23 capsular polysaccharides is shown in Figure 13.1. The same sequence of unit operations and equipment is used for the manufacture of each serotype. The sequence of unit operations is classified into six process modules, and the objective of each process module is the same for all 23 serotypes. Due to differences in the physicochemical properties of the different polysaccharides, there are minor differences in some unit operations and in some of the process parameters used in the different unit operations. While these differences are not discussed in any detail here, they drive the design of the matrix validation plan, and this is discussed in more detail in the next section.

The capsular polysaccharides can be fully characterized using state-of-the-art analytical techniques. This ability to fully characterize the polysaccharides was also a critical factor for developing and validating the new process. Since the goal was to rapidly develop a state-of-the-art process to produce the same product, analytical characterization of the current process polysaccharides formed the basis for the selection of the final product quality attributes and their associated acceptance criteria. Analytical characterization of the polysaccharides also led to the grouping of the polysaccharides into different groups of unique structural attributes, shown in Table 13.1.

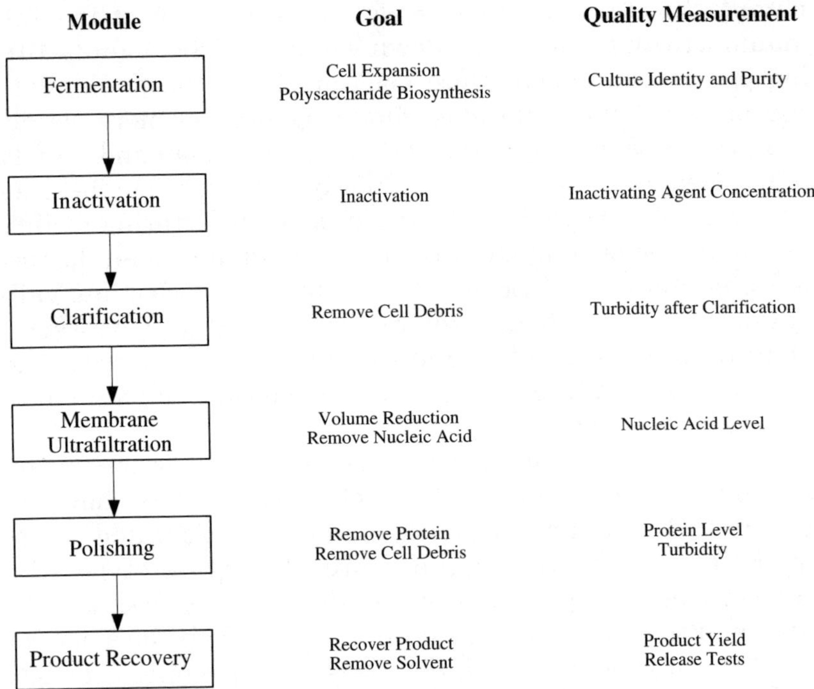

Figure 13.1 Flow diagram of the new process Pneumovax®23 fermentation and purification processes.

13.4.2 Matrix Validation Plan

At the outset, critical process parameters (CPPs) and critical in-process measures (or critical quality attributes [CQAs]) were identified along with their respective acceptance criteria. CPPs are a subset of all operational process parameters that are central to achieving the goal of a given process step or module (a module is defined as a series of steps that collectively achieve the same goal, e.g., centrifugation followed by polishing depth filtration for clarification). CQAs are important quality measures that enable monitoring of the output of a process step or module. CQAs include tests for both process intermediates and final bulk powder.

The similarities in process design for the 23 polysaccharides allowed the definition of a universal set of CPPs and

TABLE 13.1 Illustration of Matrix of Polysaccharide Characteristics

	Molecular Weight	Negative Charge	Neutral Charge	Linear	Branched	O-Acetate	Pyruvate	Phosphodiester (Backbone)	Phosphodiester (Side Chain)
3 Lots per Serotype									
Serotype A		X		X					X
2 Lots per Serotype									
Serotype B		X		X			X	X	
...		X			X			X	
...			X		X			X	
...		X			X	X			X
1 Lot per Serotype									
Serotype C			X	X				X	
...		X		X		X		X	
...		X			X	X		X	
...		X		X		X		X	
Total Lots									

CQAs across all serotypes. The extent of the commonality between CPPs and CQAs for process validation of the 23 polysaccharides is illustrated in Figure 13.2. With minor exceptions, the CPPs and CQAs for each of the 23 polysaccharides are the same. Furthermore, the ranges for the common CPPs and the acceptance ranges for the common CQAs, presented in Figure 13.2, are either identical or are have the same basis. These similarities in the process, and consequently the CPPs and CQAs, further set the stage for a matrix approach to process validation. Before embarking on the details of the actual matrix validation plan utilized for this process, it is instructive to illustrate the concept of matrix validation with specific process examples. Three examples are provided. The first example is that of the membrane ultrafiltration module, which demonstrates that even a single lot of each serotype provides adequate data and information to demonstrate process robustness and consistency of this particular process attribute. The second example of a nuclease treatment step shows that for process attributes shared by a smaller set of serotypes, it is possible to group them and demonstrate validation of the step within this group with a reduced number of lots. A third and final example demonstrates a similar grouping based on the structural characteristics of the polysaccharides.

Example 13.1:
Membrane Ultrafiltration Module

The goal of the membrane ultrafiltration module, which is common for all serotypes, is to reduce the volume of the clarified fermentation broth and remove a large majority of the nucleic acids from the clarified broth. Two different membrane molecular weight cutoffs (MWCO) are used depending on serotype — 15 serotypes use 100-kDa MWCO and the remaining eight use a 500-kDa MWCO. The clearance of DNA across this step and more generally throughout the process is shown in Figure 13.3. The CQA for this step is the DNA level at the end of the ultrafiltration module, as a representative of the total nucleic acid level at this stage. Due to similarities in the process and consequent

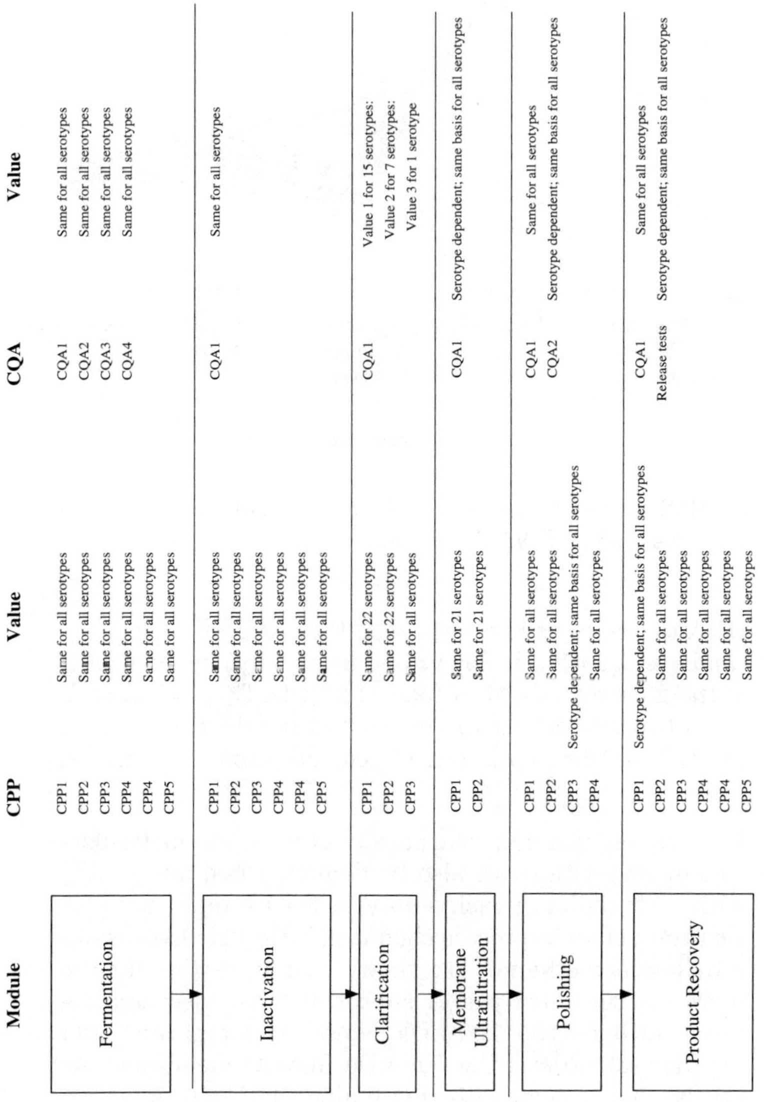

Module	CPP	Value	CQA	Value
Fermentation	CPP1	Same for all serotypes	CQA1	Same for all serotypes
	CPP2	Same for all serotypes	CQA2	Same for all serotypes
	CPP3	Same for all serotypes	CQA3	Same for all serotypes
	CPP4	Same for all serotypes	CQA4	Same for all serotypes
	CPP4	Same for all serotypes		
	CPP5	Same for all serotypes		
Inactivation	CPP1	Same for all serotypes	CQA1	Same for all serotypes
	CPP2	Same for all serotypes		
	CPP3	Same for all serotypes		
	CPP4	Same for all serotypes		
	CPP4	Same for all serotypes		
	CPP5	Same for all serotypes		
Clarification	CPP1	Same for 22 serotypes	CQA1	Value 1 for 15 serotypes:
	CPP2	Same for 22 serotypes		Value 2 for 7 serotypes:
	CPP3	Same for all serotypes		Value 3 for 1 serotype
Membrane Ultrafiltration	CPP1	Same for 21 serotypes	CQA1	Serotype dependent; same basis for all serotypes
	CPP2	Same for 21 serotypes		
Polishing	CPP1	Same for all serotypes	CQA1	Same for all serotypes
	CPP2	Same for all serotypes	CQA2	Serotype dependent; same basis for all serotypes
	CPP3	Serotype dependent; same basis for all serotypes		
	CPP4	Same for all serotypes		
Product Recovery	CPP1	Serotype dependent; same basis for all serotypes	CQA1	Same for all serotypes
	CPP2	Same for all serotypes	Release tests	Serotype dependent; same basis for all serotypes
	CPP3	Same for all serotypes		
	CPP4	Same for all serotypes		
	CPP4	Same for all serotypes		
	CPP5	Same for all serotypes		

Figure 13.2 Critical process parameters (CPP) and critical quality attributes (CQA).

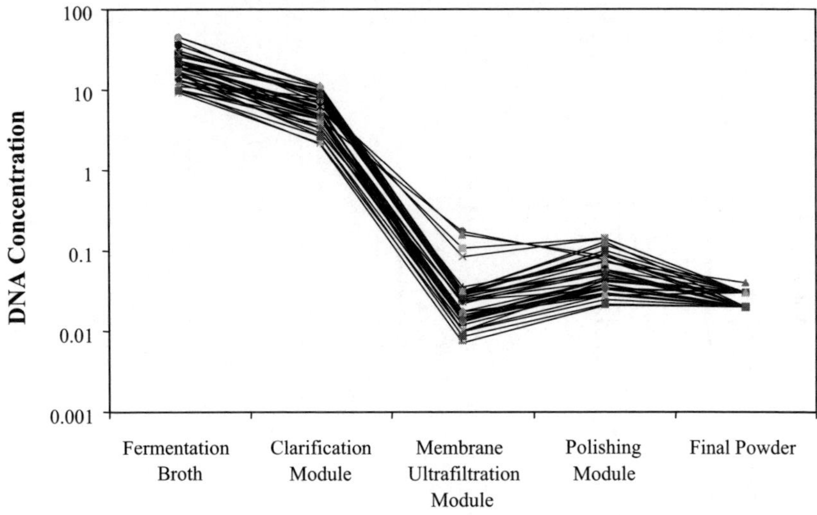

Figure 13.3 Process clearance of nucleic acids during the purification process using DNA as a marker.

DNA clearance, it is clearly seen that process consistency can be adequately demonstrated using only one lot of each of the 23 serotypes, for a total of 23 lots. Even when each of the two subsets of serotypes that utilize the two different MWCO membranes is considered, the same case can be made.

In a similar manner, clearance of other small-molecular-weight impurities can also be demonstrated adequately with a single lot of each serotype. For example, data for clearance of an in-process chemical, TRIS (tris[hydroxymethyl]aminomethane), are shown in Figure 13.4 for the more viscous serotypes. A subset of these viscous serotypes utilizes the 100-kDa NMWCO membrane and another set utilizes the 500-kDa MWCO membrane. As can be clearly seen with this limited data set, the clearance of TRIS is adequate in all cases and more importantly is similar in all cases. A single lot of each serotype,

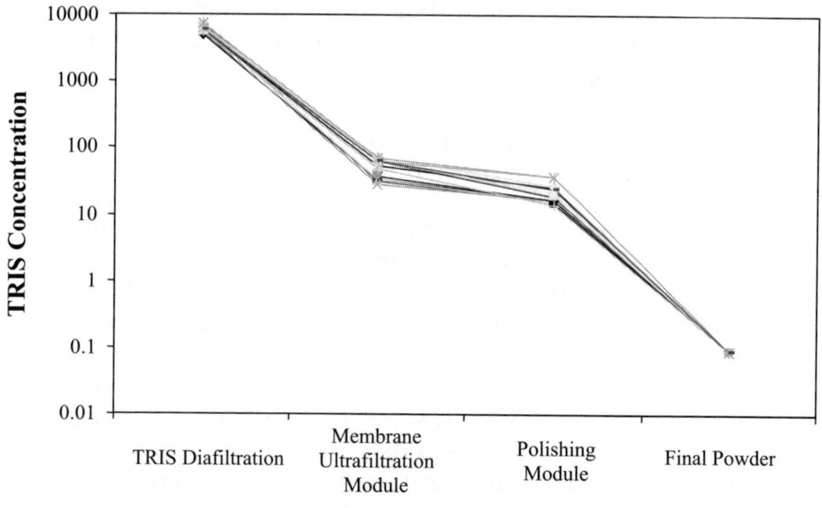

Figure 13.4   Process clearance of TRIS during the purification process for select serotypes.

for a total of 23 lots, can provide ample assurance that adequate clearance of TRIS can be achieved consistently.

Example 13.2: Nuclease Treatment Step

Nuclease treatment is carried out in the case of two of the 23 serotypes. The objective of this step is to digest cellular nucleic acids so that they can be adequately cleared during the purification process. These two serotypes, in contrast to the other 21 serotypes, have unique charge properties — the highest charge density in one case, and the presence of a positive charge center in the other case — that necessitate an additional nuclease treatment step for robust nucleic acid clearance. A related objective for the rest of the purification process is to demonstrate adequate clearance of the added nuclease. Demonstration of process consistency for both objectives can be performed by a combination of lots from the two serotypes, due to the similarity of the step. In this case, two lots of each serotype were proposed in the process validation study, thus providing assurance of the nuclease treatment and subsequent removal of the nuclease over *four* lots.

Example 13.3: O-Acetate Side Group and Phosphodiester Bonds

Similar to processing characteristics, the matrix validation plan had to capture differences in structural and physicochemical characteristics, the underlying factor causing the differences in the process characteristics. Some of the 23 polysaccharides contain potentially labile groups such as O-acetate and phosphodiester bonds. These serotypes provide test cases for validation of molecular stability over the manufacturing process. In all, ten serotypes contain the O-acetate group, six serotypes contain a phosphodiester bond in the backbone, and four serotypes contain a phosphodiester bond in the side chain. The stability of these moieties has been established independently, and of the three entities, O-acetate is considered to be the least stable.[11] Backbone phosphodiester bonds in serotype 19A, 19F, and 10A have been shown to be the most susceptible to hydrolysis.[11] A combination of one lot of each of these serotypes, for a total of 20 lots, provides adequate data to demonstrate stability of all three entities. Inclusion of data from duplicate lots of specific serotypes provides further assurance.

To summarize, as described in the previous illustrations, due to the common equipment, similar processing steps, and the monitoring of identical validation parameters across the serotypes, even one lot of each of the 23 polysaccharide serotypes would provide a large amount of data to support the conclusion that the process and all associated manufacturing systems are consistent and well controlled. Nevertheless, the matrix validation strategy proposed was to manufacture a single lot of the majority of the serotypes, duplicate lots of a select set of serotypes, and a triplicate lot of one serotype. In addition to manufacturing a single lot of each serotype, validation of process consistency was supported by duplicate lots for select serotypes, chosen to represent a range of specific process and physicochemical characteristics. In total, seven serotypes were chosen for duplicate lots because of their unique processing or physicochemical characteristics. Finally, a single serotype was chosen to be run in triplicate to satisfy confirmation of intraserotype process reproducibility and to provide a bridge to the standard validation practice for monovalent products. The single serotype chosen had a number of physicochemical and processing characteristics found in a majority of the 23 serotypes, such as negative charge, linear structure, O-acetate, moderate molecular size, and moderate viscosity.

To illustrate the concept of matrix approach, a matrix of the number of lots for each serotype, along with their respective key processing and physicochemical characteristics, was created. An example of such a matrix is shown in Table 13.1 and Table 13.2. Table 13.1 includes physicochemical characteristics — for example, charge, molecular size, branching, O-acetate, phosphate, etc. Table 13.2 includes process characteristics — for example, membrane and filter pore sizes, filter area, alcohol type, etc. These tables illustrate that there are multiple serotypes that represent each processing and physicochemical characteristic considered in the manufacturing process demonstration. By grouping serotypes based on similarities in these characteristics, the results of a validation study for a serotype in a group are representative for the other serotypes within the grouping. As a result, process validation data for each processing and physicochemical characteristic were obtained from a large number of lots.

This matrix validation strategy resulted in 32 full-scale validation lots, about an order of magnitude greater than the number for a conventional process validation of a single product, and less than half of the 69 lots that might be arrived at using conventional process validation for each of the 23 polysaccharides.

13.4.3 Regulatory Buy-In and Study Execution

This unique approach for this multivalent product was presented to CBER in a Type B meeting and to EMEA via the CPMP scientific advice procedure, well in advance of the filing

TABLE 13.2 Illustration of Matrix of Serotype Specific Process Characteristics

	Glucose in Fermentor	Clarification Train 1	Clarification Train 2	UF Concentration Factor 1	UF Concentration Factor 2	UF Membrane Pore Size 1	UF Membrane Pore Size 2	Nuclease Use	Alcohol for Fractionation 1	Alcohol for Fractionation 2	Polishing Filter Area 1	Polishing Filter Area 2
3 Lots per Serotype												
Serotype A		X			X	X				X		
2 Lots per Serotype												
Serotype B	X				X		X	X	X			
…		X			X	X	X		X			X
…		X			X		X		X			X
…			X	X			X		X		X	
1 Lot per Serotype												
Serotype C		X			X	X			X		X	
…		X			X						X	
…			X		X	X					X	
…		X			X						X	
Total Lots												

for licensure of the process. The concept was accepted by the regulatory agencies and was facilitated by: (1) the large body of experience with the currently produced product, as well as laboratory- and pilot-scale experience with the new process, (2) the analytical characterizability of the product, and (3) data from a clinical trial comparing the safety and immunogenicity of a subset of the 23 polysaccharides. Furthermore, the acceptance of the concept of matrix validation was greatly facilitated by a constant dialogue with the regulatory agencies.

The validation study was successfully executed and met the objective. The process was shown to be consistent and well controlled by the extensive data collected over the large number of lots. The concept of chemical comparability between the final product polysaccharides made from the current and new process was a central theme in this validation study. Finally, during this matrix process validation study, the other systems in the manufacturing process (e.g., manufacturing facility, equipment, analytical assays, operations, training, documentation, etc.) were extensively tested and were shown to be robust, more extensively in the case of conventional process validation of three lots.

13.4.4 Conclusions

A matrix validation strategy was proposed, accepted by regulatory agencies, and successfully executed for the process validation of a 23-valent polysaccharide vaccine. Due to similarities in the process, conventional process validation would have been redundant and would also have been impractical. The matrix validation plan incorporated a single lot from all serotypes, duplicate lots from seven serotypes, and a triplicate lot from one representative serotype, resulting in a reduced number of total lots, while ensuring multiple lots for each unique processing condition and physicochemical characteristic reflected in the manufacturing process. Furthermore, the large number of lots relative to that for a single product tested the common manufacturing systems (e.g., equipment, facility, documentation, personnel, quality control, etc.) much more stringently than conventional process validation. The matrix validation of the process thus provided adequate assurance that the manufacturing process for all 23 serotypes was consistent and well controlled.

A set of general principles on the concept of matrix validation can be developed from this case study for future application of matrix validation:

1. Matrix validation should be considered if conventional process validation is redundant — e.g., if there is a *set* of processes being validated *and* there are similarities in the processes being validated.
2. Matrix validation should be considered if conventional process validation is impractical — e.g., if it is prohibitively expansive as in the case of multivalent products.
3. Matrix validation for the process is applicable only if other aspects of the manufacturing systems are held constant across the different processes being validated.
4. Matrix validation of the process is greatly facilitated if the product and process are highly characterized.
5. Matrix validation should not lead to a number of lots that would be smaller than that required for conventional process validation of a single process (typically three).

These principles would apply in addition to those for process validation in general.

In summary, a matrix validation can provide a streamlined approach to validation of multivalent products while still adequately demonstrating process consistency and robustness. This kind of approach may also become relevant in the case of products using platform technologies such as monoclonal antibodies and gene therapy vectors.

ACKNOWLEDGMENTS

The authors would like to acknowledge the entire Pneumovax®23 Project Team.

REFERENCES AND NOTES

1. *FDA Guideline on General Principles of Process Validation, 1987.*

   Definition of process validation: Process validation is establishing documented evidence which provides a high degree of assurance that a specific process will consistently produce a product meeting pre-determined specifications and quality characteristics.

   Worst case — A set of conditions encompassing upper and lower processing limits and circumstances, including those within standard operating procedures, which pose the greatest chance of process or product failure when compared to ideal conditions. Such conditions do not necessarily induce product or process failure.

2. FDA/CDER/CBER/CVM Guidance for Industry, Manufacture, Processing or Holding of Active Pharmaceutical Ingredients (draft), 1996.

   p. 14, F.2., Validation of cleaning methods should encompass worst-case conditions.

3. Validation Master Plan Installation and Operational Qualification, Non-Sterile Process Validation, Cleaning Validation, April 2000 (PIC/S, Pharmaceutical Inspection Convention).

   p. 4, 1.19 (Introduction), Common sense and an understanding of pharmaceutical processing go a long way towards determining what aspects of an operation are critical.

   p. 9, 3.5.2.3 (Validation Master Plan), A common principle in validation studies is to challenge processes, systems, etc. The rationale behind any challenge and/or "worst case" situation should be explained. Consideration can be given to the grouping of products/processes for the purpose of validating "worst case" situation. Where "worst case" situations cannot be simulated, the rationale for the groupings made should be defined.

p. 23, 6.3.5 (Cleaning Validation), Cleaning procedures for products and processes which are very similar do not need to be individually validated. It is considered acceptable to select a representative range of similar products and processes concerned and to justify a validation programme which addresses the critical issues relating to the selected products and processes. A single validation study under consideration of the "worst case" can then be carried out which takes account of the relevant criteria. This practice is termed "Bracketing."

p. 23, 6.3.6, At least three consecutive applications of the cleaning procedure should be performed and shown to be successful in order to prove that the method is validated.

p. 27, 6.11.1, limits for product residues…should be practical, achievable and verifiable; 6.11.2, …grouping into product families and choosing a "worst case" product,…grouping into groups of risk (e.g., very soluble products, similar potency, highly toxic products, difficult to detect).

4. Annex 15 to the EU Guide to Good Manufacturing Practices, September 2001.

   p. 8, 39 (Cleaning Validation), For cleaning procedures for products and processes which are similar, it is considered acceptable to select a representative range of similar products and processes. A single validation study utilizing a "worst case" approach can be carried out which takes account of the critical issues.

   p. 9, 42. (Cleaning Validation), Products which simulate the physiochemical properties of the substances to be removed may exceptionally be used instead of the substances themselves, where such substances are either toxic or hazardous.

5. Guidance Document, Cleaning Validation Guidelines (Canadian Health Products and Food Branch Inspectorate), May 2000.

   p. 4, 3.5 (Principles), It is considered acceptable to select a representative range of similar products and processes.…bracketing may be considered acceptable for similar products and / or equipment provided appropriate justification based on sound scientific rationale is given.

6. Validation Guidelines for Pharmaceutical Dosage Forms, May 2000 (Canadian Therapeutic Products Programme).

p. 6 (Definitions), Process Validation — Establishing documented evidence with a high degree of assurance that a specific process will consistently produce a product meeting its predetermined specifications and quality characteristics. Process validation may take the form of Prospective, Concurrent or Retrospective Validation and process Qualification or Re-Validation.

Worst-Case Condition — The highest and lowest value of a given parameter actually evaluated in the validation exercise.

7. Draft Good Manufacturing Practices Guide for Active Pharmaceutical Ingredients, July 2000 (draft, ICH Steering Committee).

   p. 29, 12.5 (Process Validation Program), The number of process runs needed for validation should depend on the complexity of the process or the magnitude of the process change being considered. For prospective and concurrent validation, three consecutive successful production batches should be used as a guide, but there may be situations where additional process runs are warranted to prove consistency of the process...

8. The Gold Sheet, *Pharm. Biotechnol. Quality Control,* 35, 2001.

   The entire issue is devoted to process validation, with numerous references to matrix and family approaches to validation.

9. Health Products and Food Branch, Health Canada, Cleaning Validation Guidelines, May 1, 2001.

   "For biological drugs, including vaccines, bracketing may be considered acceptable for similar products and/or equipment provided appropriate justification, based on sound, scientific rationale is given. Some examples are cleaning of fermenters of the same design but with different vessel capacity used for the same type of recombinant proteins expressed in the same rodent cell line and cultivated in closely related growth media; a multiantigen vaccine used to represent the individual antigen or other combinations of them when validating the same or similar equipment that is used at stages of formulation (adsorption) and/or holding. Validation of cleaning of fermenters should be done upon individual pathogen basis."

10. Merck Prescribing Information Pneumovax® 23 (pneumococcal vaccine polyvalent), July 2003.

11. Pujar, N.S., Huang, N.F., Daniels, C.L., Dieter, L., Gayton, M.G., and Lee, A.L., Base hydrolysis of phosphodiester bonds in pneumococcal polysaccharides, *Biopolymers*, 75, 71–74, 2004.

14

Viral Clearance Validation:
A Case Study

MICHAEL RUBINO, MARK BAILEY,
JEFFREY C. BAKER, JERI ANN BOOSE,
LORRAINE METZKA, VALERIE MOORE,
MICHELLE QUERTINMONT, AND
WILLIAM WILER

CONTENTS

14.1 STRATEGY AND PLANNING

The development and planning of a viral clearance study, as stipulated in the guidance documents, is related to the potential for viruses to enter the production system from either the cell line or other sources such as raw materials [1–6]. The ICH Q5A, in fact, ranks cell lines based on the presence of viral particles or viruses [7]. This stratification of the cell line will then determine the viral clearance that needs to be demonstrated. Other documents written by the FDA or the European authorities provide general guidance and in some cases details on the design and implementation of viral clearance studies.

The activities surrounding the planning and designing for the viral clearance study for a mammalian cell-derived protein included use of the guidance documents as a source for the design. Two primary considerations were taken into account in the planning stages. First, the expression system for production of the protein is a human-derived cell line. Second, the production and purification of the protein in this study required the use of animal-sourced materials.

An analysis of the cell line provided information needed to determine the impact on the viral clearance studies. Although the cell line had not been reported in the scientific literature to contain retroviral particles or any evidence of retrovirus infection, the cell line prior to and subsequent to the production of a GMP master cell bank was tested for retroviruses, retroviral particles, and other viruses. No evidence of viral infection or expression of viral particles was detected. Based on this information, the ICH Q5A makes the cell line a Case A. The ICH Q5A then suggests that model viruses be used for viral clearance studies.

Prior to the initiation of any studies, a viral clearance strategy was formulated in consultation with outside experts. This included an external viral safety consultant knowledgeable of regulatory issues within and outside the United States. A biosafety contract laboratory was also chosen. This laboratory had excellent capability and had sufficient expertise in regulatory affairs to assist in the design of all aspects of the study. Discussion with internal and external experts in the design of the marketing application studies started more than 2 years prior to the proposed submission date.

Another key element to the study design was the identification of purification steps to be evaluated in the viral clearance studies. Clearance studies had already been conducted on the purification process. This previous data provided an insight into the level of clearance that could be expected from the steps evaluated. There are two steps in the process dedicated to viral inactivation and viral removal. Additional steps with viral clearance possibilities included two chromatography processes and one step in which there was an increase in temperature of the process solution to 40°C.

After identifying the process and purification steps to be evaluated, it was necessary to decide which viruses to use. No specific viruses had to be included because no particles were identified in the cell line. Consideration of which viruses to use was related to identifying viruses that could potentially grow in the production cell line and the use of bovine-sourced materials in production. The literature was a source of information on the viruses to which the cells were susceptible. In addition, a study was conducted in which the cell line was challenged with a subset of bovine viruses to determine its susceptibility. Because the range of viruses that grew in the cell was varied, viruses were chosen that represented a range of biochemical and morphological types.

The following six viruses were used in the initial viral clearance study: xenotropic murine leukemia virus (MuLV), bovine viral diarrhea virus (BVDV), adenovirus, pseudorabies virus, poliovirus, and minute mouse virus (MMV). BioReliance provided the virus and a certified titer for each study. These model viruses were chosen for the following reasons:

1. MuLV was previously used to support clinical trials and is a model for any potential retrovirus contamination of the cell line or the process.
2. BVDV was previously used in viral clearance studies to support clinical trials and was used again in the current study. BVDV is a common contaminant of bovine serum, and therefore there is a potential for the cell line to be exposed to this virus.
3. Adenovirus serotype 2 (Ad-2) was used in the spiking studies because the human cell line is susceptible to them.
4. Pseudorabies virus was chosen because it is a herpesvirus, a family of viruses that can grow in the cell line. It also completes the spectrum of viruses used since it is a nonenveloped DNA virus.
5. Poliovirus is a small (30 nm) RNA virus belonging to the paramyxovirus family. Poliovirus is resistant to many environmental conditions, and because it is so robust, the scientific literature has reported that it is commonly used in other viral clearance evaluations.
6. Minute mouse virus is a parvovirus, the smallest family of mammalian viruses. MMV is nonenveloped and from 20 to 25 nm in size. MMV is a ubiquitous parvovirus and has previously caused contaminations of CHO cell bioreactor runs. Because the cell line will support growth of MMV, it is important to evaluate the clearance of this virus.

The objectives of a viral clearance study were (1) to demonstrate that the cell culture and purification processes are capable of removing or inactivating viruses, (2) to determine the clearance of each process step and the clearance for the entire process, (3) to demonstrate the kinetics of inactivation in those process steps in which inactivation is the primary method of clearance, and (4) to demonstrate that the column chromatography regeneration solutions and processes can inactivate model viruses.

At the end of the strategy and planning phase, it was important to have good communication with local management, with internal regulatory and quality control personnel, and among the scientific staff. Included in this communication was an understanding of the goals or acceptance criteria by which the studies would be evaluated. It was key to the success of the studies that the strategy was strong and well developed prior to initiating the actual work.

14.2 LOGISTICAL CONSIDERATIONS

BioReliance of Rockville, Maryland, was selected as the biosafety contract laboratory and with whom the viral clearance studies would be performed. Once legal and quality contractual agreements were completed, the technical and quality staff conducted an audit of BioReliance. Communication between both parties was essential in designing the specifics of the study. The viral spiking studies of the scaled-down process occurred at Lilly in a biosafety level 2 (BSL-2) laboratory, for the chromatography and nanofiltration steps. Samples from these steps during the studies were then frozen and shipped to BioReliance at a later date for testing. Analysis of any inactivation step was done on-site at the BioReliance facilities. A written agreement of the study design had to be in place with BioReliance, which prepared a statement of work (SOW). The SOW is a detailed protocol of the study and includes a list of the model viruses and a list of the samples BioReliance would receive for testing.

Prior to starting any clearance study, the purification scientific staff had to design and validate scaled-down models of the process steps. The scaled-down process steps needed to be comparable to the full-scale commercial process. Regulatory guidance documents provided information helpful to the design of the scale steps. A table was prepared listing the process parameters such as column height and flow rate and the actual conditions used for commercial and laboratory scale, which were similar. Whenever process parameters could not be duplicated at the different scales, viral clearance studies were conducted under the worst-case conditions.

Once the laboratory-scale models were designed, protocols were written to outline the objectives of the studies, outline conditions that would be used, and the acceptance criteria for each step. Management reviewed and signed the protocols.

All clearance studies were done at least in duplicate, preferably on different days. For chromatography steps, the viral clearance was evaluated using columns packed with virgin resin and columns packed with resin that had been regenerated the maximum number of times that will be allowed in production before the resin is replaced. This measures the viral clearance robustness of the step relative to resin age. At least three separate process steps were evaluated for each virus, but they were not always the same three steps used in the evaluation of the other viruses.

As per the guidelines, process solutions used in the viral clearance studies were obtained from the full-scale process. Process solutions were ordered from both the clinical trial pilot plant and from the commercial production facility. For chromatography runs, sufficient process solution had to be ordered to support at least twice the number of planned viral runs plus sufficient amounts for preliminary runs. Prior to each chromatography run, the purification scientist conducted at least two or three preliminary runs without virus. One run included a spike with the viral suspension media used by BioReliance.

Process solutions were also obtained from the commercial-scale or pilot plant and were submitted for cytotoxicity, viral interference, and frozen viability studies. The purpose of the cytotoxicity study was to determine whether the process solutions in the viral spiking studies were toxic to the cell lines used to quantitate the viruses. The viral interference study also determined whether the process solutions would inactivate the viruses or interfere with their recovery from spiked solutions. The frozen viability studies were conducted to determine whether the model viruses were stable in process solutions when frozen at −80°C. The frozen viability studies were conducted over a period of a few weeks. Virus was spiked into the different dilutions of process solutions and then frozen. Samples were removed to determine whether the virus was stable at −80°C for that length of time. Frozen viability studies determined the length of time samples could be stored before being tested. The samples must be diluted with cell culture media at the dilution determined in the cytotoxicity studies. After being diluted, the samples can then be frozen for testing at a later date.

14.3 PROTOCOL DEVELOPMENT AND EXECUTION

The actual viral spiking studies could be initiated only after all the preliminary planning had been completed, the protocols at both BioReliance and Lilly were approved, and results had been received for cytotoxicity, viral interference, and frozen viability.

For chromatography processes, a control run in the BSL-2 laboratory was first performed with only process solution. Next, a run with process solution plus the viral suspension media was performed. This sequence was important because some components of the suspension media, such as bovine serum albumin, could interfere with the chromatography.

Either the purification scientific staff set up the chromatography runs in a BSL-2 laboratory at Lilly or Lilly personnel went to BioReliance to aid in the conduct of the batch process analysis. The overall approach included first spiking a process solution with virus of a known titer, then processing the solution using the laboratory-scale process step, and finally determining the amount of virus remaining in the product stream. An overall (global) reduction factor was calculated for each virus. The final reduction factor was the cumulative sum of the clearance seen for each step for that virus.

Small fractions were collected on the chromatography run and pooled to generate the samples submitted for viral testing. As samples were collected from the batch process or from the chromatography run, they were diluted in cell culture medium supplied by BioReliance. The dilution used was the one identified in the cytotoxicity/viral interference/frozen viability studies. Aliquots were prepared and immediately frozen at –80°C.

After all samples had been collected, they were shipped to BioReliance in a dry-ice shipper. BioReliance was notified in advance that samples were being shipped so that they would expect the shipment and make arrangements to start testing immediately. For studies that were conducted at BioReliance, samples were tested immediately.

For chromatography, the viral clearance was determined taking into account the amount of virus remaining in the chromatographic protein peak or mainstream. It was necessary to decide on the criteria to be used to define the peak before the chromatography study was initiated. Main peak collection for viral clearance is usually slightly broader for laboratory studies than for those at full scale. The broader peak collected in the laboratory represents a worst-case analysis for viral clearance.

Besides the main peak fraction, other parts of the chromatography run — from the postcolumn loading flow-through to the fractions prior to and after the peak — should be collected.

In addition, for chromatography, it was especially important to maintain accurate records on the volumes involved for the fractions that are obtained. The calculation of log reduction requires knowledge of the volume of process solution used in the studies. In the studies described here, Eli Lilly provided those volumes to BioReliance.

It was also necessary to provide data showing that the laboratory model was run in a manner similar to the full-scale systems. For batch processes, this appears to be straightforward. Solutions can be placed in containers and stirred using a stir bar over a magnetic stirrer. For the chromatography systems, demonstration of comparability is more complex. The rule is to keep the same contact time at laboratory scale and at full scale. The height of the resin bed needs to be similar or worst-case for laboratory scale. Other process parameters were kept the same between the two scales.

14.3.1 Calculation of Reduction Factors

At the conclusion of the study, BioReliance calculated the reduction factors for each individual study. The virus reduction factor is the $\log_{10}$ of the ratio of the input virus load to the output virus load. The reduction factor can be calculated as follows. If $V(i)$ and $T(i)$ represent the input volume (ml) and virus titer, respectively, and if $V(o)$ and $T(o)$ represent the output volume and output titer, respectively, then $V(i)T(i)$ is the input virus load and $V(o)T(o)$ is the output virus load. The virus reduction R is given by the following formula:

$$R = \log_{10} \frac{V(i)T(i)}{V(o)T(o)}$$

14.4 RESULTS

14.4.1 Cytotoxicity, Viral Interference, and Frozen Viability

The results of these studies are listed in Table 14.1. In some cases, the dilution needed to quench the reaction was on the order of 2–3 logs.

14.4.2 Laboratory-Scale Process Evaluation

The process steps were scaled to a size that would allow them to be performed in a biosafety facility where viral spiking studies can be conducted. All process solutions used in the laboratory studies came from the GMP large-scale process at either the pilot plant or the commercial facility. All buffers and resins were also from the GMP run or a comparable process. The resin to be evaluated for the end of use was obtained from scaled-down runs at the commercial plant.

Some problems occurred with the chromatography runs, and the runs then had to be repeated. These problems were related to the columns plugging and chromatographic runs that did not meet the process step acceptance criteria. In addition, samples sometimes did not get properly diluted as specified by the cytotoxicity data and studies had to be repeated.

TABLE 14.1 Test Article Dilutions or Quench Dilutions as Determined by the Cytotoxicity, Viral Interference, or Frozen Viability Studies

Step	Sample	Viruses Used in Studies				
		MuLV	BVDV	PRV	Ad-2	Poliovirus
Chromatography 1	Load	1:300	1:100	1:100	1:300	1:100
	Flow-through	1:300	1:100	1:100	1:300	1:100
	Prepeak	1:3	1:3	Undilute	1:10	1:30
	Peak	1:3	Undilute	Undilute	Undilute	1:3
	Postpeak	1:3	Undilute	Undilute	Undilute	1:3
Nanofilter	Load	1:100	1:10	Undilute	1:100	Undilute
Chromatography 2	Load	1:100	1:10	Undilute	1:100	Undilute
	Flow-through	1:10	1:10	Undilute	1:10	Undilute
	Prepeak	1:100	1:3	Undilute	1:10	Undilute
	Peak	1:300	1:100	Undilute	1:100	Undilute
	Postpeak	1:3	1:3	Undilute	1:3	Undilute
Viral inactivation	Load − no TX100	Undilute	Undilute	Undilute	Not done	Not done
	Load + TX100	1:100	1:300	1:100	Undilute	Undilute
Heat	Posttreatment	1:100	1:10	Undilute	1:100	Undilute

14.4.3 Viral Clearance per Individual Process Steps

A summary of the log reduction values obtained for the panel of viruses and the individual process steps are shown in Table 14.2. Further details for the input log and output log values for the individual viruses are shown in Tables 14.3–14.8. These tables provide the output load after volume and dilution corrections have been made. Therefore, the log reduction is simply the initial load minus the output load. As can be seen, depending on the virus, the titers ranged from just over 7 logs/ml for PRV to over 9 to 10 logs for adenovirus. In most cases, the standard deviation reported was under 0.5 log/ml.

14.4.3.1 Viral Inactivation Step

Three lipid-enveloped viruses were evaluated in this step including MuLV, BVDV, and PRV. Complete inactivation was achieved with the BVDV and PRV virus. Only 2.91 logs of reduction were obtained for MuLV, a result that could not be explained. In later studies, higher clearance was noted for this virus. Other viruses in the panel were not assessed because they did not have lipid envelopes.

14.4.3.2 Chromatography Step #1

For calculations of log reduction, the output load for the chromatographic peak was used and subtracted from the initial load. For chromatography step #1, log reduction values could not be obtained for lipid-enveloped viruses because the viral inactivant from the previous step was still present in the feed to the chromatography step. For Ad-2, poliovirus, and MVM, the clearances were 2.51, 3.04, and 4.57 logs of clearance, respectively.

14.4.3.3 Heat

One process step used mild heat (40°C). Although this temperature is lower than levels published to be effective, it was

TABLE 14.2 Reduction of Viruses in Various Process Steps

	MuLV	BVDV	Ad-2	PRV	PolioVirus	MVM
Virus Genome Envelope Size	RNA env 100 nm	RNA env 50–70 nm	DNA non-env 70–90 nm	DNA env 80–120 nm	RNA non-env 30 nm	DNA non-env 20 nm
Viral Inactivation	2.93[a] 2.89[a] (2.91)[a]	4.99 4.84 (>4.92)	Not done	>5.75 >5.53 (>5.65)	Not done	Not done
Chromatography Number 1	Not done	Virucidal activity: no value	2.80 1.21 (2.51)	Virucidal activity: no value	2.62 3.26 (3.04)	4.08 4.79 (4.57)
Mild Heat	2.33 2.08 (2.22)	0.09 0.16	−0.16 0.47	0.49 0.60	0.05 0.42	Not done
Nanofiltration	>3.29 >2.16 (>3.02)	>4.16 >4.05 (>4.11)	>3.17 >4.04 (>3.79)	>5.14 >4.97 (>5.06)	2.92 2.99 (2.96)	2.86 3.24 (3.09)
Chromatography Number 2	2.81 3.63 (3.39)	1.99 1.64 (1.84)	4.66 4.00 (4.44)	1.44 1.36 (1.40)	2.11 2.64 (2.45)	Not done
Global Reduction Factor	11.5	10.8	10.8	12.1	8.4	7.68

[a] Numbers in the boxes from top to bottom for viral inactivation, heat, and nanofiltration are the log reduction for Run 1, Run 2, and the average. For the chromatography steps, the numbers from top to bottom are the log reduction for new resin, used resin, and the average of the two.

TABLE 14.3   Reduction Factors for MuLV

Process Step	Initial Load ($\log_{10}$TCID$_{50}$)	Output Load ($\log_{10}$TCID$_{50}$)	$\log_{10}$ Reduction
Viral inactivation — Run 1	8.19 ± 0.43	5.26 ± 0.53	2.93 ± 0.68
Viral inactivation — Run 2	8.32 ± 0.48	5.43 ± 0.46	2.89 ± 0.66
Viral inactivation — average			2.91 ± 0.67
Heat — Run 1	9.20 ± 0.36	6.87 ± 0.43	2.33 ± 0.56
Heat — Run 2	7.70 ± 0.40	8.00 ± 0.44	−0.30 ± 0.59
Heat — Run 2, retest	8.20 ± 0.36	6.12 ± 0.32	2.08 ± 0.48
Heat — average			2.22 ± 0.51
Chromatography 2 — Run 1 (new resin)	7.95 ± 0.35	5.14 ± 0.60	2.81 ± 0.69
Chromatography 2 — Run 2 (used resin)	8.20 ± 0.43	≤4.57	≥3.63 ± 0.43
Chromatography 2 — average			≥3.37 ± 0.57
Nanofiltration — Run 1	8.43 ± 0.44	≤5.14	≥3.29 ± 0.44
Nanofiltration — Run 2	7.30 ± 0.37	≤5.14	≥2.16 ± 0.37
Nanofiltration — average			≥3.02 ± 0.40

decided to evaluate this step on the panel of viruses. Only with MuLV was there any significant log reduction (2.22 logs).

14.4.3.4 Nanofiltration

This step, which was included as a second dedicated viral clearance step, was very effective across the panel. Complete clearance to levels of detection for the assay was reported for all viruses except the two smallest. Complete clearance of MMV (20 nm) and poliovirus (30 nm) was not achieved, but 3.09 and 2.96 logs of clearance were obtained.

14.4.3.5 Chromatography Step #2

For calculation of log reduction, the output load from the chromatographic peak was subtracted from the input load.

TABLE 14.4 Reduction Factors for BVDV

Process Step	Initial Load ($\log_{10}$PFU)	Output Load ($\log_{10}$PFU)	$\log_{10}$ Reduction
Heat — Run 1	7.67 ± 0.23	7.58 ± 0.17	0.09 ± 0.29
Heat — Run 2	7.77 ± 0.07	7.61 ± 0.06	0.16 ± 0.09
Heat — average			0.13 ± 0.21
Viral inactivation — Run 1	7.94 ± 0.46	≤2.95	≥4.99 ± 0.46
Viral inactivation — Run 2	7.79 ± 0.09	≤2.95	≥4.84 ± 0.09
Viral inactivation — average			≥4.92 ± 0.33
Nanofiltration — Run 1	8.69 ± 0.10	≤4.53	≥4.16 ± 0.10
Nanofiltration — Run 2	8.58 ± 0.14	≤4.53	≥4.05 ± 0.14
Nanofiltration — average			≥4.11 ± 0.12
Chromatography 2 — Run 1 (new resin)	8.33 ± 0.07	6.34 ± 0.19	1.99 ± 0.20
Chromatography 2 — Run 2 (used resin)	8.26 ± 0.10	8.08 ± 0.13	0.18 ± 0.16
Chromatography 2 — Run 2 (used resin), retest	8.26 ± 0.10	6.62 ± 0.22	2.22 ± 0.24
Chromatography 2 — Run 2 (used resin), resubmission (repeat)	8.26 ± 0.10	6.56 ± 0.03	1.64 ± 0.10
Chromatography 2 — average			1.84 ± 0.10

Overall log reduction between viruses in the test panel varied greatly, from a low of 1.40 logs for PRV to a high of 4.44 logs for Ad-2. Samples from the BVDV study with used resin were retested after the first set of results yielded a difference of greater than 2 logs. To ensure that the second set of data was accurate, a backup sample was also submitted. The log reduction value obtained was the average of the retest and the second submitted sample.

TABLE 14.5 Reduction Factors for Adenovirus

Process Step	Initial Load $(\log_{10}\text{TCID}_{50})$	Output Load $(\log_{10}\text{TCID}_{50})$	$\log_{10}$ Reduction
Heat — Run 1	9.09 ± 0.43	9.25 ± 0.40	-0.16 ± 0.59
Heat — Run 2	9.22 ± 0.24	8.75 ± 0.36	0.47 ± 0.43
Heat — average			0.26 ± 0.52
Chromatography 1 — Run 1	10.72 ± 0.37	7.92 ± 0.40	2.80 ± 0.54
Chromatography 1 — Run 2	10.74 ± 0.51	9.53 ± 0.51	1.21 ± 0.72
Chromatography 1 — average			2.51 ± 0.64
Chromatography 2 (new resin)	9.70 ± 0.49	5.04 ± 0.41	4.66 ± 0.64
Chromatography 2 (used resin)	9.20 ± 0.32	5.20 ± 0.24	4.00 ± 0.40
Chromatography 2 — average			4.44 ± 0.53
Nanofiltration — Run 1	9.17 ± 0.36	≤ 5.13	$\geq 4.04 \pm 0.36$
Nanofiltration — Run 2	8.32 ± 0.37	≤ 5.15	$\geq 3.17 \pm 0.37$
Nanofiltration — average			$\geq 3.79 \pm 0.37$

14.4.4 General Comments on Viral Clearance

In these studies, in most cases, there was less than a 1-log difference between the two independent runs, whether it was just a repeat of the same process step or, for chromatography, new resin and used resin were used. It is customary to report overall or global log reduction values for each virus. This is accomplished by adding the log clearance achieved at each step. Log reductions of 1.0 logs or less were not included. The global reduction values from low to high were as follows: 7.68 logs for MMV, 8.4 logs for poliovirus, 10.8 logs for Ad-2, 10.8 logs for BVDV, 11.5 logs for MuLV, and 12.1 logs for PRV.

TABLE 14.6 Reduction Factors for PRV

Process Step	Initial Load ($\log_{10}$PFU)	Output Load ($\log_{10}$PFU)	$\log_{10}$ Reduction
Heat — Run 1	9.05 ± 0.10	8.56 ± 0.12	0.49 ± 0.16
Heat — Run 2	8.63 ± 0.22	8.03 ± 0.09	0.60 ± 0.24
Heat — average			0.55 ± 0.20
Viral inactivation — Run 1	8.70 ± 0.17	≤2.95	≥5.75 ± 0.17
Viral inactivation — Run 2	8.51 ± 0.22	≤2.98	≥5.53 ± 0.22
Viral inactivation — average			≥5.65 ± 0.20
Chromatography 2 — Run 1	8.09 ± 0.20	6.65 ± 0.25	1.47 ± 0.32
Chromatography 2 — Run 2	7.90 ± 0.29	6.54 ± 0.21	1.36 ± 0.36
Chromatography 2 — average			1.42 ± 0.34
Nanofiltration — Run 1	7.53 ± 0.24	≤2.56	≥4.97 ± 0.24
Nanofiltration — Run 2	7.73 ± 0.17	≤2.59	≥5.14 ± 0.17
Nanofiltration — average			≥5.06 ± 0.21

14.5 CONCLUSION

The studies demonstrated very good clearance of the model viruses by the process steps. The viruses used represented a cross section of various morphological and biological types. For each virus, at least one process step and in most cases two process steps resulted in more than 3 logs of viral clearance. There were at least three steps for each virus that provided viral clearance. The two smallest viruses, MMV and poliovirus, exhibited the lowest clearance at over 8 logs. MuLV, a retrovirus, had 11 logs of clearance. This may be lower than seen with product derived from CHO cells. Since CHO cells have retroviral particles and this cell line does not, the clearance obtained for MuLV is more than sufficient.

The viral clearance study required almost 2 years of activity from start to finish by personnel dedicated full-time

TABLE 14.7 Reduction Factors for Poliovirus

Process Step	Initial Load ($\log_{10}$PFU)	Output Load ($\log_{10}$PFU)	$\log_{10}$ Reduction
Heat — Run 1	8.90 ± 0.29	8.85 ± 0.33	0.05 ± 0.44
Heat — Run 2	7.81 ± 0.18	7.39 ± 0.23	0.42 ± 0.29
Heat — average			0.27 ± 0.37
Chromatography 1 — Run 1 (new resin)	9.72 ± 0.06	7.10 ± 0.21	2.62 ± 0.22
Chromatography 1 — Run 2 (used resin)	10.17 ± 0.39	6.91 ± 0.13	3.26 ± 0.41
Chromatography 1 — average			3.04 ± 0.33
Chromatography 2 — Run 1	8.27 ± 0.20	6.16 ± 0.19	2.11 ± 0.28
Chromatography 2 — Run 2	9.23 ± 0.41	6.59 ± 0.18	2.64 ± 0.45
Chromatography 2 — average			2.45 ± 0.37
Nanofiltration — Run 1	9.15 ± 0.07	6.16 ± 0.23	2.99 ± 0.24
Nanofiltration — Run 2	9.24 ± 0.12	6.32 ± 0.11	2.92 ± 0.16
Nanofiltration — average			2.96 ± 0.20

TABLE 14.8 Reduction Factors for MMV

Process Step	Initial Load ($\log_{10}$TCID$_{50}$)	Output Load ($\log_{10}$TCID$_{50}$)	$\log_{10}$ Reduction
Nanofiltration — Run 1	9.04 ± 0.35	6.18 ± 0.40	2.86 ± 0.53
Nanofiltration — Run 2	9.29 ± 0.37	6.05 ± 0.00	3.24 ± 0.37
Nanofiltration — average			3.09 ± 0.46
Chromatography 2 — Run 1 (new resin)	8.49	4.41	4.08
Chromatography 2 — Run 2 (old resin)	9.74	4.95	4.79
Chromatography 2 — average			4.57

to the project. Good planning and communication, especially with the contract biosafety laboratory, were vital to the success of this study. Studies of this nature require interaction between scientific staff in purification, production, quality control, and regulatory departments.

ACKNOWLEDGMENTS

The author wishes to acknowledge the expert assistance of Eli Lilly and Company employee Mark Smith for his editorial comments. Also, the author thanks Dr. Carol Marcus-Sekura for her excellent advice.

REFERENCES

1. Committee for Proprietary Medicinal Products (CPMP), Note for Guidance: Validation of Virus Removal and Inactivation Procedures, III/8115/89, 1991.

2. Center for Biologics Evaluation and Research, Points to Consider in the Manufacture and Testing of Monoclonal Antibody Products for Human Use, Food and Drug Administration, Bethesda, MD, 1997.

3. Federal Health Office and Paul Erlich Institute Federal Office for Sera and Vaccines, Notice on the Registration of Drugs: Requirements for Validation Studies to Demonstrate the Virus Safety of Drugs Derived from Human Blood or Plasma, *Bundesanzeiger*, 84, 4742–4744, 1994.

4. The European Agency for the Evaluation of Medicinal products, Human Medicines Evaluation Unit — CPMP Biotechnology Working Party, Note for Guidance on Virus Validation Studies: The Design, Contribution and Interpretation of Studies Validating the Inactivation and Removal of Viruses, CPMP/BWP/268/95 Final Version 2.

5. Center for Biologics Evaluation and Research, Points to Consider in the Characterization of Cell Lines Used to Produce Biologicals, Food and Drug Administration, Bethesda, MD, 1997.

6. International Commission on Harmonization Topic Q5D, Viral Safety Evaluation of Biotechnology Products Derived from Cell Lines of Human and Animal Origin.

7. International Commission on Harmonization Topic Q5A, Quality of Biotechnological Products: Viral Safety Evaluation of Biotechnology Products Derived from Cell Lines of Human or Animal Origin.

Index